Art Therapy Through the Lifespan

Art Therapy Through the Lifespan: A Collection of Case Studies introduces theories and models of human development highlighted by case studies written by art therapists and broken down by developmental age ranges.

Each chapter introduces vignettes written by seasoned art therapists, illuminating the clinical practice of art therapy across relevant developmental levels. Chapters cover major developmental factors through a range of theoretical perspectives, including the definition and use of art therapy, and how developmental knowledge and understanding impact art therapy practice with clients of all ages. The reader will develop an understanding of the impact of human development on assessment, treatment planning, and implementation of art therapy, and will be able to create effective art therapy interventions that coincide with factors related to events across the human lifespan that include normal and abnormal development.

The first of its kind, this book encourages and supports readers to develop their knowledge of art therapy and human development across the lifespan with a focus on safety, material quality, and artistic intent.

Peg Dunn-Snow is the owner of Children's Corner: Art Therapy for Children in Davie, Florida. She has been in practice since 2004 and specializes in seeing children of military families.

Jill McNutt is an art therapy educator at Edgewood College in Madison, Wisconsin. She also practices as a medical art therapist at Aurora Health Care and serves her local community as a founding member of the nonprofit Art Therapy House, Inc.

"This book delves into the diversified environments and ethical considerations art therapists encounter across the lifespan. A merge of human growth and development utilizing art therapy cases to exemplify unique aspects across various age groups. It is directed towards a variety of theoretical orientations that the reader can tailor to their framework. This book will broaden perspectives, improving any art therapist's practice as they expand to work with a range of developmental needs and populations across the lifespan."

Leara Glinzak, *ATR-BC, ATCS*

"*Lifespans* is a beautifully written and illustrated collection of developmental art therapy presentations. The book is the first of its kind and an invaluable tool for not only art therapists but also for psychologists. Peg Dunn Snow and Jill McNutt have edited a masterful publication, which is an important contribution to the field of art therapy."

Stephen W. Koncsol, *PhD, associate professor of Psychology,*
Barry University, Miami Shores, Florida

"*Art Therapy Through the Lifespan* is a long-awaited text that views human development through the lens of art therapy treatment. Dunn-Snow and McNutt have complied a wide-ranging resource that supports conceptualizing and implementing treatment with an eye to age appropriate and developmentally sensitive use of media in the context of psychological and art therapy theory. This book draws from the many resources that have been necessary to teach and practice art therapy from a developmental platform. Case studies are structured around a format that brings variety and clarity to the text. Those interested in investigating the human life cycle from a fresh and clinically informed perspective will appreciate the contributions of the many clinicians that have contributed to this valuable text."

Barbara J. Fish, *PhD, ATR-BC, ATCS, LCPC, HLM*

Art Therapy Through the Lifespan

A Collection of Case Studies

Edited by Peg Dunn-Snow and Jill McNutt

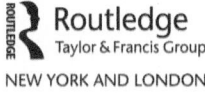

Routledge
Taylor & Francis Group

NEW YORK AND LONDON

Designed cover image: © Getty Images

First published 2025
by Routledge
605 Third Avenue, New York, NY 10158

and by Routledge
4 Park Square, Milton Park, Abingdon, Oxon, OX14 4RN

Routledge is an imprint of the Taylor & Francis Group, an informa business

ISBN: 978-1-032-34993-0 (hbk)
ISBN: 978-1-032-34992-3 (pbk)
ISBN: 978-1-003-32480-5 (ebk)

DOI: 10.4324/9781003324805

Typeset in Sabon
by Deanta Global Publishing Services, Chennai, India

This book is dedicated to our students, past, present, and future. We appreciate all the insights, interactions, and challenges. This work would not have happened without you.

Contents

Foreword

After reading this tome, edited by Peg Dunn-Snow and Jill McNutt, with contributions by numerous standouts from the Art Therapy field, I wished that I had access to this book much earlier in my career and when I was training future art therapists. Alas, nothing akin to this existed. In fact, when I started writing, researching and working clinically in 1976, the closest thing to discussing developmental stages in art was the infamous "Bible of Art Education" by Lowenfeld and Brittain (1975). But that fell short for me and apparently many of these authors herein. That is because not only had Lowenfeld and Brittain stopped discussing artistic developmental stages of development at adolescence but also failed to compare their developmental stages to other theoretical concepts, and in fact had not even considered what a Brian-Injured stage might look like from Traumatic Brain Injury or childhood-birth anomalies. I talked about this in many of my publications and books (Horovitz, 2021, 2020, 1981, 1980) and suggested not only considering Brain-Injury, or an Adult Stage of artistic development but also an Artistic Stage of development. Indeed, like other authors herein, I also suggested comparing developmental stages to other theorists such as Erikson, Fowler, Piaget, Kohlberg, and Gantt and Tabone.

Alas, I don't mean to fault Lowenfeld and Brittain, for we have evolved in our own thinking and currently utilize other theorists' works and insert them into our own clinical practice (e.g., EMDR, hypnosis, somatic training, such as yoga and polyvagal trauma training, etc.). But this compendium offers all art therapists a theoretical and applicable clinical platform to consider art therapy treatment on a much broader scale. Indeed, I might suggest that this book presents current and future art therapists with a much-needed compendium for our own field, no longer hanging onto the coattails of Lowenfeld and Britain's Art Education "Bible".

Not only does this edited book cover the "lifespans" from a developmental and educational perspective, toddler through age 99, but the clinical cases are rich, diverse, gripping, introspective, and informative. While more comorbid clinical cases could have been added, what has been amassed has an encyclopedic feel to it, and I imagine with many editions to come, it will become just that.

While I didn't have this book 48 years ago when I was an incipient art therapist, 50 years later, I am grateful to have this in my library now. There were so many excellent ideas from bibliotherapy references to therapeutic applications that I know I will turn to this in my own private practice for ideas and inspiration.

Table 0.1 Stages of Development

Eras/age	Erikson	Piaget	Kohlberg	Lowenfeld/Brittain	Fowler	Gantt and Tabone	Horovitz
Infancy (0–1.5 years)	Basic trust vs. basic mistrust (hope)	Sensorimotor stage		Scribble stage: Beginning of self-expression (0–2 years)	Stage 0: Primal or undifferentiated (0–2 years)	Rating 0: Cannot be rated	
Early childhood (2–6 years)	Autonomy vs. shame and doubt Initiative vs. guilt (purpose)	Preoperational or intuitive	Preconventional level 1. Heteronomous morality	Preschematic stage: First representations (4–7 years)	Stage 1: Intuitive-projective (3–7 years)	Rating 1: Scribbles/masses Rating 2: Geometric shapes (4–6 years)	
Childhood (7–12 years	Industry vs. inferiority	Concrete operational	2. Instrumental exchange, conventional level 3. Mutual interpersonal relationships	Schematic stage Formed concepts (7–9 years)	Stage 2: Mythic-literal (mostly in school children)	Rating 3: Latency, age/logical and proportionate	Adult stage Formation in the world (8 to adulthood)
Adolescence (13–21 years)	Identity vs. role confusion (fidelity)	Formal operational	4. Social system and conscience	Gang age: Dawning realism (9–12 years)	Stage 3: Synthetic/conventional (12 to adulthood)	Rating 4: Adolescence/realism	Artistic stage: Formed art any age (generally in adolescence through adulthood)
Young adulthood (21–35 years)	Intimacy vs. isolation (love)		Postconventional principled level 5. Social contract, individual rights	Pseudonaturalistic stage: Age of reasoning (12–14 years)	Stage 4: Individualitive-reflective (mid 20s–late 30s)	Rating 5: Adult/some artistic sophistication	
Adulthood (35–60 years)	Generativity vs. stagnation (care)			Adolescent art: Period of decision (14–17 years)	Stage 5: Conjunctive (mid-life crisis)		
Maturity (60+ years)	Integrity vs. despair (wisdom)		Universal ethical principles		Stage 6: Universalizing (enlightenment)		

(Used with permission from Horovitz, 2021).

So, thank you, Peg and Jill for amassing this compilation and to all the authors who enriched us with their knowledge, stories, and hearts. May we continue to develop, share, and inform each other as we evolve as a field. This book, epigenetic in its structure, lays the foundation to do just that.

Dr Ellen G Horovitz, ATR-BC, LCAT, E-RYT500, C-IAYT

Yogartherapy.com

References

Horovitz, E. G. (1981). Art therapy in arrested development of a preschooler. *Arts in Psychotherapy, An International Journal*, 8(2), 119–126.

Horovitz, E. G. (1980). Case study: Developing the body image of a visually handicapped child. *American Journal of Art Therapy*, 20(October), 19–24.

Horovitz, E. G. (Ed.). (2020). *The art therapists' primer: A clinical guide to writing assessment, diagnosis, and treatment* (3rd ed.). Charles C Thomas.

Horovitz, E. G. (2021). *Head and HeART: Yoga therapy & art therapy interventions for mental health*. Handspring Publishers.

Lowenfeld, V. & Brittain, W. L. (1975). *Creative and mental growth* (6th ed.). Macmillan.

Preface

In the winter of 2010, I began teaching in one of the first, long-distance, graduate art therapy programs housed at Saint-Mary-of-the-Woods College in Terre Haute, Indiana. The course I taught each year was entitled *Art Therapy Throughout the Lifespan*. During the third year I taught the course, the graduate program had increased its student population and a new faculty member was hired. This is when I first met Jill McNutt. One of her new teaching assignments was to teach an additional section of the lifespan course. That winter, we decided to co-teach all the students together during the residency weekend and then teach our separate section of students online during the rest of the semester. We revised the course each year that we taught together as new information in the fields of trauma and neurology became relevant to the course. In order to cover the subject thoroughly, we required our students to purchase several books. We often wished there had been one comprehensive book that was available in the field to cover an overview of the topics covered in the course.

It was at the annual Art Therapy Association Conference in Miami in 2018, that Jill first suggested that we edit a book together based on our collective teaching experience. Then at the annual conference in 2019, we talked again about this project. Finally, during the summer of 2021, we got serious about the idea. We outlined our book and decided to create a companion website with the book, in order to keep current with the subject matter, knowing how quickly books go out-of-date after publication. We then decided to invite credentialed art therapy colleagues to write client case studies that would illustrate the use of art therapy throughout the life-span and develop a case study template that would provide consistency in the case study format throughout the text. We then wrote our own case studies to test and make edits to the template. Later in the fall of 2021, we submitted our book proposal to the Routledge/Taylor & Francis Group Publishing Company, and in early March of 2022 our proposal was accepted unanimously by its board.

This book was written for students, faculty, and administrators of art therapy training programs, and practicing art therapists from recent graduates to seasoned professionals. It is anticipated that this book will demonstrate the efficacy, values, and advantages of art therapy. The book will also report how art therapy works within a variety of learning and developmental theories, psychotherapy perspectives, and in a variety of clinical settings and delivery models with diverse populations throughout the lifespan.

Peg Dunn-Snow
Children's Corner: Art Therapy for Children, Owner

Contributors

Casey L. Burke, LCAT, ATR-BC
Cedar Crest College, Allentown, PA

Samantha Castellano, MA, LPAT, LPC, ATR-BC, NCC
North Caldwell, NJ

Natashia P. Collins, PhD, LPC, LPAT, ACS, ATCS, ATR-BC, NCC
Antioch University, Keene, NH

Mia de Béthune, PhD candidate, ATR-BC, LCAT, ISP/SEP
New York University, Lesley University, Hasting-on-Hudson, NY

Tami Joe DeLisle, LPC, ATR-BC
UnMasked Expressive Therapies, Reeseville, WI

Heather Denning, MA, ATR-BC, ATCB, LSW
Mercyhurst University, Erie, PA

Gabrielle Gingras, PhD candidate, RCAT-ATPQ
Université du Québec en Abitibi-Témiscamingue, Montreal, Québec, Canada

Tami Harris, PhD, MAAT, MFA, LMHC, ATR-BC, TF-CBT, FCC
Fishers, IN

Erin Hein, MS, LPC, ATR-BC
Aurora Health Care, New Berlin, WI

Kara-Leigh Huse, MA, ATR-BC
Ramona, CA

Katherine Jackson, PhD, ATR-BC, RYT
Ursuline College & Beachwood Counseling Center, Cleveland, OH

Jinnie Jeon, PhD, RCAT, RCC
Adler University Vancouver British Columbia, Canada

Valeria Koutmina, MPS, ATR-BC, LCAT
Pleasantville Wellness Group, Scarsdale Psychology Associates, Valley Cottage, NY

Amanda Lightner, LPC, ATR-BC
Madison, WI

Rebecca Miller, PhD, LPC, ATR-BC, ATCS
Ursuline College, Lakewood, OH

Dixie Moore, MA, ATR
The Neutral Ground Collective, New Orleans, LA

Rebecca Reinholz
Aurora Health Care, Port Washington, WI

Maria Riccardi, PhD candidate, ATR-BC, RCAT-ATPQ
Université du Québec en Abitibi-Témiscamingue, Montréal, Québec

Susan Ridley, PhD, LPC, NCC, CPS, CPRP, ADC, REAT, ATR-BC
West Liberty University, West Liberty, WV

Emily Sharp, LCAT, ATR-BC
NY Art Therapy, Brooklyn, NY

Lisa Thompson-Gibson, MA, MA, LCPC (IL), LPC (MO), NCC
New Sage Art Therapy and Counseling, PLLC, OFallon, IL

Molly Tomony, MA, LPC, ATR-BC
Edgewood College, Madison, WI

Editors

Peg Dunn-Snow, PhD, LPAT, LMHC, ATR-BC, is an art therapist and mental health counselor with post-graduate training in trauma and sandtray therapies. She has authored and co-authored several articles and has given numerous workshop presentations and keynote addresses in the United States and abroad on art therapy with children and adolescents. Dr. Dunn-Snow is the former director of the graduate art therapy program at Barry University in Miami Shores, Florida and a former faculty member with the graduate art therapy training program at Saint-Mary-of-the-Woods College in Terre Haute, Indiana. She has been in private practice since 2004 as the owner of Children's Corner: Art Therapy for Children in South Florida, specializing in working with children of military families.

In 2014, Dr. Dunn-Snow introduced the profession of art therapy to students, faculty, and the community at large through a series of workshops while working at the University of Akureyri in Iceland as a Senior Fulbright Scholarship recipient. Dr. Dunn-Snow has also served as the conference chair and president of the American Art Therapy Association and the Florida Art Therapy Association.

Jill McNutt, PhD, LPC, ATRL, ATR-BC, ATCS, is an art therapist, professional counselor, supervisor, and educator. Her art therapy practice has centered in medical art therapy, specializing in cancer care where she has written and presented professionally in art therapy and in medical venues. Dr. McNutt has been an art therapist at Aurora Health Care in Milwaukee, WI for several years. McNutt has earned two Doctorates of Philosophy, the first in Expressive Therapies from Lesley University and the second in Counseling Education and Supervision from Regent University. Dr. McNutt's work in education includes directorship, faculty, designing programs, accreditation, and licensing with various states across the US. Her current role is as Director of Graduate Art Therapy and Counseling at Edgewood College in Madison, Wisconsin. Dr. McNutt was also a founding member of the Art Therapy House, Inc., a non-profit in Brown Deer, Wisconsin. Dr. McNutt has been an active member of the American Art Therapy Association where she served as the Chair of the Research Committee for four years, and the Wisconsin Art Therapy Association where she has served as president, and currently serves as governmental affairs chair.

Introduction

Art Therapy

Art therapy is grounded in psychological theory and requires art therapists to have a working knowledge of human development. This text works to demonstrate the effectiveness of art therapy in light of these theories within art therapy relationships. Art therapists view art as the first language in human development (Eubanks, 1997), and this strong language component allows art therapy to advance the work of talk therapy. Through the following case studies, this relationship will become evident and demonstrates the efficacy of art therapy. Twenty-two authors from various backgrounds, with various developmental expertise and continuing educations in a variety of supplemental, therapeutic interventions, illustrate the benefits of art therapy with diverse populations within a variety of therapeutic settings and have contributed to make this text relevant.

Art therapy benefits people who are challenged with medical and mental health problems and with people who seek emotional, creative, and spiritual growth. It supports the "lives of individuals, families, and communities and is used to improve cognitive and sensory-motor functions, foster self-esteem and self-awareness, cultivate emotional resilience, promote insight, enhance social skills, reduce and resolve conflicts and distress, and advance societal and ecological change" (American Art Therapy Association; AATA, 2023). Art Therapy "enriches the lives of individuals through active art-making, the creative process, applied psychological theory, and the human experience within a psychotherapeutic relationship" (AATA, 2023).

Development

For the purpose of organization, development is presented in this book using the traditional, linear stage-age developmental theory (Lowenfeld & Brittain, 1987; Lansing, 1969; McFee, 1970; Chapman, 1978; Salmone & Moore, 1979; Gardener, 1990). However, each stage is fluid as illustrated among the case studies in each of the chapters, and some scholars in areas of artistic and creative development no longer believe in universal developmental theories (Anderson, 1992; Felman, 1980; Wilson & Wilson, 1981). Instead, they believe other factors, besides age, have a stronger influence on the development of the individual. This is especially true in the area of artistic development. Anderson (1992) suggested, "there may not be a universal developmental continuum in children's artistic development that

DOI: 10.4324/9781003324805-1

transcends culture" (p. 138). Wilson and Wilson (1981) concluded that developmental stages in art do not address cultural, instructional, or peer influence; do not acknowledge graphic development as markedly different based on norms created more than 70 years ago; and do not consider artwork done between defined stages of graphic development. Understanding of developmental stages also often ignores emotional and aesthetic aspects of the artwork.

Chapters

Introductions

An introduction to each chapter includes the developmental markers for that age range, followed by a preview of some of the case studies featured in the chapter. The markers included the areas of physical, emotional, cognitive, social, and artistic development while the previews of the case studies covered characteristics of the developmental stages the clients exhibited and how that impacted their therapy. Some previews included clients' choices in media and what level(s) of the Expressive Therapies Continuum their artwork represented (ETC; Lusebrink, 1990; Hinz, 2019).

Case Studies

Case studies are included in the second part of each chapter. Case studies are units of information with which therapists reveal theoretical models and approaches that inform their practice with patients and clients (Yin, 2018). Written by seasoned and credentialed art therapists, these case studies will illustrate the practical application of how art therapists have assessed and provided treatment goals to a diverse client population in a variety of settings. Each case study will include goals based on selected developmental markers, learning theories and other therapeutic approaches complementary to art therapy. Each case study may also include family structures, culture diversity, trauma background, and/or socio-economic status as factors that would influence the therapists' work with each client. Pseudonyms were given to all the clients in these case studies.

References

American Art Therapy Association. (2023). About Art Therapy. https:/arttherapy.org/about-art-therapy/pdf

Anderson, F. (1992). *Art for all the children: Approaches to art therapy for children with disabilities* (2nd ed.). Charles C Thomas Publisher.

Chapman, L. (1978). *Approaches to art in education.* Harcourt, Brace, Jovanovich.

Eubanks, P. K. (1997). Art is a visual language. *Visual Arts Research, 23*(1), 31–35.

Felman, D. H. (1980). *Beyond universals in cognitive development.* Ablex Publishing Corporation.

Gardener, H. (1990). Art education and human development. (Occasional Paper number 3). *The Getty Center for Education in the Arts.*

Hinz, L. D. (2019). *Expressive therapies continuum: A framework for using art in therapy* (2nd ed.). Routledge.

Lansing, K. (1969). *Art, artists, and art education.* McGraw-Hill.

Lowenfeld, V., & Brittain, W. L. (1987). Creative and mental growth (8th ed.) Macmillan.

Lusebrink, V. B. (1990). *Imagery and visual expression in therapy.* Plenum Press.

McFee, J. (1970). *Preparation for art.* Wadsworth Publishing Company.

Salmone, R. A., & Moore, B. (1979). *Development of figure concepts in the graphic artwork by children from different countries.* International Film Bureau, Inc.

Wilson, B., & Wilson, M. (1981). The use and uselessness of developmental stages. *Art Education, 36*(2), 4–5.

Yin, R. K. (2018). *Case study research and applications: Design and methods* (6th ed.). Sage.

Chapter 1

Toddlerhood and Early Childhood

Artistic and creative development is integral, fostering imagination, problem-solving, and self-expression.

Introduction

Developmental Markers

Human development through age nine is a complex interplay of various factors, including biological, social, ecological, cognitive, artistic, emotional, neurological, creative, spiritual, moral, and cultural influences. Biological development is marked by genetic and hormonal influences, contributing to physical growth and maturation. Brain development, particularly the growth of the prefrontal cortex, which governs decision-making and impulse control, is especially significant during this period (Barresi & Gilbert, 2023). Social development, as emphasized in Bowlby's (1969) attachment theory, underscores the importance of early relationships in forming emotional bonds and secure attachments. Bronfenbrenner's (1979) Ecological Systems Theory further highlights the impact of microsystems (family, school, and peers), mesosystems (interactions among microsystems), exosystem (community), and macrosystem (culture and society) on a child's development.

Cognitive development, as proposed by Piaget and Inhelder (1969), involves the progression through stages of cognitive growth including *sensory-motor (0–2), pre-operational (2–7)*, and *concrete operational stages (7–11)*. The concrete operational stage enables logical thinking and understanding abstract concepts (Piaget & Inhelder, 1969). Artistic and creative development is integral, fostering imagination, problem-solving, and self-expression (Lowenfeld & Brittain, 1987).

Emotional development, as described in Erik Erikson's psychosocial stages, is crucial. Children work towards achieving emotional milestones and forming a sense of identity (Erikson, 1967). Typically, children ages three to nine, as covered in this chapter, would be in stage three, *initiative vs. guilt*, and stage four, *industry vs. inferiority*. Clients in this chapter would typically fall into Kohlberg's (1969) *preconventional* level defined by punishment and obedience, and instrumental relations to themselves.

Additionally, cultural influences, as emphasized in cultural psychology, shape a child's beliefs, behaviors, and identity. Cultural norms, traditions, and values profoundly impact development (Haggis & Schech, 2002). Spiritual development involves the exploration of existential questions and values, often influenced by family beliefs, religious practices, and

DOI: 10.4324/9781003324805-2

exposure to diverse worldviews (Fowler, 1995). Children in this chapter exemplify stage one, intuitive-projective (imitates parental figure's beliefs and attitudes; and literal understanding of good and evil), and stage two, mythical and literal (symbolization through story; and moral rules including fairness and justice are literal and concrete).

Setbacks

Child development from birth through age nine can face numerous setbacks, with trauma being a significant factor. The Adverse Childhood Experiences (ACEs) study sheds light on how adverse experiences in childhood can impact development and long-term well-being.

The ACEs study, (Felitti et al., 1998), identified ten types of adverse childhood experiences, including abuse (e.g., physical, emotional, sexual), neglect, and household dysfunction (e.g., substance abuse, mental illness, divorce, incarceration) (Felitti et al., 1998). These experiences can significantly disrupt healthy development.

Traumatic experiences, such as abuse or neglect, can impair the development of trust, attachment, and emotional regulation (Bowlby, 1969). Children exposed to trauma may struggle with forming secure relationships, managing emotions, and developing a positive self-identity. Trauma can interfere with cognitive development, impairing attention, memory, and problem-solving skills (Perry, 2009). These setbacks may affect academic achievement and intellectual growth. Trauma often leads to emotional and behavioral challenges, including anxiety, depression, aggression, and withdrawal (Maynard et al., 2019). These difficulties can persist into adulthood if left unaddressed.

Resilience and Protective Factors

It is essential to note that not all children exposed to trauma experience severe setbacks. Resilience and protective factors, such as supportive relationships, can mitigate the impact of ACEs and promote healthier development (Felitti et al., 1998). Early intervention and support are crucial for children who have experienced trauma. Trauma-informed care, therapy, and social services can help children and families navigate the challenges posed by adverse experiences and work towards recovery.

Case Studies

The age of children in this chapter ranged from three to nine years old. The therapy settings included in the home, in private practice, and in an art therapy studio-based program at a local art museum. Art therapy was delivered within individual sessions, family sessions, or a combination of both. Although there was a wide range of presenting problems, all the case studies were trauma-focused, and safety was among the major goals for these children. The presenting problems included children witnessing a violent attack on a family friend; the death of a sibling; experiencing a temporary foster care placement; having a sibling with epilepsy; the kidnapping by a father and paternal grandmother; physical abuse, neglect, and abandonment; bullying at school; and the death of a kindergarten classmate followed by repeated losses of school friends in the first, second, and third grades.

Art therapy was especially effective for these children who had experienced trauma because during this age range children's language development is limited and they do not always have the words to explain what has happened to them. With preschool children, art therapy, play therapy, and drama therapy are often combined; as examples, two children created puppets to help them tell their story. While young, school-aged children's drawings and paintings illustrate what they know rather than what they see and their pictures help them to tell their stories.

It is not surprising that all these case studies were described as trauma-focused with safety being a major goal for these young clients. In recent years, trauma has been redefined in broader terms beyond the battlefield (van der Kolk, 2014). This change in defining what trauma is together with the understanding of how trauma affects everyone has led to the development of trauma-based protocols by art therapists and other related professionals in the field of mental health. The authors of these case studies were trained in and described the use of several of these protocols (Chapman, 2014; Dana, 2020; National Child Traumatic Stress Network, 2023; Schwartz, 1995; Tinnin & Gantt, 2013) that helped these clients and their families overcome traumatic experiences. Other theories and approaches to therapy that helped these children and complemented art therapy and a trauma-based approach included: constructivist theory (Gergen, 2015); polyvagal theory (Porges, 2011); object relations theory (Robbins, 1994); expressive therapies continuum (Hinz, 2019); play therapy (Schaefer & Cangelosi, 2016); person-centered therapy (Rodgers, 1951); narrative therapy (Dunne, 2016), cognitive behavior therapy (Beck, 2020); sandtray therapy (Homeyer & Lyles, 2022), and bibliotherapy (Lu, 2008).

Setbacks to development from birth through age nine, especially those associated with trauma as highlighted in the ACEs, can have profound and long-lasting effects on a child's physical, emotional, and cognitive development (Felitti et al., 1998). Recognizing and addressing trauma early, while providing a nurturing and supportive environment, is essential for promoting resilience and healthier development in children facing adversity.

These case studies also illustrated a range of success. When working with minors, art therapists also work with their families or guardians. When art therapists can engage parents and other family members or caregivers to participate in the child's therapy, the outcome is always more successful.

CASE STUDY OF DEE: GRIEF IN TODDLERHOOD

MOLLY TOMONY

Setting and Approaches

The first 15 years of my career as an art therapist, I did hospice work. Due to my own life transitions, this work was done in three different states. My job title was "bereavement counselor" and my co-workers were trained as social workers. As the only art therapist, I was often asked to meet with those who communicated non-verbally. Typical referrals included gruff older adults who grunted to express feelings, angry teens who hid behind walls figuratively and literally, and preschool-age children who were just gathering words for expression. These individuals were formative in my understanding that non-verbal gestures often have greater meaning than words. Working in a home setting can provide a wealth of information but also presents challenges with boundaries and privacy. The materials used in these home settings were transportable in a crate on wheels, with developmental and medical needs considered as well as individual interests. These needs could vary from an elderly patient desiring to do a life review to children sublimating frustration through transformative art projects, such as breaking terracotta pots and making something new with the pieces to represent their feelings of their world being shattered.

Intake Session

Dee was a month shy of three years old when I met her, or as she informed me, "almost free". Dee's parents were in their late twenties and lived in a rural town. They had just given birth to their second child who had several serious health issues, and the life expectancy was weeks to months. The family hoped to keep their infant comfortable and bring the baby home so they could have as much family time as possible. Hospice was used to provide education, physical, emotional, and spiritual support during this transition. A nurse on the hospice team was going to meet Dee's parents and the baby. It was determined that it would be beneficial to have someone from the children's bereavement team accompany her to meet with Dee during this meeting. I agreed and in preparation packed my crate with paper, crayons and markers, play dough, puppets, small dolls and fidgets, bubbles, lunch bags, collage materials, and some books about life cycles and feelings including, *Lifetimes* (Mellonie, 1983) and *Double Dip Feelings* (Cain, 2001).

As the nurse and I drove to the family's home, it was clear that due to Dee's young age, the nurse did not expect me to provide bereavement support. She asked that I "occupy" Dee so that she could have privacy with the parents and Baby T. Walking into the family's small, cozy home gave me a snapshot of their lifestyle. The home was filled with family photos, children's artwork, plants, hand-knitted baby blankets, and a medium-sized friendly dog. The hardwood floors were worn and Dee's toys were plentiful and strewn about. Men's work boots, a hard hat, and a crucifix hung by the door. These observations and brief small talk provided most of the answers to the typical intake assessment.

The family was a white working-class Christian family with traditional gender roles. The couple had met in high school and married in their early twenties. Dad worked in construction, and the mom stayed at home with Dee. They had just brought their baby home from the hospital and instead of it being a joyous occasion filled with family and photo opportunities, they were nervous, sad, and flanked by strangers and medical equipment. They welcomed us into their home, but there was an awkwardness entering one's life as a stranger during such an intimate milestone. They wanted support but also wished that there was no reason for us to be there.

As the nurse began to examine Baby T, I introduced myself and asked how Dee was adjusting. They explained that she was proud to be a big sister and was gentle and sweet but was having temper tantrums and demanding lots of attention. The mom stated, "She knows that T is sick but other than having six fingers on one hand she looks like a regular baby. We have not talked about where this is likely headed, and we are still praying for a miracle". The mother began to cry, explaining they just wanted as much normal family time as possible. I asked what kind of support they had. The parents spoke of a close, large, extended family in the area and that parishioners from their Catholic church were bringing meals. I showed the parents some of the books and play items I brought and explained that I was a family bereavement counselor and was available to meet with Dee when the nurse came. I spoke of other children I had worked with that were Dee's age who found art and play to be comfortable languages to express feelings and fears about changes in their families. The parents asked some developmental questions about how to talk to Dee about the situation, and I wondered aloud with the nurse and parents about coming up with a different word for Baby T's condition other than the word "sick", as they mentioned. We talked about how everyone will be sick at some point, but Baby T's condition was different, and a distinction seemed important. The nurse suggested "serious illness or trisomy 13". The parents agreed, recognizing the importance of differentiating this from the common cold or other non-threatening issues, and our teamwork began.

I asked mom if she thought Dee would be comfortable playing with me in the nearby kitchen while they met with the nurse in the living room. She glanced at my crate of toys and art materials and stated, "She loves doing art and will talk your ear off". Using a turtle puppet from my crate, I playfully introduced Tommy the turtle to Dee, who had been watching Sesame Street and asked her if she wanted to see what other surprises I had in my box. My turtle puppet became a favorite of mine to introduce myself to young children as its head can be moved in and out of the shell to represent shyness and a need for protection. Dee and I worked at a round kitchen table. She sat on a booster seat and tried Tommy the turtle on. She practiced poking her finger in and out of the head to hide it or pop the head out to say hello. I then offered her some paper and drawing materials and she began to draw circles naming them as family members. Dee's use of drawing materials, controlled mark-making, and random use of color showed her to be between the scribble and pre-schematic stages of Lowenfeld's developmental model. She exaggerated the things that were noteworthy. For example, "my Dad has a beard" while adding "hair" around the entire circle representing his head (Figure 1.1).

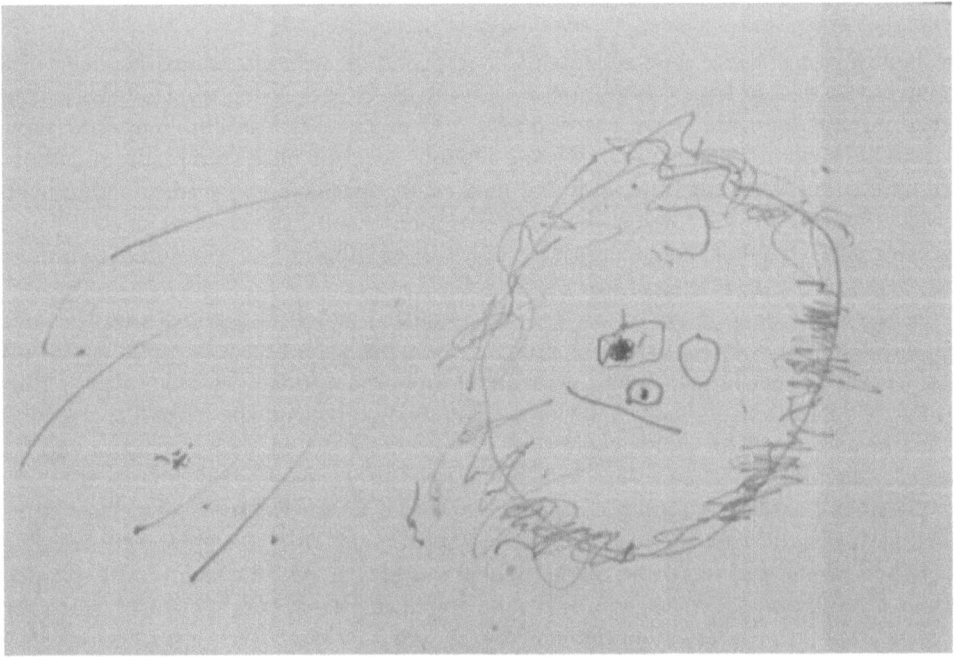

Figure 1.1 Dad's head

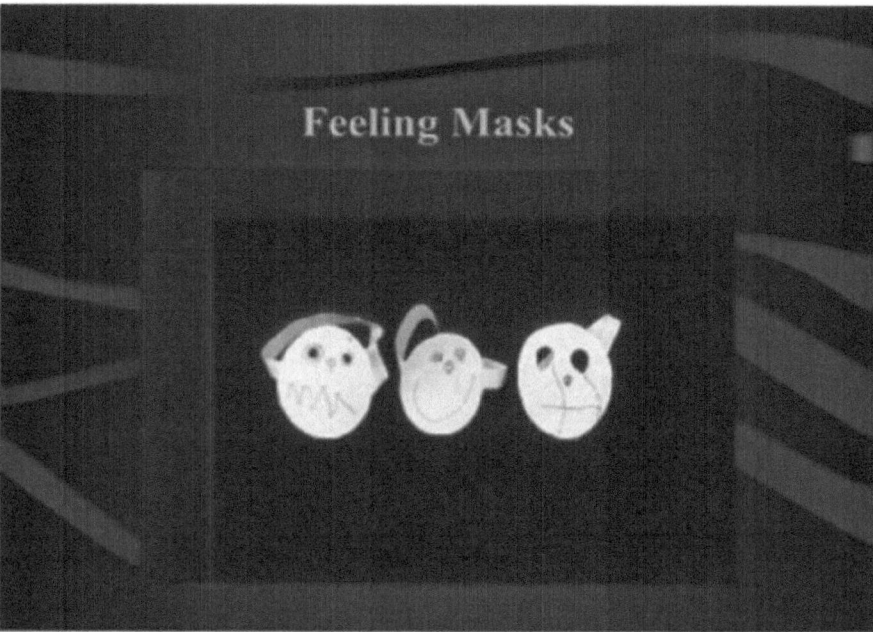

Figure 1.2 Feeling Masks

While Dee drew, I cut out shapes like hers to represent feeling faces. I asked Dee to help me draw faces that represented mad, happy, and sad on each of the shapes. As we created them, we role played the feelings. Growling for mad, big smiles for happy, and loud crying for sad (Figure 1.2). We turned these faces into masks and continued to put them on and *become* the feeling as we did so. This made a game out of "feeling identification" using art and play paired with the words.

Early Sessions

The nurse and I continued to visit Dee's family in this format for weeks. Dee and I played "family or house" using puppets and the feeling masks. We read books about feelings and wore our masks based on how the characters in the books were feeling. We blew bubbles and used beanie babies on our bellies to practice deep belly breathing while developing ways to regulate feelings. On a couple of occasions, Dee would not play alone in the kitchen with me. She sat next to her mom on the couch melting into her side as her mom fed Baby T. Dee showed me T's cute toes and counted the baby fingers noting with pride that she had six fingers. Dee showed me how she can *hold* T and nursed her own baby doll on her belly.

During the second month we met, Dee would separate from her Mom and often wore the "mad mask", growling. She rarely sat and we began to do some of our sessions outside including movement and play. When she drew her family with chalk on the driveway, her mom was often made with two circles on top of each other like a snow person. There were faces drawn on each, one representing her Mom and one for Baby T. It became evident that her Mom and Baby T were like one person in Dee's drawings and in real life too, as her Mom always seemed to be holding Baby T.

One day as we worked, I wondered if she wanted to make her own puppets using lunch bags. Dee suggested we make a family of bunnies. We proceeded to cut out bunny ears and tape them at the top of the lunch bags. Two ears for a Mom bunny puppet, two for a Dad, and big sister. Dee insisted that the baby bunny have three ears (Figure 1.3). She often put the smaller paper-bag puppet inside the Mom puppet. These puppets stayed in the crate and week after week we got them out during many sessions and played with them. We made various items for the bunnies as instructed by Dee. "They need food, beds, books, and a pool". Using the puppets during our house play, Dee would often create scenarios in which the baby bunny, with the extra appendage-like Baby T, would remain in the crate while the

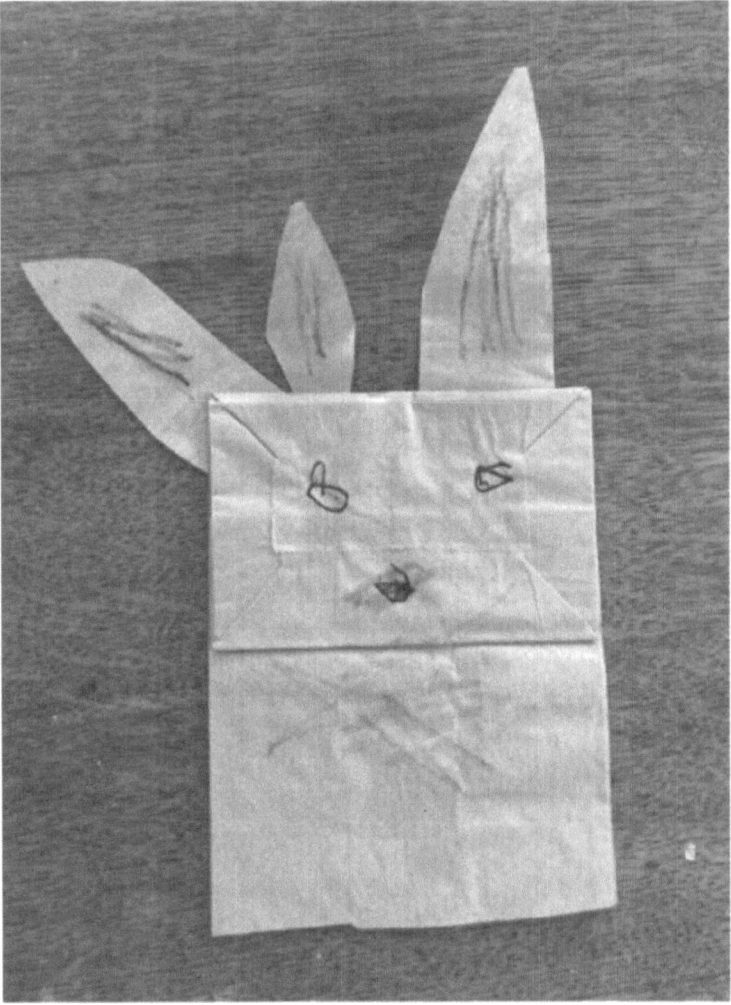

Figure 1.3 Paper-bag Bunny Puppets

older kid bunny got to play with the Mom bunny by herself. Dee instructed the play, "You be the mom and I am the kid, the baby has to sleep, and the dad is at work". The mom and kid bunny puppets baked play dough cookies and carrots, and hopped to the zoo to visit friends. As I played the role of the Mom bunny, I would try to introduce parallel supportive educational comments like, "It is fun to play with you", "I love the baby but I can't bake cookies with him", or "Even though big sister bunnies think the baby bunny is cute, sometimes they want them to go away so they can be with their parent alone". On one such occasion, Dee took the baby bunny puppet out of the crate and responded, "Sometimes they even wish the baby bunny was dead!". Dee then ripped up the baby bunny puppet into pieces and said, "It is dead" (Figure 1.4). Dee's Dad then entered the kitchen to get a drink and gave me a stern, hurt look that indicated he heard what Dee said. The play paused as

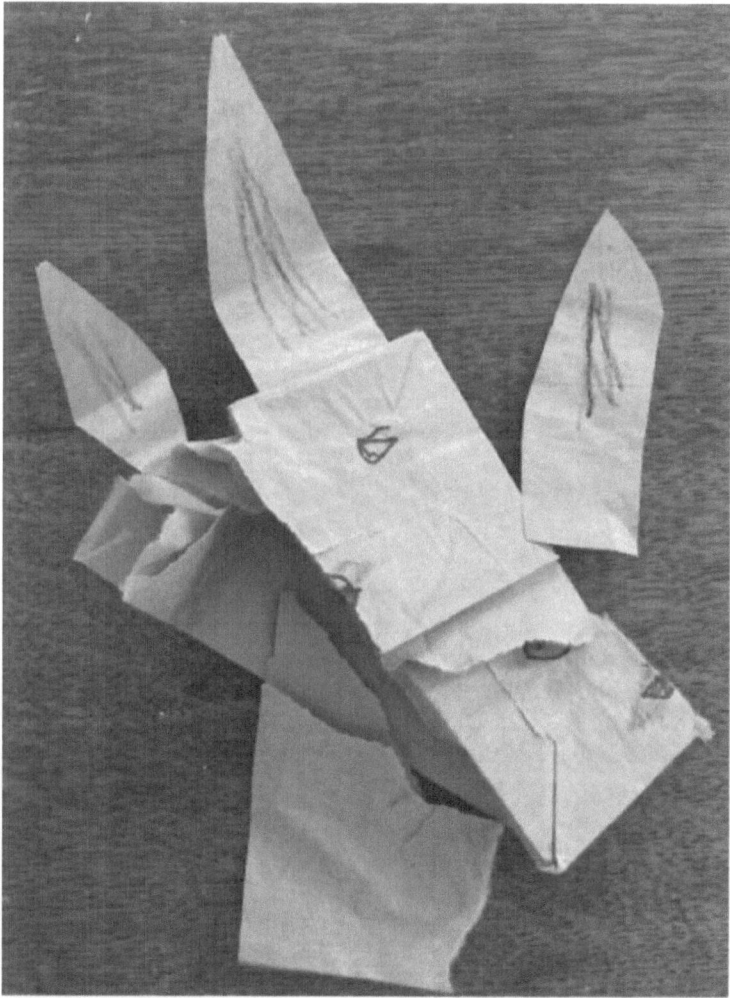

Figure 1.4 Paper-bag Bunny Puppets

her Dad left and I was reminded of some of the difficulties of doing therapy in the home and not having privacy. Though I was concerned about Dad's feelings, I knew Dee was waiting for my response. Using the Mom bunny, I stated "You sound mad, would you like to go outside and hop around or throw balls?" Dee broke from the play and said, "Let's go outside for real", and we ended our session playing in her backyard. I went back to the office and set up a supervision appointment.

What I was learning was that much more was happening than "just occupying" or babysitting. Preschool-age children can use play and art to express many things they are experiencing. I recognized how important it was to "stay in the play" and not to say the "aha moments" aloud. The work was happening and I needed to trust the process. It was clear, even though she knew Baby T had a serious illness, Dee was also experiencing typical sibling feelings of jealousy, deeply missing her parents, and had anger about the situation. Knowing that she was in the developmental stage of magical thinking, I feared that Dee may later think that her very normal feelings of wishing Baby T would go away made it happen.

When I met with my supervisor, she suggested I speak with the parents before my next session and let them know it seemed that even though they had not directly told Dee about the seriousness of Baby T's illness, she seemed to sense it was terminal. My supervisor believed foreshadowing what was likely to happen could make Dee feel more secure, trust her parents, and on some level understand her wishes could not make terrible things happen. Simply stating, "Usually doctors can treat illnesses and make people get better but sometimes the illness is so serious that even doctors cannot fix it and the person dies" would help Dee to grieve the impending loss.

Though I found the work with Dee to validate my belief in art therapy, I also used supervision to share my insecurities. I had much experience working with young children and felt comfortable working with Dee. However, at that time I did not have my own children and I felt unsure about giving parenting advice.

I spoke with Dee's mom and dad, and they supported me in answering Dee's questions about Baby T through our play and art. The Dad expressed his shock at the play he had overheard and stated, "I did not even think Dee knew what dead was," he added, "She has not had someone die in her life". We talked about ways she had experienced death and life cycles in nature like bugs, and a dead bird in their yard. I shared a book called *Lifetimes* (Mellonie, 1983) that simply talked about the life cycles of organisms from simple to complex. It explains that all living things have a birth and a death, with a lifetime in between. Insects' lifetimes may be days to weeks, animals' months to years, and people can live many years if they are healthy and do not have a serious accident. I spoke with them about just simply talking about living and lifetimes when the subject arose. I wondered what their beliefs were about what happens after someone dies. They shared their thoughts about afterlife and heaven and, through tears, mentioned that Baby T would be buried with a Catholic funeral.

Later Sessions

Dee and I continued to meet twice a week for a half hour. We read books about life cycles, played games around feeling identification, and did art. As we read *Double Dip Feelings* (Cain, 2001), we talked about how you can lick several flavors of ice cream and taste all the flavors at the same time, just as one can experience many feelings at the same time, i.e., scared, excited, and proud to start preschool, or happy and mad to be a big sister.

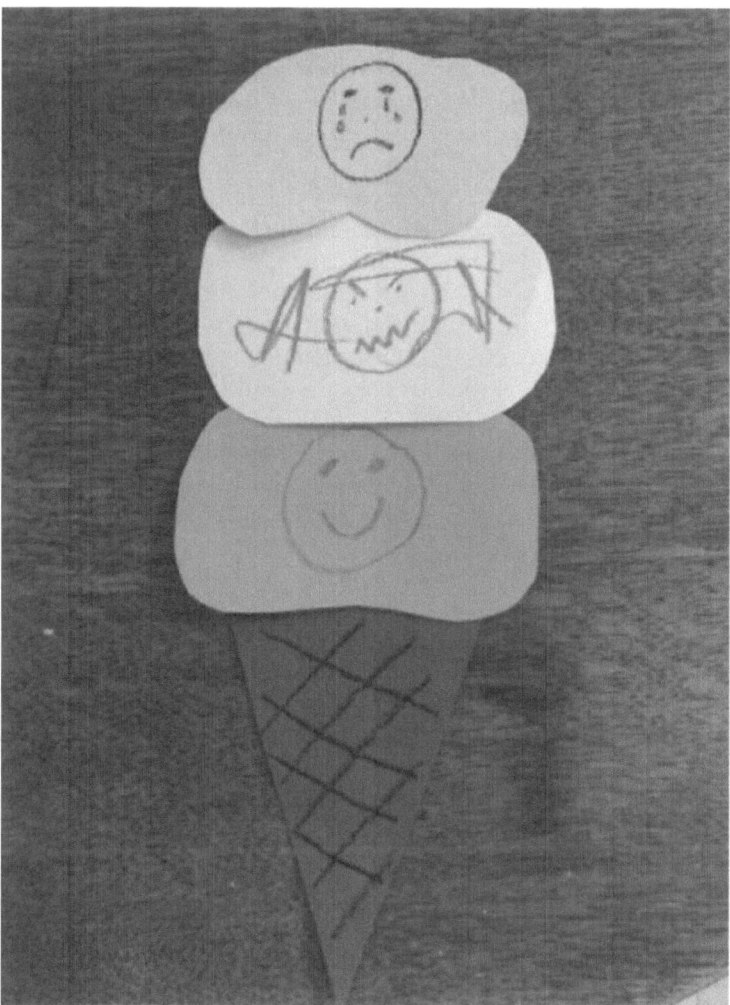

Figure 1.5 Double Dip Cone

We made double dip ice cream cones cut out with construction paper that had scoops of ice cream with feeling faces on them that extended from the floor to the ceiling (Figure 1.5).

After rapport was developed, I could tell she was receptive to these topics. When we were in attunement, Dee had temper tantrums when I told her it was time to clean up and say goodbye. I would give her a five-to-ten-minute warning, let her choose our last activity, and still she would often rip up art she had made out of anger. We began to make these ripped pieces into "mad balls" and used the garbage can as a basket to clean up and share what we were mad about. She yelled "Goodbyes!"

Outcomes

Baby T's condition was worsening, and the family was told that he had days to live. When I would arrive at the home there were often other family members present and Dee was easily distracted by the activity and change in her routine. Dee dug through my crate of materials and quickly played with a toy or art material, and then thrust it aside and moved on to the next. She found the family of bunny puppets we had made in our earlier session, and we began to play with them again. She asked where the baby bunny puppet was, and I reminded her that she ripped it up and said it was dead. I found the pieces, showed her, and stated when something is dead it stays dead. It can't breathe, hop, or eat carrots anymore. I put the Mom puppet on my hand and began to pretend the puppet was crying. The Mom bunny said, "I feel sad and miss the baby bunny, but I can still take care of my kid bunny". Dee giggled a bit at my dramatic crying and asked what we should do with the dead bunny. I explained that we needed a special box or casket to bury the dead bunny puppet in the ground. I dug through my crate of materials and found a small checkbook box. We lined the box using paper towels for blankets and wrapped the bunny puppet carefully in the box. We then went outside in the yard, dug a hole, had the bunny family bury it, and shared stories about the baby. I asked Dee if she wanted to say a prayer and she said, "God take care of my baby". We then played in her backyard.

Baby T died a week or so later. I offered to attend the wake and provide art materials for the children in attendance. Several children between the ages of two and twelve stopped by the "family room" where I posted mural paper to make a "picture for Baby T". I also provided cookies and milk. Dee ran in and out of the room, often drawing, but also visiting with cousins and friends and enjoyed the attention and activity. She would ask the kids if they wanted her to go with them to see Baby T and explained, "She can't breathe anymore or cry because she died. She can't feel". Sometimes she would add "God will take care of her now".

Conclusions

By bringing Baby T home with hospice, Dee's family created memories. Dee and I continued to meet weekly, and then monthly, for 13 months after Baby T died. We made a memory book, practiced healthy ways to cope with grief, and spent time with her parents making art and playing. The family had not had time to play together for a long time. Dee and her family also participated in our family grief-groups held once a week for parents and children who had a family member die. Dee taught all of us that preschool-age children are very aware of changes in their caregivers and routines. She reminded us of the importance of finding a comfortable language for them to explore their feelings and fears. For Dee, making art, reading books, and puppetry were a natural fit. Other preschool-age children may prefer Legos, movement, or music. The important thing is to develop rapport and provide creative opportunities for expression, support, and exploration. Dee will revisit her grief and the meaning of this loss at each new developmental stage (Lowenfeld & Brittain, 1987). Dee's memory book entitled "My Baby T". will serve as a reminder of her role as a big sister and all the double dip feelings that go with it.

AN IN-HOME TRAUMA-INFORMED ART THERAPY APPROACH IN THE CASE OF A TODDLER IMPACTED BY EXPERIENCES OF VIOLENCE AND LOSS

REBECCA MILLER

Setting

Home-based art therapy was provided in a designated space within Carla's home. Before sessions started, an informed consent process involved careful review of policies and procedures concerning home-based art therapy, such as liabilities, privacy concerns, use of space and materials, and other factors. Carla was three years of age and one or both of her parents were at home for all sessions. The parents stayed in a separate room, with the exception of the intake and family sessions. The client's mother completed the intake with me and, during one of the last sessions, both parents participated in the client's creative process. The majority of materials were transported by me to the client's home. Some personal items (photographs) were contributed by the family for use with the final project. I reproduced the photos in color for a decoupage box before returning the originals. Artwork created throughout the course of art therapy was kept in a portfolio that remained with me and then was given to the client, via the care of her parents, at the last session.

Approaches

My theoretical approach in this case was developmentally focused and trauma-informed. It incorporated consideration of early childhood development and the impact of the significant loss over the death of her grandmother. The loss had affected Carla's socio-emotional and overall functioning. The primary focus of art therapy was to allow the client a safe space for exploration of the loss of her grandmother that was compounded by an unexpected traumatic event, witnessing an act of violence in a park. Because Carla's parents requested a brief duration of therapy not lasting longer than ten sessions, the *SELF* (*Safety, Emotions, Loss,* and *Future*)compass of the Sanctuary model, a trauma-informed philosophy and model of treatment (Bloom, 2013; Bloom & Farragher, 2013), was used to inform the structure and chronology of art-based directives and activities. Originally developed by Dr. Sandra Bloom and colleagues for use with adults in short-term psychiatric settings, the model has since been adapted for use with children, adolescents, families, and caregivers within a wide variety of health and human service settings all around the globe (Bloom, 2013; Clarke, 2013; Elwyn et al., 2015; Rivard et al., 2003). Since 2008, the National Child Traumatic Stress Network (2023) has continued to include it among their list of empirically supported trauma-informed treatment and service approaches.

A core component of the Sanctuary model, the *SELF* compass is a useful framework for guiding art therapy practice when working with children and adolescents who have experienced trauma and losses. Rather than stages, *SELF* is conceptualized as a compass, implying that the therapist must be ready to pivot focus to any of these areas based on the client's presenting needs. In this case, using the *SELF* compass, art and play-based interventions targeted these four areas deemed critical in helping trauma survivors heal and maintain a sense of hope and optimism. This systemic lens was incorporated and a key consideration for including family members in treatment.

Client

Carla was of Puerto Rican, Dominican, and Native Hawaiian/Japanese descent, living in a densely populated urban area apartment with her biological parents, and a middle-school aged sister. Her mother, a woman in her late 30s was pregnant and expecting her third child, requested home-based art therapy for Carla following a series of difficult events that had resulted in observable behavioral and somatic changes in her youngest daughter, including anxiety and nightmares. One month prior to intake, Carla's beloved paternal grandmother died unexpectedly. Within days after the grandmother's death, Carla witnessed a violent assault on her mother's friend, a man stabbed her as they walked through a city park. Her symptoms included increased worry, anxiety, fear, hypervigilance, nightmares causing difficulty sleeping, and eating less than usual. As the family paid for art therapy out of pocket, a mental health diagnosis was not given.

Intake Session

The intake session occurred in the home with Carla and her mother, following arrangements made for home-based therapy during a telephone consultation. Carla remained in another room for the first part of the intake, and then joined towards the end. The focus of the intake was to better understand the contextual factors pertaining to the relational loss, traumatic events, and the negative impact mom saw in Carla relative to normative functioning for her age. We discussed family and cultural factors, identified goals for short-term art therapy, completed the informed consent paperwork, and I assessed interest in receiving additional psychoeducational resources to aid in coping with loss and trauma. Lastly, and of critical importance, I spoke to Carla in a developmentally appropriate way to assess her view of the concerns, ensured she understood the basic purpose and goals for art therapy, and gained her assent to working with me.

We scheduled weekly 50-minute sessions to take place within a predefined "rainbow rug" space while the mother remained in a separate room. We agreed to have at least two family sessions within the course of treatment to provide a forum for facilitating communication with Carla and her family concerning the focus and goals of our work together. Carla's dad worked during the day and her sister was in school, so it was mainly Carla's mom who attended, though Carla's dad was able to come for a brief time to one of these sessions. Carla's mother was also aware that she could contact me at any time by telephone, and that I would send reminder messages prior to each weekly session.

Early Sessions

Using the *SELF* compass as a guiding framework, the first few sessions were oriented around the focus of *Safety*. At the start of our first session, Carla was at the door with her mom. Carla appeared excited to see me and my friend "Camilo", a green stuffed lizard that she had met the week before during the intake. She was clutching the transitional object I had left with her until our first session, a small, multicolored "koosh" toy. Before Carla's mom left to go into a separate room, I checked in with her to see if she had any questions, and provided psychoeducational materials and resources to aid in coping with loss and trauma. Carla then led me into the corner of the living room where we would work, and together we unfurled the "rainbow rug", a rainbow-colored blanket I brought to define the art therapy working space.

At the start of each session, to create a sense of safety through ritual and promote positive coping with anxiety and stress, we began with several short somatically focused warm-up activities. In this first session, we did bubble blowing to promote deep breathing and we squished modeling clay into a balloon to create a stress ball. In the next session, I introduced a modified version of progressive muscle relaxation, focusing on the upper body where we imagined the clay was an orange that we were squeezing. Following the ritual of warm-up activities, we moved into the main activities.

The first session focused on favorite things that helped us to feel safe, and I asked if she might like to use the modeling clay to create what some of those things are for her. Immediately Carla began to transform the modeling clay into a variety of foods, first pancakes, then pizza, and finally grapes. As Carla worked on forming grapes, she asked Camilo to help. We jumped into the persona of the friendly lizard and made a small mountain of grapes. Maintaining the theme of safety and holding, I squealed in Camilo's delighted voice, "Wow, so many yummy grapes, maybe we should make a bowl to hold them?" I demonstrated how to make a simple pinch pot, Carla mirrored my process and made a bowl of her own. She also created and personalized her own "safe space" portfolio-box where all of her work could be safely kept. Carla added a picture of Camilo and the koosh toy, suggesting movement towards positive attachment with me via the conduit of the plush lizard and transitional object. We ended this first session, just as we would all subsequent sessions, with the ritual of the "clean up song", followed by more bubble blowing, and then packing up the "rainbow rug".

In the next few sessions, a focus on *Safety* continued, especially through our opening and closing rituals creating a "sandwich of safety", while also shifting the compass towards the areas of *Emotions* and *Loss*. In the second session, Carla associated colors with a simple range of emotions (i.e., happy, mad, sad, scared), and then used a template of a body outline to indicate where in her body she felt each of these emotions. In the third session, we read the book *A Terrible Thing Happened* (Holmes et al., 2000), using the story as a springboard for making art and directly discussing any feelings and memories that were elicited about the violent assault she witnessed. In response, she made a drawing reflective of her age and developmental level that depicted what the character Sherman's "terrible thing" might have been (Figure 1.6). She said that it was "a baby and a daddy in a car", with "lots of blood all around".

In a prior drawing, Carla had similarly used a red marker to draw an image of "scary pirates" that were trying "to get her", as well as "lots of blood". Although these drawings didn't reflect the exact nature of the violent act, metaphorically, they characterized feelings of fear, along with the literal depictions of spilled blood Carla had observed. During later sessions Carla told Camilo details about the assault on her mom's friend as they played "tea time", a play activity involving aspects of comfort and warmth that counterbalanced the violent details she described. Carla shared that a man assaulted her mom's friend with a knife, resulting in serious injury, and "a lot of blood". Also, "the man ran away" before the police and ambulance arrived to bring the friend to the hospital. In the next session, Carla reflected on the feelings and emotions she had felt when it happened and how "hard" it had been to share about it with me while we worked on forming a coil pot she decided could be a "nest" for Camilo. She added eggs to the nest that Camilo needed to sit on to protect, and made sustenance for him in the form of paper leaves and lollipops made of wax and pipe cleaners (Figure 1.7). In this way, the needle on the compass shifted fluidly between the domains of *Safety*, *Emotions*, and *Loss*. Carla's mother had joined us when Carla most

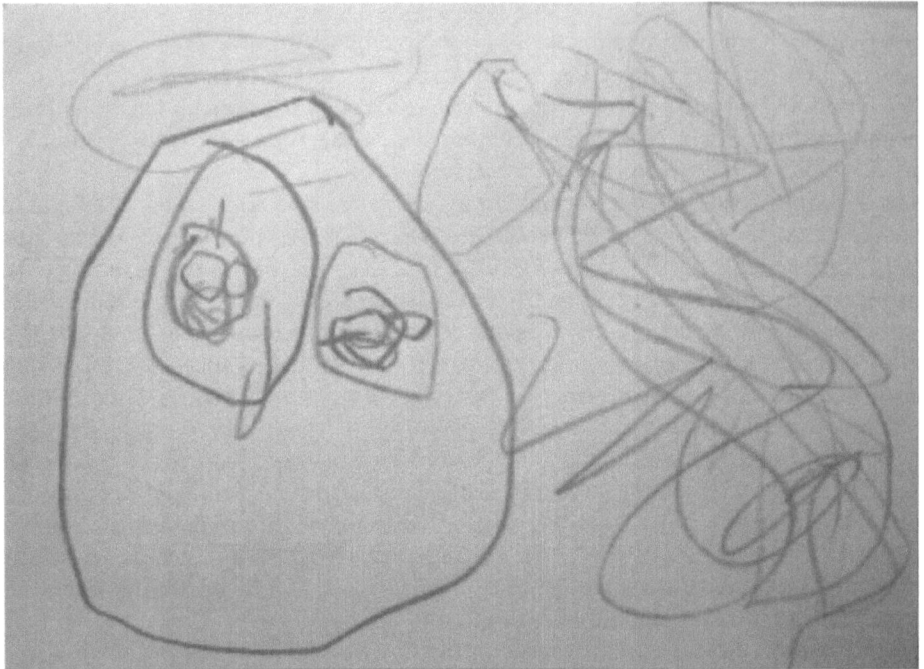

Figure 1.6 Untitled Drawing from Carla

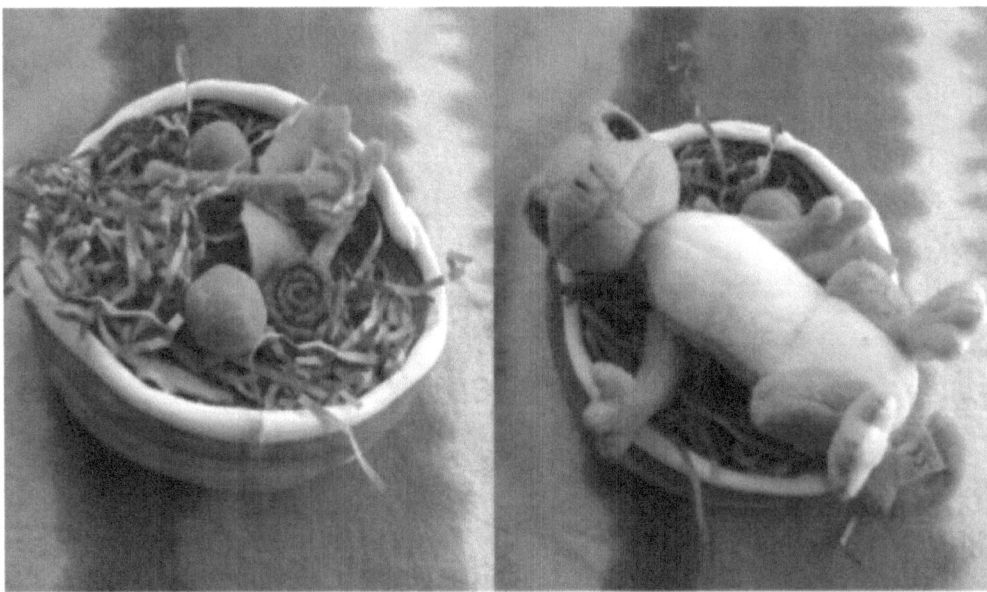

Figure 1.7 Camilo's "Nest" on the "Rainbow Rug"

directly shared about the traumatic event, and Mom supported Carla and actively encouraged her to draw and talk about the experience.

In the next session, Carla worked on creating a hand puppet friend for Camilo. I used this opportunity to begin talking about supportive relationships, including friends and family to turn to for emotional comfort and support. This provided a segue to address the loss of her grandmother, and include her family in the culminating art-making activities.

Later Sessions

Later art therapy sessions continued to target the area of *Loss* with direct attention to the death of her grandmother. They encompassed *Future* through exploration around themes of family, culture, belongingness, and resilience. As per the fluidity of the compass model, themes of *Safety* and *Emotions* were also an inherent part of this exploration.

In our sixth and seventh sessions, Carla created a family constellation using iridescent stickers of stars and planets to symbolize and place important family members in relation to her symbol, the sun. She included her recently deceased grandmother, referred to as "Tutu", the diminutive word for grandparent in Hawaiian. We also read together the book, *I Miss You: A First Look at Death* (Thomas & Harker, 2001). Both these activities provided a forum for creative and verbal expression of feelings related to Tutu's death. The book also served to validate and normalize the wide variety of feelings and thoughts that children may experience when someone close to them dies. Carla's mother joined us again, and during this time we discussed a plan for the last three sessions.

I presented several options for a creative, culminating project that would facilitate memory work. Art can be an important way to engage in memory work because it allows grief and mourning to become visible. According to Worden (2018), mourning helps individuals learn to accept the reality of the loss, work through the pain of grief, adjust to an environment where the deceased is missing, and emotionally relocate the deceased and move on. Mom provided photographs of the family with Tutu, I made color reproductions, and Carla chose to make a decoupage memory box.

In the remaining sessions, Carla sponge-painted the exterior of her box using green and purple paint. As she worked, we talked about her memories of Tutu, many of which related to Tutu's love of brightly colored flowers and music. Prior to our next session, I obtained a variety of small stickers and decals of flowers, musical notes, and other items. Mom joined the next session to assist in the emotionally significant part of adding photos and mementos to the memory box (Figure 1.8).

The engagement of Carla's mom facilitated positive reflection around meanings and stories for various photos and cultural mementos. For example, in one photo Tutu wore a kimono, and this allowed mom to explain to Carla about her Japanese and Hawaiian cultural heritage on her dad's side. Mom also shared stories behind the photos where Tutu held Carla, and Carla chose to put these images on the top of the box. This process allowed positive reminiscence and reflection on Tutu, while promoting the trusting relationship with Mom. Towards the end of this session, Carla reflected aloud, "We used to love Tutu", to which her mom responded, "We still love Tutu". Witnessing this tender and poignant exchange between Carla and her mom, I acknowledged the contradiction between the finality of death and the continuation of memories, replying that "When people die, they are not here anymore, but our memories of them are still here with us, so we can still love them".

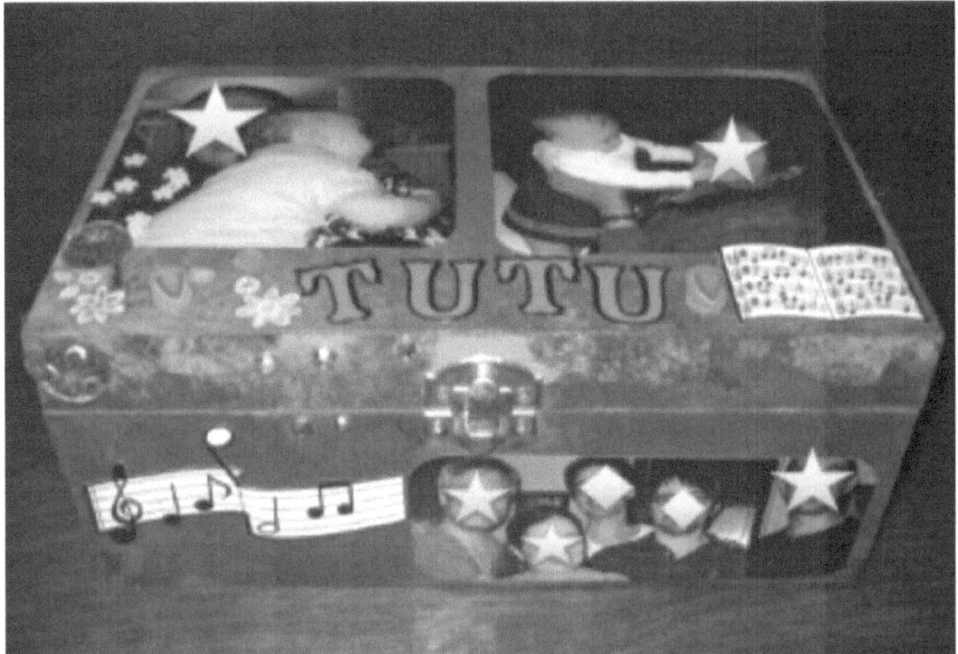

Figure 1.8 Carla's Memory Box

They were not able to fit every image onto the box, but decided they could be contained within it, along with anything else in the future that Carla might find.

Toward the end of the final session, Carla's dad joined us and Carla proudly reflected on the pictures and her process of creating the memory box. Dad said little as he listened attentively to his daughter, and before returning to his work, wiped tears from his eyes and thanked me. In this session, Carla and I did our opening and closing rituals for the last time, and in between reflected on her progress while playing a game involving Camilo. I relayed the strength and resilience I saw in her, along with the love and closeness I observed in the family as they worked on the memory box.

Outcomes and Conclusions

Using the *SELF* compass of the Sanctuary model as a guide, the primary goal of my art therapy work with Carla had been to provide a safe space for processing the experience of trauma and loss, to aid in positive coping, and remediate negative symptoms. This was achieved by grounding the sessions in the domain of *Safety* through use of rituals that built positive coping skills, defined clear boundaries in the physical space, and built a strong therapeutic alliance. Play-based interventions were a significant aid as well, just ask Carla's plush-green-lizard friend, Camilo! The "sandwich of safety" created through these means allowed Carla to directly address the areas of *Emotions* and *Loss* in connection with the assault witnessed and the death of Tutu. About halfway through the course of therapy, shortly after we directly processed the assault, Carla's mom reported the nightmares had stopped and Carla's anxiety and fearfulness seemed to lessen. Art therapy had also served to facilitate positive grieving and loss integration through the culminating memory box. Given Carla's young age, further use of the box might continue to provide a safe space for containing additional memories as they arise. Pertaining to the area of *Future*, the support Carla received from both parents while working on the box reflected strengthening bonds of support, love, connection, and resilience that they could draw on as they moved forward as a family.

COMPOSITE CASE STUDY OF PRESCHOOL-AGED YOUTH IN FOSTER CARE

CASEY L. BURKE

Setting

Home-based, individual art therapy sessions were conducted in foster families' apartments throughout a large metropolitan area in the northeast. All families were connected to the same foster care agency, which was located in the region. Most sessions occurred in a central location in the foster families' home, such as a coffee table, on the floor in the families' living room, or at a kitchen table. Foster parents and foster siblings were often present in the home during the time of the sessions, and occasionally joined in the sessions or participated in discussions with the client and myself. I typically brought materials to the home in a large bag, which could include, construction paper, markers, crayons, oil pastels, water color paints, acrylic paints, paint brushes, Play Doh, Model Magic, feathers, beads, yarn, glitter glue, and occasionally natural materials such as sticks, leaves, and pine cones. These materials would vary from week to week.

Approaches

Individual art therapy sessions were conducted with an integrative approach, in which both psychodynamic and strengths-based models were implemented. All clients were treated through a trauma-informed lens, with special attention to attachment-based issues stemming from their separation from their biological parents. In certain circumstances, despite their young age, these clients may have already transitioned through multiple caregivers. The fact that the sessions were conducted in the clients' foster homes where they were living at the time allowed for a deeper understanding of how they were connecting with their environment and the people in it. Winnicott (1971) stated, "A description of the individual cannot be made entirely in terms of the individual, but that in certain areas ... the behavior of the environment is part of the individual's own personal development and must therefore be included" (p. 53).

Clients

This is a composite case study summarizing my work as an art therapist with several preschool youth ages three to five in a foster care system. Many of the clients I worked with were in kinship foster care, meaning that they were placed with a family member such as a grandparent, aunt, or uncle. The children I worked with were Black, Hispanic, and mixed-race individuals. They tended to come from lower socioeconomic families, while the foster families they were living with during the time of services typically ranged from the lower to lower-middle class status. Biological siblings would sometimes be placed in the same foster home with my clients, while other clients had siblings living with other relatives or in other foster placements. Some of the children's biological parents were experiencing homelessness or incarceration.

Presenting Problems

The clients I worked with ranged in their developmental levels and needs. Some of the children were developing typically, while others had been either diagnosed with Pervasive Developmental Disorder or Oppositional Defiant Disorder according to the DSM-5-TR (APA, 2022). Some of the children had also been born with positive toxicology screens, which may have been the reason for their removal from their biological mothers, and this had led to both cognitive and emotional delays. None of the children I worked with specifically had any physical developmental delays that were evident at the time. One set of preschool-aged siblings who I worked with were living with a deaf grandmother in a kinship foster care arrangement, neither of the children had hearing losses.

Early Sessions

My initial sessions were about introducing myself, and my role as an art therapist. Early sessions were also about beginning to earn the trust of both my clients and the foster families where they were placed. My primary focus included building rapport while creating appropriate boundaries with the clients and their foster families.

The clients demonstrated their early attachment traumas in the ways they connected with me in our first sessions together. Some clients reflected their earlier experiences in their resistance to eye contact, conversation, or to participating in art therapy in general. Others displayed intense separation anxiety when I announced it was time for the session to end, or would blur boundaries by trying to sit in my lap during a session or asking to come home with me.

The foster families they were placed with had often endured their own traumas and hardships. Sometimes the navigation of a complex foster care system could be frustrating. Foster families often showed their own resistance to entrusting me with the children in their care or sharing information that may be helpful to treatment.

Short-term treatment objectives often included increased tolerance of frustration, accurately identifying emotions, and decreasing the frequency of tantrums or outbursts. Longer-term goals involved developing emotional regulation tools, working collaboratively and effectively with the foster families, and forming healthy relationships.

Later Sessions

The most crucial element to breaking through resistance with these clients, and to supporting them to feel seen and heard while maintaining clear boundaries, was engaging them through art and play. Due to the fact that much of the trauma that was experienced by these clients occurred in their preverbal stages of development, their ability to process trauma in a non-verbal format was extremely important. Mahler et al. (1975) were the first to establish the concept of separation-individuation. They defined the separation-individuation process as

> the establishment of a sense of separateness from, and relation to, a world of reality, particularly with regard to the experience of *one's own body*, and to the principal representative of the world as the infant experiences it, the *primary love object.*
>
> (p. 3)

I often found when working with these children that part of my role as an art therapist was to guide them back through a separation-individuation process that they had not fully experienced before, or had been forced through previously in a disruptive manner.

When clients had difficulty connecting with me, as evidenced in their closed off body language or limited verbal communication, sensory experiences with Play-Doh and Model Magic were helpful because it diffused some of their anxious energy. I often used metaphors to communicate with clients. For example, exploring the story of two birds drawn by one client including the relationship between the birds, and where they lived, was less threatening than asking the clients direct questions about their relationship with their biological parents.

For the children who threw themselves on the floor, or began crying and screaming when I announced it was time to clean up, I noted the importance of a consistent routine. For one child in particular, this routine involved utilizing a "magic wand" that we had created in one of our sessions using a wooden dowel, paint, ribbons, and gems. At the end of each session, I would announce that it was time to clean up, and the client would take out their magic wand. They would then point the magic wand at each of the materials that we had used that day, and when they pointed at the materials I would make them "disappear" into my bag. The act of cleaning up became a game that the client looked forward to, and over time the tears and tantrums over my imminent departure ceased.

Outcomes

Boundary testing continued throughout my work with these clients, as was developmentally appropriate for their age range, and at times there were regressions in their behaviors. Sometimes those regressions would occur within our sessions, while other times they would be reported to have occurred in the home throughout the week, or in school or daycare settings. Overall, I did generally see progress in terms of the treatment goals established. I noted that the clients were able to identify their emotional states more easily, and employ the regulation tools provided to them when they became overwhelmed. Later in treatment, I would often come to the homes and be presented with a stack of drawings that the clients had created throughout the week. Art became an outlet for these clients, and the foster families began to see the value of allowing the children in their care the space to express their emotions in a creative way. Robbins (1994) explained,

> For a fortunate few, the world of creativity becomes a major source of externalization. Here in the safety and confines of a sphere when they are completely in charge, the individual dares to bring forth and concretize the early representations of past conflicts.
>
> (p. 39)

In this new creative exploration that the clients engaged in, they began to resolve early conflicts and heal wounds from traumatic experiences from their pre-verbal and early verbal lives.

Because the foster care system is unpredictable, and due to the fact that both the clients and the providers are often at the mercy of the courts, proper termination was not always possible. I would sometimes receive notice a day or two before I was scheduled to see a child that our sessions would not be continuing, as the child had returned to their biological parents. When I did have proper notice of a looming termination date, or in the cases where I myself was ending the relationship to go on maternity leave, I typically created a transitional object with the clients. This was my way of both honoring the losses and separations these clients had already experienced, as well as the relationship we had created together. These transitional objects were typically small, such as a rock that we painted together, or a small teddy bear that the child would help to decorate and fill with stuffing and which I would sew together. They were easily held and transported by the child, with the knowledge that this may not be their last time transitioning to a new home or to a new therapist.

In certain cases, I was able to help transition the children to their new art therapists prior to my departure, if those therapists were a part of my agency. When possible, having a transition session in which I was present alongside the new therapist helped to make for a smoother hand-off, and allowed the clients as well as the foster families to feel more comfortable allowing this new person into their homes. When my role shifted to a supervisory position within my agency, I would sometimes receive updates on children I had worked with previously from my supervisees. Changes in treatment objectives and reunification plans had often occurred over time on the side of the foster care agency, and these changes impacted the overall well-being and presentation of the clients. Generally, the reflections of the ongoing art therapy sessions I received from my supervisees demonstrated clients' willingness to continue engaging in art therapy and progress towards establishing healthy relationships.

Conclusions

I learned a great deal from working with this population as an art therapist as well as a supervisor. I was continually reminded of how formative the early years are, and how trauma from unhealthy attachment experiences can so deeply impact a child's ability to connect with others in a meaningful way. I also observed the reparative nature of art and play. Winnicott (1971) stated, "It is in playing and only playing that the individual child or adult is able to be creative and to use the whole personality, and it is only in being creative that the individual discovers the self" (p. 54). Art therapy can be a method of creative play that bridges the divides created by trauma. I was able to help the children I worked with understand themselves and the environment they lived in through routine, use of metaphor, and safe exploration. Although I was not ultimately able to remove all of the challenges and environmental stressors from these clients' lives, I do believe that the tools they developed through art therapy will help them with understanding and managing their emotions surrounding their circumstances, as well as in navigating future relationships.

FAMILY CARE: FINDING VOICE THROUGH PUPPETRY

JILL MCNUTT

Self-Expression Through Art was a recurring, six-week, hour-and-a-half session for families impacted by epilepsy. There were two sessions each week, the earlier for children under 12, and the afternoon for teens. The programming occurred in the studio space within the local art museum, once in the fall and once in spring. Sessions were designed with one project that was built from the foundation during the earlier sessions through completion during the fifth and sixth sessions and included some kind of display or closure that invited other family and community members to attend.

The groups were grant-funded through the Forest County Potawatomi Foundation and occurred through a partnership with the local Epilepsy Foundation, the art museum, and me as the art therapist. I also brought art therapy interns into the program regularly. Youth with epilepsy and their families attended the sessions.

The studio space was well-stocked except for plumbing. Each session, we brought in five-gallon pails of water for use during the studio and subsequent clean-up. The sessions on which this report was written featured sock puppets. Materials laid out for the creation of sock puppets included paper and drawing materials for sketching and planning, adult-sized colored athletic socks, cardboard circles of various sizes to create puppet mouths, hot glue guns, yarn, thread, fabric, felt, buttons, sequins, and a collection of found objects.

The therapeutic approach used in this case aligns with humanistic and person-centered principles, as it encourages self-expression, creativity, and the development of personal growth and insight. Socialization, self-esteem, and quality of life were overarching goals for these groups.

Client

Tommie attended the morning sessions with his family. Tommie's older brother had epilepsy. He and his brother attended sessions along with his mother and grandfather. Tommie at the age of six had just started the first grade. He did not engage with other members of the group during the first five weeks of sessions. Instead, he spoke silently only to his mother and grandfather. Mom was clearly the primary caregiver, and Papa was a valuable substitute when Mom needed to tend to Tommie's brother's medical needs. Tommie's family is of Hispanic origin, and they frequently shared traditions and celebrations within the context of the group.

Sessions

During the first session, Tommie stayed very close to his mother, hiding behind her skirt and avoiding eye contact with anyone except his immediate family. During check-in, he whispered to his mother, who shared his name and favorite color, pink. Following check-in, we introduced the sock puppet project for the upcoming six weeks and invited families to use paper and drawing utensils to create a plan for their puppets. Parents and other family members were encouraged to participate independently, creating the art processes on their own. Papa, Tommie, and his brother each drew puppet plans while Mom chose to sit back and observe.

Tommie's drawing plans for his puppet were at the preschematic level (Lowenfeld & Brittain, 1987), which is typical for children of three and four years of age. Figures drawn at this level are called encephalopods. Tommie's puppet plan included a large head with arms extending from the top, ears extending from each side, and legs extending from the bottom. The face included a smile with an extended tongue, two eyes, and a button nose.

The second week, colored socks and mouth circles were chosen by each participant. In the absence of a pink sock, Tommie chose a blue one. Participants were given directions on folding the cardboard circles for making mouths and hot gluing them into the interior of the sock. Fiberfill was provided for stuffing the head above the cardboard mouth. Tommie was assisted by his mother in securing the mouth, but was able to fill the head with fiberfill. When the basic sock puppets were formed, participants were invited to start to play with the puppet and dialogue with it to help determine what materials would be necessary for the completion of the puppets. Tommie and his mother collected materials to replicate his drawing including felt, pipe-cleaners, googly eyes, sticks, and a miniature pair of black boots. They also collected raffia to make hair, and some fabric to make clothing.

The next session, the puppet assembly began. Tommie quickly drew hand shapes on the felt and began to cut them out. His movements were quick, and he accidentally cut three of the fingers off the felt hand. Mom recognized his anticipation and made an agreement with Tommie that they would make his puppet together. From this point forward, Tommie and Mom became a team, and they spent the next two sessions following Tommie's original design. During these sessions, Tommie spoke to no one except his immediate family. Papa and Tommie's brother continued working independently on their puppets. The fifth session was spent creating a dramatization for the puppets to interact. Tommie's brother agreed to be a part of a three-puppet song and dance show with two other youths with epilepsy. Tommie wanted his mother to be his partner, but she explained that she did not have a puppet. Papa graciously agreed to partner with Tommie. The two (three, including mom) developed a scene like *The Princess Bride* (Reiner, 1987), where the grandfather came to sit with the grandchild who was unable to go to school. In the plans for this puppet play, most of the dialogue was Papa reading a story.

The final session was a puppet show. Staff had built a wooden puppet show frame and used a curtain rod to secure a red curtain so that the puppets would have a space to be introduced to the rest of the group. When it was Tommie's turn to present, Papa took a chair behind the stage, and Tommie chose to stand. The puppets rose from behind the screen and Tommie's puppet started chattering. Papa had difficulty getting a word in edgewise and never got to read the proposed story to Tommie's puppet. When his turn was over, Tommie's puppet did not leave Tommie's hand. Tommie began to engage with it out from behind the curtain. Tommie's puppet started introducing itself to other children and parents who had spent the last six weeks with Tommie in silence. Another parent asked Tommie about the puppet, and Tommie responded directly to her without the interface of the puppet. His smile was as wide as his face as his mother escorted him to his seat to watch the remaining puppet shows. During the remaining shows, Tommie interacted with the puppets on stage when prompted and applauded loudly following each performance.

Conclusions

Tommie, a six-year-old male, came to a family art therapy group with extreme shyness and reluctance to speak, except with his immediate family. Tommie's brother has epilepsy, which seemed to contribute to his social withdrawal. In the six-week art therapy group, Tommie and his family engaged in five weeks of creating sock puppets, culminating in a puppet show. During the final session, Tommie used his puppet as a transitional object (Winnicott, 1971) to communicate and interact with others, breaking his silence. Subsequently, he has become more engaged and communicative.

Outcomes

Tommie's progress indicated the effectiveness of art therapy in helping him overcome his shyness. By using the puppet as a transitional object, he gained confidence and a voice. Tommie's family returned for the next three offerings of Self-Expression Through Art as Tommie continued to develop his communication skills and cope with the challenges related to his brother's epilepsy. This case illustrates the power of art therapy in helping children overcome emotional challenges and highlights the importance of a family-centered approach to addressing the needs of siblings in such situations.

CHILDREN'S CORNER: ART THERAPY FOR CHILDREN CASE STUDIES

PEG DUNN-SNOW

Setting

The therapy setting is a small, but comfortable office suite located in the southeast. The practice serves children ages five to 12 and their parents or guardians. Parents or guardians are required to participate in the therapy sessions with their children who are dealing with a wide range of challenges. These presenting problems can include severe anxiety, conflicts with others, serious medical conditions, issues of grief and loss, and other traumatic injuries. The office has two comfortable chairs for parents and the older clients to use. There is also a small table and chairs for the smaller clients. A variety of art materials as well as a sandtray, sandtray figures, puppets, a dollhouse, dolls, a library of books for bibliotherapy, and therapeutic games are available to facilitate art therapy goals and objectives with the children.

Approaches

Approaches to therapy are tailored to the clients' needs and can include: Constructivist Learning Theory (Gergen, 2015), Internal Family Systems (Schwartz, 1995), Cognitive Behavioral Therapy (Beck, 2020), Narrative Therapy (Dunne, 2016), Polyvagal Theory (Dana, 2020; Porges, 2011), Sandtray-Play Therapy (Homeyer & Lyles, 2022), and Instinctual Trauma Response (ITR; Tinnin & Gantt, 2013). The three case studies below will specify the approaches used with the clients.

Brian and Faye: Inter-Family Kidnapping

Siblings Brian and Faye were seen in weekly art therapy sessions for 12 months before their mother was transferred to a new military assignment and the family moved out-of-state. The children were seen in individual sessions, dyads, and in family sessions with their mother. Their mother also participated during the last 15 minutes of the children's individual and dyad sessions.

Intake Sessions

The children were first seen in the month of December and a preliminary diagnostic impression of post-traumatic stress disorder (PTSD) acute, was made based on the following information. It was reported that two months earlier, just prior to Halloween, the children were kidnapped by their father, his girlfriend, and their paternal grandmother. The children were taken across state lines for approximately six weeks where they lived with their father and grandmother until authorities returned them to their mother. In the intake sessions, the mother reported the children had been abused and neglected, and were in poor health when she regained custody of them. During the time the children attended art therapy sessions, their mother was granted full custody of her son and daughter.

Early Sessions

When the children were first seen in art therapy, they both exhibited physical symptoms. Brian experienced having more physical symptoms than his sister, including headaches and stomach aches. Both children had nightmares and wet the bed once they were living with their mother again. Neither child slept alone throughout the entire night. Faye continued to wet the bed during the year she was in therapy and frequently got up in the middle of the night to sleep with either her mother or her brother.

During early art therapy sessions, their father called them on video every month. The calls were approximately eight to 12 minutes long, and initially only Faye spoke to their father. During one call, the children reported that their father told them their mother was dying and too sick to take care of them, and the reason she wanted them to live with her was because she received extra money for having them with her. Immediately afterwards, all phone calls with the father stopped. The issue of their mother's possible death became the topic of concern in many future art therapy sessions. Faye asked many times about her mother dying during her individual sessions. Neither child asked about their mother receiving money because they were living with her.

The first goal was safety. For several months, visual schedules were created and used at the beginning of each of the children's sessions, providing a sense of control for these siblings over their environment as they knew ahead of time what was going to happen to them in the therapy room. Allowing children to have some predictability of the future helps to build safety (Dana, 2020; Redfield & Onderko, 2016).

Safety as a metaphor carries with it a physiological state (Porges, 2011). If children feel safe, they have the ability to play. In a therapy setting, play is defined as a neutral exercise allowing children to mobilize their nervous systems to reduce traditional stress responses (i.e., fight, flight, freeze, or fawn) or other defense systems with face-to-face social interactions. Play allows children the ability to integrate their conflicting thoughts and feelings about themselves in relation to their experiences and develop stronger coping strategies. Goals charts were also created in early art therapy sessions and used at home to track their behavioral and academic accomplishments.

Assessments and Treatment Plans

Assessments were ongoing throughout the children's time in art therapy. Initially informal assessments included free drawings, self-portraits, and play therapy activities such as an altered *Magic Wand* technique (Schaefer & Cangelosi, 2016). This activity helped to better understand each child's emotional state and self-concept. The Magic Wand is a drawing directive that provides a child three magic wands that correspond to themselves, another person they know, and the world in general. The task asks them to illustrate a change they would make in each of these three areas. The siblings were also asked to complete a protocol designed specifically to identify their responses to their kidnapping experience and what followed afterwards. What is most important in addressing trauma is helping the client understand his or her responses to the traumatic event versus the trauma itself (Porges, 2011).

Psychiatrist Louis Tinnin and art therapist Linda Gantt (2013) developed and published their work on trauma therapy which they call The Instinctual Trauma Response (ITR). This protocol is a combination of art therapy, narrative therapy, and parts work as described in writings about the Internal Family Systems (IFS) approach to therapy (Schwarz, 1995, Spiegel, 2017). Other examples on the use of the ITR protocol can also be found in the writings of other art therapists (Arrington, 2007).

Art Therapist Linda Chapman (2014) developed the Chapman Art Therapy Treatment Invention (CATTI). Working with children and adolescents who require trauma therapy, the CATTI protocol is similar in design to the ITR. Although the CATTI was not administered to these siblings, I referenced Chapman's work frequently when working with these clients, especially her writings on helping to promote safety during early therapy sessions.

Long term goals included expanding the family's support system, resolving the siblings' fear of losing their mother, reducing the siblings' physical symptoms caused by trauma, resolving the siblings' loss of their father and grandmother, forgiving family members who hurt the children, and restoring the siblings' sense of self-worth.

A first set of short-term objectives included providing a safe place and developing a trusting relationship with the siblings and their mother, encouraging age-appropriate activities for the children, and providing a safe way to have the children tell the story of their kidnapping and abuse. A second set of short-term goals included having the children identify their physical reactions, thoughts, and feelings about their traumatic experience as well as identifying ways they began individual self-care. A third set of short-term objectives included correcting any false beliefs the siblings may have connected to their traumatic experiences, reducing any excessive anger or displays of aggression caused by their trauma, and helping the siblings regulate their nervous system to stress by developing other coping strategies to express their thoughts and feelings.

Later Sessions

With the exception of formal and informal assessments, the siblings' ongoing sessions were non-directed with each child given the opportunity to select what they wanted to do during therapy. Children must experience success in order to improve their self-esteem and self-confidence (Leary & Baumeister, 2000). Developmental levels also influenced these non-directed art therapy sessions.

Developmental Considerations

The differences in the children's ages, stages of art development, and cognitive, language, and fine motor development were deciding factors in what art materials, and, subsequently, the art task, they chose during sessions. Developmental consideration also influenced the types of coping strategies they used initially in response to their traumatic experience of being kidnapped, and later abused and neglected.

There was also evidence that developmental considerations influenced the differences in the children's understanding and memories of the traumatic experience. Brian's language and vocabulary development gave him the ability to understand more accurately what had happened to him and his younger sister. Brian, age ten, was also able to talk about their experiences and how those experiences related to the meaning of his artwork. Faye, age five, was reluctant to talk about her experiences and expressed her conflicted feelings about her father and grandmother using non-verbal sandtray therapy and play therapy.

With his fine-motor skills, Brian was able to manipulate clay and frequently created monsters (Figure 1.9), explaining they represented his anger and fear toward his father. He also used the sandtray depicting battles of good and evil forces to represent his own good and bad parts. Brian often discussed his conflicting thoughts and feelings about his dad, grandmother, and himself.

Like most younger children, Faye was unable to put into words her thoughts and feelings about what had happened to her and her older brother. In the beginning of therapy, Faye used the sandtray exclusively, creating three-dimensional scenes depicting a grandmother figure who was nurturing, perhaps as a way of illustrating her conflicted feelings about

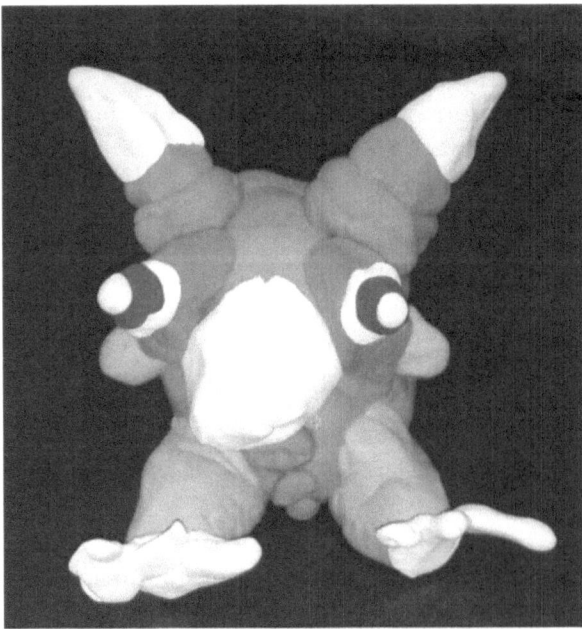

Figure 1.9 Brian's Monster

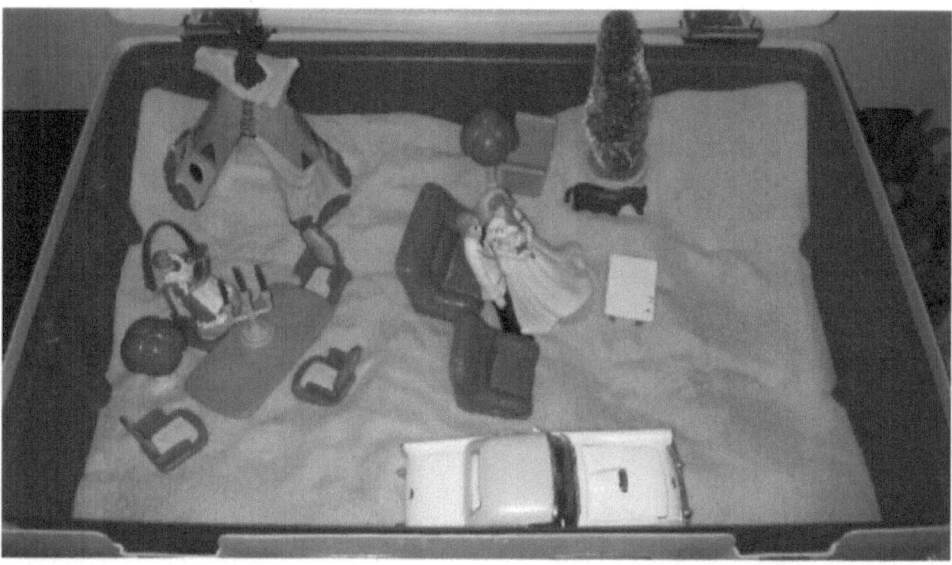

Figure 1.10 Faye's Nurturing Grandmother

her own paternal grandmother (Figure 1.10). Faye also laughed in sessions that were not always socially appropriate, which could also indicate her inability to currently use words to reveal her thoughts and feelings. Through play therapy in later sessions, Faye used dolls and a dollhouse to talk about what life was like living with her mother again.

Because both children enjoyed reading and listening to stories, bibliotherapy was added to their treatment plans during some sessions. Echoing their family, ritual, weekly board games, *Kids' World Inside & Out: A Psychotherapeutic Game* was also added to the treatment plan (Mones, 2017). This board game is specifically used in therapy sessions to help young clients identify and understand their feelings and behaviors as defined as partswork within the IFS approach to therapy (Schwartz, 1995; Spiegel, 2017).

Outcomes

Cognitive and Emotional Growth

Throughout the school year both children did well academically, but emotionally they both exhibited anger in school by getting into fights with classmates or not following classroom rules. It was difficult for them to make friends, especially for Faye. Both Brian and Faye were very attached to their mother and at times continued to express their fears about losing her. Safety continued to be a primary topic for discussion for both children through the year they were in therapy.

Ambivalence Toward Their Father and Grandmother

Both children exhibited different degrees of ambivalence toward their father and grandmother. Even before the video calls with their father were stopped, Brian had already decided he did not want to talk to their father. During the course of therapy, both children continued to integrate conflicting thoughts and feelings about their father and grandmother. It was near the end of therapy that both Brian and Faye began to accept and integrate the experience of being kidnapped as well as thoughts and feelings toward their father. Brian stated that he forgave his father for inflicting physical abuse on his sister and himself. Faye asked, on more than one occasion, if "Daddy" was better now, was it okay to still love him?

Termination

After a year of therapy, termination sessions were conducted for both children, as their family was preparing to move out-of-state after the December holidays. There was an expectation that both children would experience a period of regression after they moved to start a new life in a new state, and attend a new school during the middle of a school calendar year. It was recommended that the children start therapy sessions again once they were relocated and settled in their new home.

Post-Terminations Sessions – A Setback

A week after the children stopped coming to art therapy sessions, their mother contacted me to schedule some family sessions. Prior to their move, their father had insisted on having a supervised visit with the children in early January. It was reported by the mother that as soon as the children were told about this visit, Brian began having nightmares again. During these post-termination sessions, a detailed explanation was given to the children about the steps that would be taken to schedule a four-hour supervised visit. Both children were anxious about this visit as evidenced by the many questions they had and the statements they made in their sessions. When told that their father would have to follow certain rules before the visit could take place, Brian stated, "My dad doesn't follow rules. He speeds when he drives his car". Faye stated, "Dad just wants to snatch us again".

It was also discussed with the children who a guardian ad-litem was and how she would be with them supervising their visit with dad. They were told where they would meet their dad and how close by their mother would be during the visit. They were also told their visit was only scheduled with their dad, and if they saw their grandmother or their father's girlfriend, they were to immediately tell their guardian ad-litem and the visit would end. The children were again told their father had to follow directions which included contacting their guardian ad-litem's supervisor several days in advance to schedule the visit and if he did not do this, the visit would not be scheduled. The visit took place without incident.

An Update in 2021

As reported by the children's mother, both Brian and Faye are thriving and living happy and productive lives as students.

Hi Dr. Peg

I would love to tell you how Brian and Faye are doing since they last saw you. Brian turns 14 tomorrow and is going into 9th grade in the fall. He has been an honor student every year and has matured into an amazing young man. He loves to help people and empathizes more than one expects of a teenage boy to do. Faye skipped a grade and is moving on to 6th grade this fall. She is also growing into a beautiful, strong, independent young lady. She is a Level 5 Junior Olympic Gymnast and is hoping to move to Level 7 in a few months.

They do not have contact with their father, but he has done four supervised visits since the kidnapping and abuse. The kids have been doing better and better each year but are saddened by their father's lack of effort to call or see them more often. We talk about it less and less. They are happy and loved and the longer time goes on the more it all seems like a distant memory to them. I don't think we would have had such a good foundation to recover and move on if it weren't for you. Thank you for helping us.

(Personal communication with their mother, May 17, 2021)

Conclusions

Brian's and Faye's ability to make art, play, tell their stories, and discuss responses to trauma experiences helped them understand, integrate, and in some discussions, celebrate their responses to past traumatic experiences. Their work in art therapy illustrated both their survival and healing power of what happened to them. The year these children were seen in therapy resulted in strengthening resilience, flexibility, sense of safety, stability, and self-esteem.

Amy: Custody Issues Following Loss

Case Study

I worked with Amy for almost nine months, from September to June during an entire school year. When I first met Amy, she was seven years old and beginning the second grade in a new school, in a new state, and living alone with her mother for the first time. Previously, she had lived with her dad, stepmother, and younger half-brother who had special needs. Before living with her dad, Amy lived with her mother and her maternal grandmother. Amy's mother reported Amy was having difficulties adjusting to her new living arrangements. It was also reported that the main reason for Amy's latest move was because her stepmother had died, and her dad could not take care of both of his children alone while facing deployment.

Intake Sessions

During the intake sessions, a preliminary diagnostic impression of adjustment disorder with mixed disturbance of emotions and conduct was made based on the following information. Amy had to move twice in a short period of time. These moves were initiated after her stepmother died and her dad was deployed overseas. Amy also had to give up her cat when she moved from her father's home. Amy first moved out-of-state to live temporarily with her maternal grandmother. Later that year, Amy moved out-of-state again to live with her mother permanently. It was also reported that Amy was struggling academically in school this year, as she was several months behind her classmates in reading comprehension skills. During this session, Amy was friendly but exhibited anxious behaviors. She was unable to sit still, picked at her fingers, and had a hard time making eye contact. During this session,

Amy's mother also reported concerns about Amy's angry outbursts at home. It was noted that none of these outbursts were happening at school. With information reported about the number of losses Amy had recently experienced, it was determined that her initial therapy would be trauma-based and include the ITR protocol (Tinnin & Gantt, 2013).

Early Sessions

During the course of early art therapy sessions, Amy completed art therapy directives designed specifically to address past traumatic experiences that included the death of her stepmother, the loss of her cat, and being separated from her dad.

Amy's Graphic Narratives

Safe Place: Amy's safe place was on the base on the East Coast where her dad worked and she went to school. Amy felt happy in her safe place, and she believed "No one bad could get on the base. If someone bad did get on the base, the alarm would go off".

THE SAD STORY

(Note: Amy was living with her brother, dad, and stepmother.)

> Amy, age six, was with her baby brother Andy, age three, and they were wearing bathing suits. They were with Amy's stepmother Nancy who was looking for a water park. That day Nancy had a cold. Amy, age six, was feeling happy and thinking she will have fun at the water park.
>
> Two weeks later Amy was living with her maternal grandmother (mom-mom). Amy, age six, was outside crying. Amy, age six, was feeling sad and thinking she was very sad for Andy, age three, because Nancy was his mother and she got very sick and died.
>
> Amy, age six, was at mom-mom's house and she was downstairs in the basement. Amy, age six, was feeling very sad and was thinking she did not like that mommy Nancy died.
>
> Amy, age six, went to hug mom-mom. She was feeling nauseous. When Amy, age six, was sad she sometimes became nauseous, and her stomach hurt. Amy was thinking when she went outside, she was afraid she would be sad again when she thought about mommy Nancy, especially when she remembered seeing Nancy in the hospital in her bed.
>
> Later, Amy, age six, went outside in mom-mom's yard. She was feeling the breeze and was playing on the swing in the tree. She was thinking I will try and forget about mommy Nancy. Amy, age six, was feeling in-between sad and happy. Amy, age six, continued to swing and she was feeling nothing and had forgotten everything for a while.
>
> Amy, age six, took care of herself by breathing in and out a lot of times. She was feeling happy and thinking I will try to forget about mommy Nancy so she wouldn't get sad again.

Later Amy turned seven years old and she was still living at daddy's house. She was thinking she would get to play a lot at daddy's house and she was feeling very happy. THE END

SAD CAT

(Note: Amy was still living with her father after her stepmother died, and had to give up her cat when her dad was deployed and she had to go live with her grandmother.)

Amy, age seven, was playing with her cat. She was feeling happy and was thinking she was going to have Lucky forever.

Amy, age seven, was fighting with her dad because she wanted Lucky to stay. Amy, age seven, was sad and thinking I don't want Lucky to leave. Amy, age seven, and Lucky were both crying.

Amy, age seven, gave up, she was sad and began to take care of herself by thinking someday when she was older, she will have another cat. Next Amy, age seven, took care of herself at school. One day she imagined dad was crying too, was feeling sad, and was thinking he did not want Lucky to leave. In her imagination, Amy, age seven, was talking to dad and dad told her he was sad that Lucky had to leave. After Amy, age seven, [imagined she] talked to her dad she was feeling sad but also thinking daddy felt the same way she did which made her happy. Amy, age seven, was also trying to take care of herself by not thinking about Lucky. Amy, age seven, was feeling sad and thinking "Just forget about it".

Now Amy, age seven, was at a new school and she made a new friend named Sharon. Amy, age seven, was feeling happy and thinking I made a new friend. The story entitled Sad Cat has a beginning, middle, and end and it is over. THE END.

DADDY GOING AWAY STORY

(Note: Amy was living with her grandmother when her daddy was deployed and then later moved again to live with her mother.)

Amy, age seven, was feeling happy she was back at mom-mom's house. She was thinking I am going to the pool soon with mom-mom and my cousin Ann. Dad came to grandma's house and told Amy he had to leave some day and go on his ship. Amy, age seven, was thinking she would be very sad when daddy leaves and she was feeling sad now too.

Amy, age seven, was crying and feeling very, very sad. Amy, age seven, started to take care of herself by saying when daddy returned, she would give him a big hug. When bad things happened, Amy felt better when she could hug her daddy. Amy, age seven, was thinking daddy will be gone for three years but he will come home for holidays. She was crying and dad was a little sad too.

Now Amy, age seven, is going to art therapy. Amy, age seven, continues to take care of herself by talking about her sad feelings about missing her dad. The story entitled The Daddy Going Away Story had a beginning, middle, and end and it is over. THE END.

Intermediate Sessions

Amy's mother had previously reported her daughter's angry outburst at home and Amy's graphic narratives also revealed that she used her avoidance and anger protective parts (Figures 1.11, 1.12, 1.13). These parts were her major coping strategies when she experienced upsetting events in her life. Through parts work Amy began to understand how avoidance and anger can sometimes try to protect her from feeling sad, but in doing so, her avoidance and angry behaviors did not give her the opportunity to express her sad thoughts and feelings with words and images or discover whether her sad part was holding onto any false beliefs that she might have developed through her recent experiences of loss.

During her second graphic narrative, Amy started using color. Among art therapy researchers, the use of color to create images was equivalent to a client's ability to begin to express feelings and emotions (Hiscox & Calisch, 1998; Levick, 1983; Robbins, 1994; Wadeson, 1995). Others also believed that behavior changes first show up in a client's drawings. Children's actions in certain situations can sometimes be predicted through their drawings. So by the time Amy created her last graphic narrative, she was directly expressing her sad part through her drawings, storytelling, and discussions with me about missing her dad.

As Amy began to understand the relationship between her angry and sad parts, she was introduced to the "Turtle Technique". The "Turtle Technique" is a strategy taught to young children, like Amy, on how to control and use their angry part productively (Lentini et al. 2019). Other sessions during this stage in Amy's therapy addressed some of her struggles academically with reading skills. Bibliotherapy was included in some of Amy's therapy sessions. Bibliotherapy introduces books to a child wherein the main characters in the story

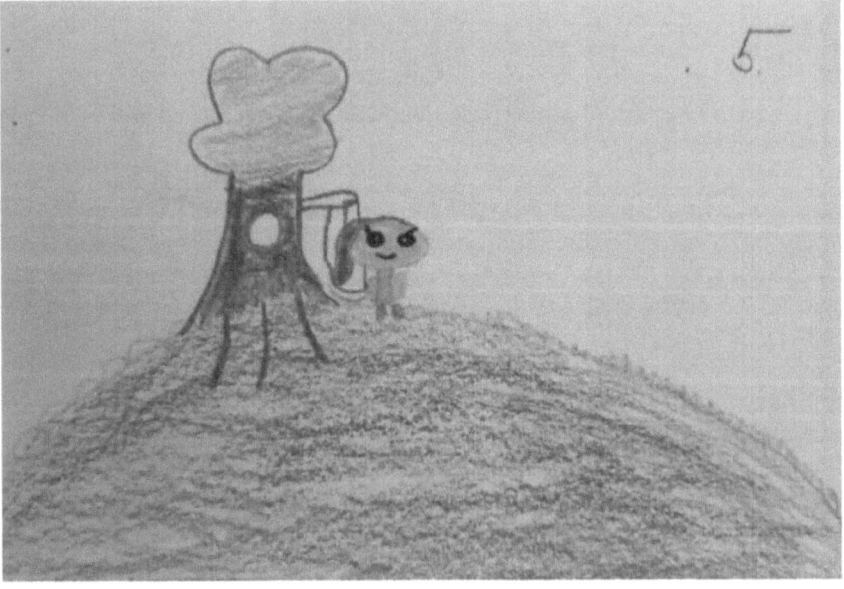

Figure 1.11 Avoidance, Playing on the Swing

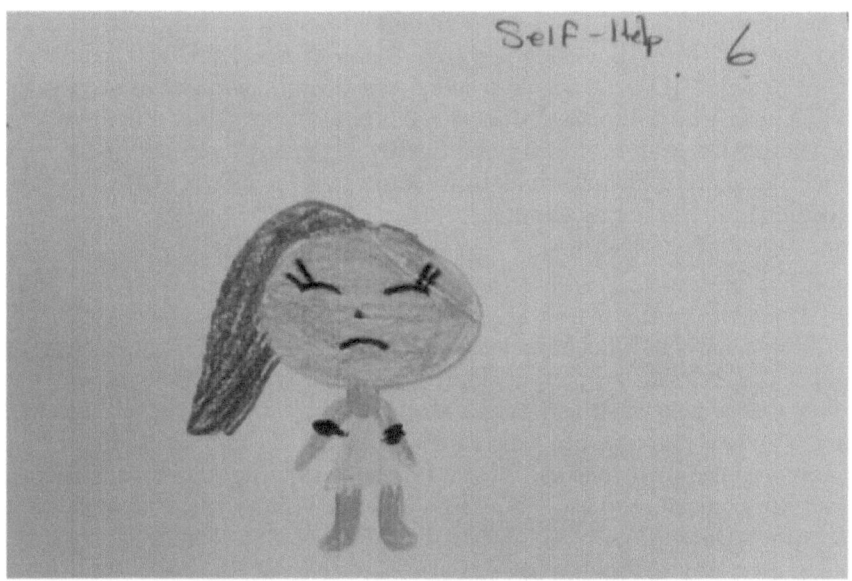

Figure 1.12 Avoidance, Feeling Happy and Thinking

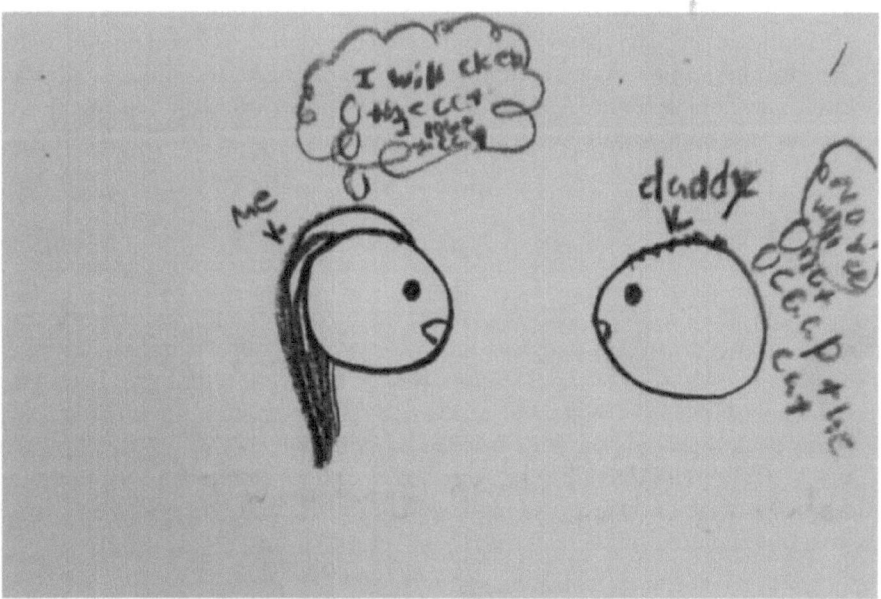

Figure 1.13 Anger, Fighting with Dad

are having similar life experiences and challenges. The reading of the story supports and helps the child identify and acquire an understanding and insight that their experiences are universal and not just theirs (Lu, 2008). In other sessions, the Language Experience Approach (Jones & Nessel, 1981) to teaching reading, using Amy's own stories she created from story cards, pictures, and photographs, was introduced. This provided Amy opportunities to practice reading out loud to improve her fluency in reading and subsequently her reading comprehension skills. Teaching children to read using their own words increases their focus, motivation, and interest in learning.

Outcomes

In February, just before her eighth birthday in March, Amy was told she would be going back to live with her dad, her half-brother, and new stepmother and step siblings. Dad had remarried. It was not clear whether it was Amy's mother or father's idea that Amy return to her dad's home. However, around this time Amy's mother was complaining that it was too difficult for her to raise Amy by herself. Then I learned from the mother that one of her neighbors reported her to social services, and a series of home visits began. The school had been notified and Amy's teacher had been interviewed. The mother asked if I would agree to be interviewed and I said yes, though the interview never happened. Like her daughter, Amy's mother was a likable woman and was consistent in bringing her daughter to therapy each week. However, at the end of my work with Amy, I suspected that her mother had serious problems of her own and was unable to care for her daughter without daily support. Formal termination sessions began with Amy during the middle of May, in anticipation of Amy's next out-of-state move that would take place as soon as the current school year ended.

When Amy was told in February, she would be leaving her mother and going back to live with her dad, half-brother, and a new stepmother and two younger step siblings, she was ambivalent. During our final sessions, Amy continued to say how excited and sad she was at the same time. She was happy to live with her dad again but was sad to leave her mom.

Conclusions

Academic Development

Amy was a bright and likable young girl who struggled throughout the school year academically in reading comprehension and had difficulty verbally expressing her thoughts and feelings sequentially. Although Amy made progress in her reading skills this year, she was still approximately three months behind at the end of the school year in reading fluency that impacted her comprehension skills in other school subjects. During March of this school year, Amy's teacher had already recommended that Amy repeat the second grade. In mathematics, Amy's favorite subject, she made good progress and was on grade level at the end of the school year.

Social Development

Amy made friends easily at her new school and had playdates with some of her classmates outside of school. She was cooperative in the classroom and got along well with her teachers and other staff members at school.

Emotional Development

Amy was compliant in her art-making and appeared to benefit from her time in therapy. She created a number of graphic narratives to address the many losses she had experienced over the last year. Being able to express her anger in a more appropriate way and to understand that being angry was not equivalent to being "bad". This was a significant lesson for Amy to learn. Also significant was Amy's ability to talk about her sad feelings and not avoid those feelings. Her improvement in her reading skills over the course of the school year also seemed to improve Amy's self-confidence. I hope this last move for Amy will become a stable home where she can grow up and feel safe.

Recommendations

At the request of the father, I provided a summary of my sessions with Amy and the following list of recommendations for her before school started again in the fall.

Emotional Development and Stability

1. Based on clinical judgment and information provided from the art therapy sessions, it is strongly recommended Amy begins seeing a new art therapist (not to be confused with play therapy) as soon as possible once she is relocated and settled in her new home.
2. Schedule daily contact for Amy with her mother through phone calls and FaceTime.
3. Scheduley early visits for Amy during the holidays and/or summer vacations with her mother and maternal grandmother, both of whom are a big part of Amy's support system.

Academic Development

1. Amy should have the opportunity to read books from the local library on her independent reading level during this summer. Students who do not read during summer breaks can lose as much as three months of their reading skills obtained during the previous school year (Allington et al., 2010).
2. Amy could also benefit from weekly tutoring sessions during this summer so she can reach her grade level in Reading skills before the next academic year begins in a few months.

Livie: Patterns of Losses and Bullying

I was contacted in mid-fall following COVID-19 by parents of a former client, asking if I could begin seeing their younger daughter. The parents had concerns about Livie, age nine, who was enrolled in fourth grade at the beginning of that school year. I saw her for 12 individual art therapy sessions, including the intake session. At least one parent, and sometimes both parents participated during the last 15 minutes of each session.

Intake Sessions

Livie was first seen at the beginning of a new school year close to the Halloween holiday, which turned out to be a significant event for this client. During the intake session, a preliminary diagnostic impression of adjustment disorder with anxiety was made based on the following information. It was reported that Livie had experienced losing her best friend at school earlier in September. Her friend had moved out of the neighborhood and was assigned to another public school in the district.

In the intake session, Livie's parents also reported that she was being picked on by her 4-H Club leader. The reported events bordered on bullying. Initially, Livie did not disclose this information to her parents because Livie's mother and her 4-H leader were both working with the children in the club. This 4-H Club provided opportunities to care for a group of horses and learn to ride.

Livie's parents were concerned with the decrease in Livie's confidence and her self-esteem as evidenced by her negative self-talk. They were hearing Livie frequently say out loud that she was "stupid and dumb". Before the intake session ended Livie was asked about other sad events in her life. She was able to construct a timeline of these events and a pattern emerged showing that Livie had lost a best friend at the beginning of each school year. Livie's most traumatic loss of a best friend was in kindergarden, when her friend that year was struck and killed in an automobile accident while trick or treating on Halloween night.

Assessments and Treatment Plan

With information given in the intake session, including the parents' wishes for brief therapy for their daughter, it was determined the major treatment for Livie would be trauma-based and the ITR would be used (Tinnin & Gantt, 2013).

Early Sessions

During the intake session, it was also reported that Livie began to display an increase in angry, tearful outbursts at home over her homework as well as an increase in arguments with her older sister. There is a five-year age difference between the girls that was becoming more significant as her sister wanted to spend more time with friends and less time playing with Livie. Livie was expressing feelings of rejection from her older sister. At school, she reported having trouble getting along with some classmates, and it was hard for her to sit still and focus during classroom instruction. In the earlier therapy sessions, Livie also found it difficult to sit still even when she was engaged in artmaking.

During the first session, Livie talked more about her timeline and losing best friends during the beginning of each school year. She talked mostly about her friend who died when they were in kindergarten. During the second and third sessions, using the ITR protocol, Livie completed her graphic narrative. The protocol began with Livie being asked to draw one of her safe places as a grounding activity before she began her graphic narrative. Next, Livie drew sequential pictures of the event, as she remembered them, followed by a story about the death of her kindergarten classmate, Helen. The story was directed through a series of questions that Livie answered in the third person that included her thoughts, feelings, and what her body was doing as part of her memory of the event. At the end of the session, I read Livie's story to her. It was within her drawings and story, Livie identified her responses to the death and loss of her friend and what followed afterwards. What is most important in addressing trauma is helping the clients understand their responses to the traumatic event versus the trauma itself (Porges, 2011). Stories can be an integral part of the healing from trauma (Davis, 2019). In the third session, Livie reviewed her drawings and story for any missing pictures or story details. Satisfied that her graphic narrative was accurate and complete, Livie was given a copy of her story and drawings to take home to keep and reread.

Livie's Graphic Narrative

SAFE PLACE

Livie, age nine, reported one of her safe places is on the couch in the living room cuddled up with her dog. When in her safe place, Livie feels happy and thinks about the next TV show she will watch.

THE HALLOWEEN NIGHTMARE

Livie, age five, was out walking and trick-or-treating in her neighborhood. Livie, age five, was thinking and hoping to get more candy than her sister. Livie, age five, was feeling happy that she was getting candy.

Livie, age five, came home after trick-or-treating and was told by her mom that her friend Helen had died. Livie, age five, lit a candle for Helen and was thinking she had lost one of her best friends. Livie, age five, was feeling sad as her body slumped downward.

Livie, age five, helped herself by hugging her cat, Jiminy. Livie, age five, was crying and was sad. Livie, age five, was thinking I am not going to see Helen in school tomorrow. Later that night, Livie is lying in bed with her mom and thinking I won't be able to sleep because my friend is not here anymore. Livie, age five, had stopped crying but her face was red, and her nose was sniffling.

Other ways Livie, age five, took care of herself was by playing outside and playing on her computer. She was feeling sad but thinking she needed to distract herself from thinking about Helen and start having some fun.

Now Livie is nine years old, and she likes to play with her new friend who moved into the neighborhood about a year ago. She likes to play on the big swing in her friend's yard. Livie, age nine, is thinking about how much fun she is having with her friend and feeling happy that she is playing and having fun.

The story entitled *The Halloween Nightmare* had a beginning, middle, and end, and it happened many years ago and it is over. THE END.

Intermediate Sessions

During the fourth session, Livie was given an explanation of parts work, as defined by Schwarz (1995) and Spiegel (2017). Using her graphic narrative, Livie was able to identify how she cared for herself during the time her classmate was killed. She was able to illustrate healthy coping skills as she took comfort in hugging her cat (Figure 1.14), playing outside, and on her computer (Figure 1.15). But a more important discovery, after Livie completed her external dialog with her five-year-old sad part, was realizing that her five-year-old sad part falsely believed she would never have another friend after Helen's death. This was a breakthrough moment for Livie when she recognized her five-year-old self was influencing her thoughts and feelings about friends in the present. Her mother reported during the next

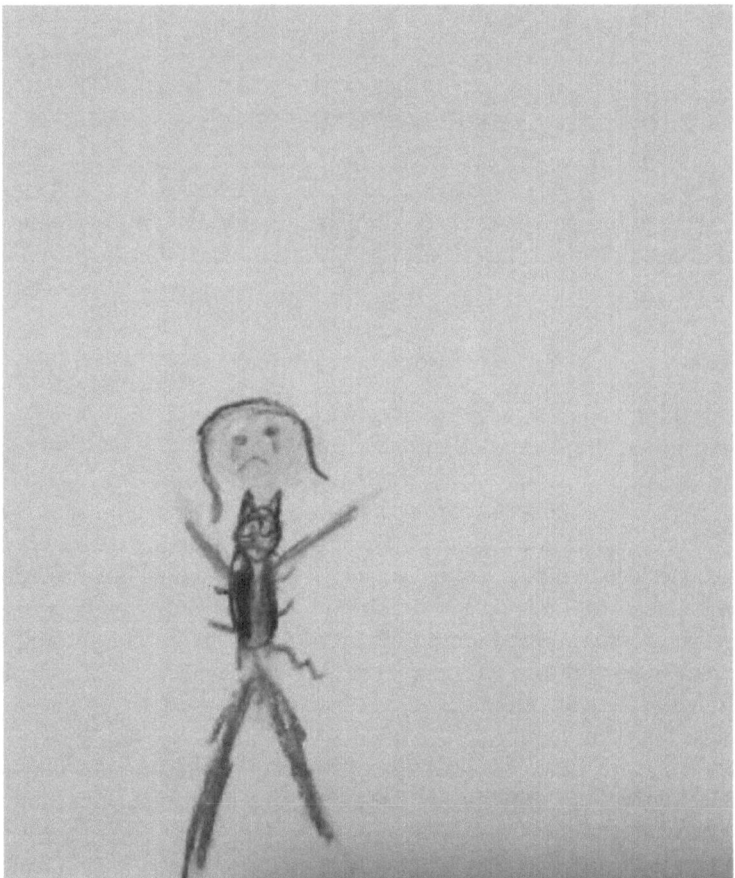

Figure 1.14 Livie Hugging Her Cat

session that Livie was having fewer angry outbursts at home, and she was hearing fewer negative and self-deprecating comments from her daughter.

Later Sessions

During the remainder of the time I saw Livie in therapy, there were two major issues that were covered during these sessions. The first issue was with Livie's 4-H Club leader whose behavior toward Livie got worse. This issue was also complicated because Livie's mother and her 4-H club leader were also in conflict with each other. Livie's mother finally intervened and defended her daughter, so Livie felt safe again attending her 4-H meetings.

The second issue covered was about a classmate who had been verbally bullying Livie in the classroom. Again, Livie did not tell her parents about this situation but once Livie's mother heard about this problem during an art therapy session, she again intervened on

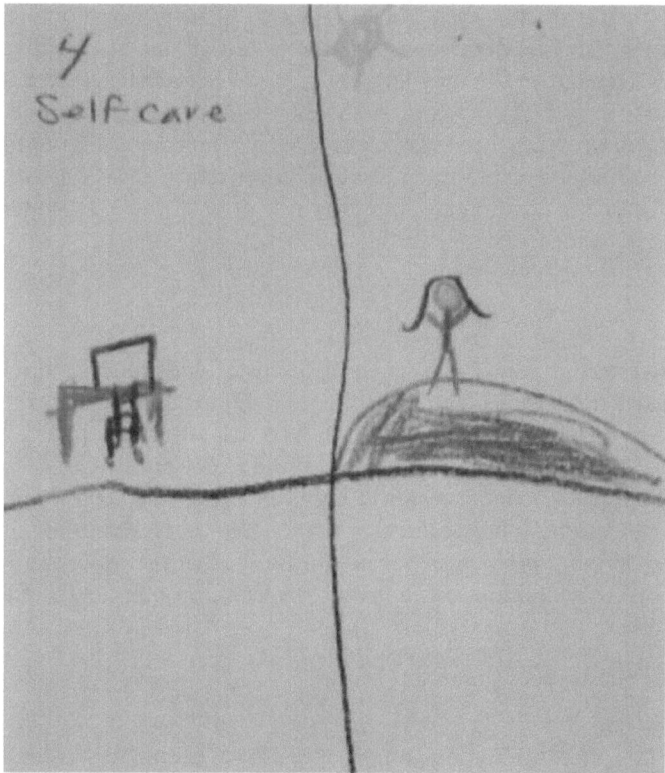

Figure 1.15 Livie Playing Outside and Working on Her Computer

behalf of her daughter. From these events, it appears that Livie was learning it was safe to ask for help with a challenging problem from a trusted person in her life.

During this time Livie's self-esteem and self-confidence continued to be bruised. I suggested that she create a self-portrait collage using words and pictures from the magazine collection in the room. Livie was asked to illustrate her positive experiences and characteristics. She was pleasantly surprised to find out how easy it was to identify so many happy events she had already experienced in her life. Children must experience success to improve their self-esteem and self-confidence (Leary & Baumeister, 2000).

Because the parents had asked that I see Livie for a limited number of sessions, directed art therapy tasks were selected for this client. Developmental levels also influenced the tasks that were suggested as well as art materials that Livie was familiar with and felt confident using.

Developmental Considerations

Livie's vocabulary was advanced for her age, and she was articulate while participating in discussions in therapy. Her language and vocabulary skills gave her the ability to accurately understand what was happening between her and her 4-H leader and her classmate. With her fine-motor skills, Livie was able to recall details about the death of her classmate Helen while completing her graphic narrative of that event, helping her to identify her thoughts and feelings about that sad event in her life. Livie was also able to talk about her positive experiences and how those events related to the meanings in her artwork as she created a self-portrait collage of words and images. As my time with Livie was coming to an end, the mother reported (without Livie present) there was trouble in her marriage. I listened to her concerns and suggested she find a good family therapist. After that discussion with the mother, I unfortunately did not see Livie again and was not able to have a proper termination session with her and her mother.

Outcomes

Livie was compliant and was invested in her art-making and discussions during her brief art therapy experience. It appeared that she benefited from her time in therapy when she had a chance to challenge her false belief that she would never have friends. Livie also had the opportunity to identify some of her positive characteristics and experiences. Children like Livie are resilient and flexible and if communication between Livie and her mother continues, her prognosis appears to be good. However, therapy for Livie was unfinished. It is possible that another major, underlying problem reported during the last therapy session (i.e., the parents' marital problems) may continue to contribute to feelings of anxiety and a lack of safety for Livie in the future.

Conclusions

Livie came to therapy because of her notable anxiety, and it appears the theme with all her conflicts, both in the past and the present, involved not feeling safe. In the past, after the death of her classmate Helen, it was not safe to have friends. In the present at school, after having conflicts with others whether adults or peers, it was not safe to have discussions and ask for help. In the present at home, after having conflicts with her sister and perhaps observing conflicts between the parents, it was again not safe to have discussions and ask for help.

Livie was a bright and energetic girl with an advanced vocabulary for her chronological age and she had strong comprehension skills as evidenced by her academic success in school. Although Livie's cognitive skills were advanced, it appeared her social and emotional skills were underdeveloped. She learned in therapy that she had developed some healthy coping skills but one of her primary coping skills, that was not helpful, was avoidance. This coping skill seemed to be how she was handling her recent challenges. I believe it wasn't until Livie felt safe enough in therapy sessions to discuss with her mother her thoughts and feelings, caused by the continuing conflicts she was having with others, that her anxiety began to decrease. Seeing her mother take immediate actions to defend and help her also contributed to Livie's well-being.

References

Allington, R. L., McGill-Franzen, A., Camilli, G., Williams, L., Graff, J., Zeig, J., Zmach, C., & Nowak, R. (2010). Addressing summer reading setback among economically disadvantaged elementary school students. *Reading Psychology*, *31*(5), 411–427.

American Psychiatric Association Publishing. (2022). *Diagnostic and statistical manual of mental disorders: Dsm-5-Tr*. Washington, DC: American Psychiatric Association.

Arrington, D. A. (2007). *Art, angst, and trauma*. Charles C. Thomas Publisher.

Barresi, M., & Gilbert, S. (2023). Developmental biology (13th ed.). Oxford University Press.

Beck, J. S. (2020). *Cognitive behavior therapy* (3rd ed.). Guilford Press.

Bloom, S. L. (2013). *Creating sanctuary: Toward the evolution of sane societies* (Revised edition). Routledge.

Bloom, S. L., & Farragher, B. (2013). *Restoring sanctuary: A new operating system for trauma informed systems of care*. Oxford University Press.

Bowlby, J. (1969). *Attachment and loss* (volume 1). Basic Books.

Bronfenbrenner, U. (1979). *The ecology of human development*. Harvard University Press.

Cain, B. (2001). *Double dip feelings*. American Psychological Association.

Chapman, L. (2014). *Neurobiologically informed trauma therapy with children and adolescents: Understanding mechanisms of change*. W.W. Norton & Company.

Clarke, A. (2013). Sanctuary in action. *Children Australia*, 38, 95–99.

Dana, D. (2020). *Polyvagal exercise for safety and connection: 50 client-centered practices*. W.W. Norton & Company.

Davis, N. (2019). *Therapeutic stories to heal and empower*. Therapeutic Stories, Nancy Davis, PhD.

Dunne, P. (2016). *The narrative therapist and the arts* (2nd ed.). Possibilities Press.

Elwyn, L. J., Esakin, N., & Smith, C. A. (2015). Safety at a girls secure juvenile justice facility. *Therapeutic Communities: The International Journal of Therapeutic Communities*, 36, 209–218.

Erikson, E. (1967). *Identity and the life cycle*. W.W. Norton & Company.

Felitti, V. J., Anda, R. F., Nordenberg, D., Williamson, D. F., Spitz, A. M., Edwards, V., Koss, M. P., & Marks, J. S. (1998). Relationship of child abuse and household dysfunction to many of the leading causes of death in adults: The Adverse Childhood Experiences (ACE) study. *American Journal of Preventative Medicine*, 14(4), 245–258.

Fowler, J. W. (1995). *Stages of faith: The psychology of human development and the quest for meaning*. HarperSanFrancisco.

Gergen K. J. (2015). *An invitation to social contraction* (3rd ed.). Sage Publications.

Haggis, J., & Schech, S. (Eds). (2002). *Development: A cultural studies reader*. Wiley-Blackwell.

Hinz, L. D. (2019). *Expressive therapies continuum: A framework for using art in therapy* (2nd ed.). Routledge.

Hiscox, A. R.. & Calisch, A. B. (Eds). (1998). *Tapestry of cultural issues in art therapy*. Jessica Kingsley Publishers.

Holmes, M. M., Mudlaff, S. J., & Pillo, C. (2000). *A terrible thing happened*. Magination Press.

Homeyer, L. E., & Lyles, N. (2022). *Advanced sandtray therapy: Digging deeper into clinical practice*. Routledge.

Jones, M. B., & Nessel, D. D. (1981). *The language approach to reading: A handbook for teachers*. Teachers College, Columbia University.

Kohlberg, L. (1969). Stage and sequence: The cognitive-developmental approach to socialization. In D. A. Goslin (Ed.). *Handbook of socialization* (pp. 347–480). Ran McNally.

Leary, M. R.. & Baumeister, R. F. (2000). The nature and function of self-esteem: Sociometer theory. In M. Zanna (Ed.). *Advances in experimental social psychology* (volume 32, pp. 1–62). Academic Press.

Lentini R., Giroux L. N., & Hemmeter, M. L. (2019) *Tucker turtle takes time to tuck and think: A scripted story to assist the teacher with the turtle technique*. National Center for Pyramid Model Innovations (NCPMI) Office of Special Education

Levick M. L. (1983). *They could not talk and so they drew: Children's styles of coping and thinking*. Charles C. Thomas Publisher.

Lowenfeld, V., & Brittain, W. L. (1987). *Creative and mental growth* (8th ed.). Macmillan.

Lu, Y. (2008) Helping children cope: What is bibliotherapy? *Children & Libraries*, 6(1), 47–49.

Mahler, M., Pine, F., & Bergman, A. (1975). *The psychological birth of the human infant.* Basic Books.

Maynard, B. R., Farina, A., Dell, N. A., & Kelly, M. S. (2019). Effects of trauma-informed approaches in schools: A systemic review. *Campbell Systematic Reviews, 15*(1–2).

Mellonie, B. (1983). *Lifetimes.* Random House Publishing Group.

Mones, A. G. (2017). *Kids words: Inside & out: A psychotherapeutic game.* Stoelting Company.

National Child Traumatic Stress Network (2023). *Intervention fact sheets: Sanctuary model.* https://www.nctsn.org/treatments-and-practices/trauma-treatments/interventions

Perry, B. (2009). Examining child maltreatment through a neurodevelopmental lens: Clinical applications of the neurosequential model of therapeutics. *Journal of Loss and Trauma, 14*(4), 240–255.

Piaget, J., & Inhelder, B. (1969). *The psychology of a child.* Routledge.

Porges, S. W. (2011). *The polyvagal theory: Neurophysiological foundation of emotions, attachment, communication, and self-regulation.* W.W. Norton & Company.

Redfield, R., & Onderko, K. (2016). *Polyvagal theory and the social engagement system with Stephen Porges* [Audio podcast]. Integrated Listening System.

Reiner, R. (1987). *The Princess Bride.* Twentieth Century Fox.

Rivard, J. C., Bloom, S. L., Abramovitz, R., Pasquale, L. E., Duncan, M. E., McCorkle, D., & Gelman, A. (2003). Assessing the implementation and effects of a trauma-focused intervention for youths in residential treatment. *Psychiatric Quarterly, 74*(2), 137–154.

Robbins, A. (1994). *A multi-modal approach to creative art therapy.* Jessica Kingsley Publishers.

Rogers, C. (1951). *Client-centered therapy: Its current practice, implications, and theory.* Houghton-Mifflin.

Schaefer, C. E., & Cangelosi, D. (2016). *Essential play techniques: Time-tested approaches.* Guildford Press.

Schwartz, R. C. (1995). *Internal family systems therapy.* Guildford Press.

Spiegel, L. (2017). *Internal family systems therapy with children.* Routledge.

Thomas, P., & Harker, L. (2001). *I miss you: A first look at death.* Sourcebooks Explore.

Tinnin, L., & Gantt, L. (2013). *The instinctual trauma response dual-brain dynamics: A guide for trauma therapy.* Gargoyle Press.

van der Kolk, B. (2014). *The body keeps the score: Brain, mind, and body in the healing of trauma.* Penguin Books.

Wadeson, H. (1995). *The dynamics of art psychotherapy.* John Wiley & Sons, Inc.

Winnicott, D. W. (1971). *Playing and reality.* Basic Books.

Worden, J. W. (2018). *Grief counseling and grief therapy: A handbook for the mental health practitioner* (5th ed.). Springer.

Chapter 2

Middle Childhood and Early Adolescence

Youth progress from the virtue of competency into fidelity, and social networks expand beyond the family to include peers and broader community connections.

Introduction

Developmental Markers

This chapter covers the developmental levels of ages nine to fifteen. As with early childhood development, there is a complex matrix of developmental perspectives. This period marks significant changes across multiple domains. It highlights the complex and multifaceted nature of human development during adolescence. Biologically, puberty marks pivotal changes with rapid physical growth, hormonal changes, and the onset of sexual maturation (Baressi & Gilbert, 2023). Brain development continues, particularly in areas related to reasoning, impulse control, and emotional regulation.

Socially, adolescents experience increasing independence and autonomy that lead to shifts in peer relationships and a growing desire for social acceptance. Psychological development in this age range starts in Erikson's *Industry vs Inferiority* crisis and transitions to the *Identity vs Role Confusion* crisis (Erikson, 1967). Youth progress from the virtue of competency into fidelity, and their social networks expand beyond the family to include peers and broader community connections (Broffenbrenner, 1979). Youth awareness of social and ecological issues and a developing sense of responsibility towards the environment and society are also rooted in this age.

Adolescents' abstract thinking, problem-solving, and critical reasoning begin blossoming during these years (Piaget & Inhelder, 1969). Abilities to express themselves through artistic means increase, along with interests and desires to explore themselves through creative outlets. Self-perception and understanding are priorities at this level of development (Winner, 2000).

As the adolescent brain continues to develop, emotional volatility due to hormonal changes and maturation of the limbic system emerge (Baressi & Gilbert, 2023). Learning emotional regulation and understanding complex emotions are at the heart of the developing adolescent (Pollak et al., 2019). Neurological development supports improved decision-making and social cognition.

Early adolescence marks a period of exploration of personal beliefs, values, and spirituality, often influenced by cultural and family contexts (Fowler, 1995). Moral reasoning and

DOI: 10.4324/9781003324805-3

ethical understandings include aspects of fairness and justice (Kohlberg, 1969; Gilligan, 1982). Awareness and understanding today also includes ethnic, racial, and cultural diversity, gender identity, and sexual orientation (Branje et al., 2021).

Setbacks

Potential setbacks during these years continue to be impacted by Adverse Childhood Experiences (ACEs) such as abuse, neglect, or household dysfunction that can lead to emotional disturbances including anxiety, depression, and PTSD, among others (Felitti et al., 1998). Trauma can hinder cognitive development, affect memory, attention, and executive functioning. This impairment might lead to academic difficulties and problems with decision making.

ACEs also correlate with social difficulties during this age range, including peer relationships, social withdrawal, aggressive behavior, and substance use or abuse (Felitti et al., 1998). These challenges can further hinder the development of social skills and secure relationships (Bowlby, 1969). Long-term physical health consequences are also linked to ACEs, including an increased risk of chronic disease, obesity, and autoimmune disorders (Felitti et al., 1998).

Life trauma can affect brain architecture and neurodevelopment, particularly the stress response system (Porges, 2011). This potentially leads to long-term alterations in brain structure and function. Interventions during these times are especially important to reduce lasting effects on future educational and career opportunities. Lower academic achievement, school drop-out, and learning difficulties could be indicators (Maynard et al., 2019).

Adolescents who experience ACEs are also at an increased risk of developing mental health disorders later in life, leading to ongoing emotional struggles and potential disruptions in functions (Felitti et al., 1998). Addressing setbacks related to trauma and ACEs during this critical period involves early intervention, trauma-informed care, and comprehensive support systems that encompass mental health services, social support networks, and educational interviews (Maynard et al., 2019). By providing timely and targeted interventions, it is possible to mitigate the long-term impacts of adverse experiences and promote healthier development during adolescence.

Case Studies

The case studies in this chapter include clients ranging in age from 12 to 22 and the majority of the art therapy settings were in private practice. Other settings include a grief center, a community-based art therapy studio, and a school-setting at a public middle school. Sessions included individual, dyads with a parent, and family therapy. Most of the clients in this chapter received long-term therapy and in one case the client was seen for a decade. The clients' major issues in this chapter include traumatic events, including abandonment, abuse, and the death of a parent or another family member. Attempted suicide, selective mutism, anxiety and depression, the inability to self-regulate thoughts, feelings, and actions, and a lack of self-confidence and independence brought other clients to therapy. The primary approaches used with art therapy included the following theories and therapies: Polyvagal Theory (Porges, 2011), Objects Relations (Robbins, 1987), Psychoanalytic Theory (Johnson, 1989), Attachment Theory (Beeb & Stelle, 2013), Psychoanalytic Therapy (Jordan, 2017), Narrative Therapy (Dunne, 2016), and models including the Expressive

Therapies Continuum (ETC, Hinz, 2019) and Internal Family Systems (IFS, Schwartz, 1995). In one case, the therapist's unique approach to therapy used the literal space of the art therapy setting to develop rapport and set boundaries with her client.

Together with their art therapy education and training, these art therapists came from a variety of educational backgrounds and skill sets and use all their proficiencies for the benefit of their clients. Some of these authors applied their knowledge of Reiki and yoga practices, Somatic Experiencing (Levine, 2010), Eye Movement Desensitization and Reprocessing (EMDR, Shapiro, 2014), Family Therapy (Bowen, 1982), and trauma-based therapy approaches such as the Instinctual Trauma Response (ITR, Tinnin & Gantt, 2013).

This age group is a challenge for parents and therapists alike due to the normal changes that take place during this time of development. The changes clients experience include adjusting to physical changes, shifting approval from parents to peers, needing to fit in with friends and classmates, experimenting with new roles, including all components of sexuality, and discovering talents and intellectual interests, while adjusting to expected and additional responsibilities at school and at home (Erikson, 1967). These changes all culminate into a new identity at the brink of adulthood.

During this age of development, clients were not always able to regulate their thoughts, feelings, or actions. They were angry, confused, and sometimes felt unsafe and misunderstood. In more severe situations, they felt abandoned. Consequently, trust is something these clients struggled with too (Perry, 2009).

Parents were also challenged during this age in their children's development, especially if they discovered their parenting skills might be lacking. With benevolence, some parents struggled to find a balance between accepting and protecting their children at this age. In these cases, some of the authors worked with both the client and the parents or guardians in parallel therapy sessions. In one case, the therapist provided psychoeducational therapy to help a guardian understand the developmental needs of children diagnosed with autism, as well as how severe, traumatic events can affect the development of young children. Unfortunately, not all parents were able to act on the discoveries made in therapy about their parenting skills. In one case, it was evident that the client and parents would benefit from family therapy in the future.

When therapists work with this age group, resistance is a common factor (Baressi & Gilbert, 2023). As one author wrote, sometimes when therapists question whether they are really helping, they need to remember it is a victory when clients simply stay in the therapy room. Discussing the aesthetic of an artwork before asking about the symbolic meaning of the art, and drawing a portrait of the client, are two other strategies to resistant behaviors. Including clients in the planning of their goals and objectives and letting them know that therapy would proceed on their timeline are other strategies. Another challenge therapists faced was their inability to provide art therapy in a consistent and timely manner, which sometimes led to clients regressing and prolonging their need for therapy. Therapists also found themselves making adaptations in order to provide therapy online during the pandemic. The flexibility exhibited by the therapists was key to overcoming these situations.

Therapists recommending services out of their scope of practice was another key to success with clients. Convincing parents to arrange for their children to be tested was an important part in helping some of them. These tests included traditional psychological tests as well as art therapy assessments. Good examples of termination sessions were also reported, which gave the therapist an opportunity to recommend resources and services for the client's family in the future. This is a challenging age group to work with, but experiencing successful results is rewarding for everyone involved.

ART-BASED ATTUNEMENT AND AFFECT
REGULATION IN CHILD ART THERAPY

AMANDA LIGHTNER

Setting

The following case study was conducted in a private practice setting. The practice is in a Victorian era house located in an American Midwest capital city, near the downtown area. Approximately a dozen other therapists make up this co-op style practice in which each therapist practices out of a room in the house. The room this case was conducted in is a medium-sized room with wood floors and large windows.

The space contains an art table that seats up to four people, a comfortable chair, a locked file cabinet to secure documents, and an additional large, locked cabinet for patients' artwork. A wheeled cart with a range of art materials is available for participants: oil pastels; watercolor pencils, markers, and crayons; colored markers, pens, and pencils; and graphite pencils (2H-6B). A glue stick and erasers including gum, pink rubber, artist kneaded, and vinyl were also available. A range of papers were available: mixed media, watercolor, drawing, tracing, colored construction, colored tissue paper, and small to medium-sized canvases. Watercolor and tempera paint were available with access to a bathroom sink for water. Collage materials, polymer clay, and clay tools made up the remainder of the general studio supplies.

This case, like many of my clients, was a self-referral. I receive emails or telephone calls directly from parents or a potential patient. An important aspect in working with children of separation or divorce is to obtain consent for treatment from both parents. In this study, consent was obtained by the father in the absence of the mother. When the mother joined the treatment process two years later, her consent was also obtained.

When working with children, each case is different and should be evaluated as such. For Katherine, I elected to provide individual sessions with separate individual parent sessions due to the parents' relational discord. Sessions with parents were provided to discuss strengths and problem areas, alongside exploration of helpful parent behaviors. The final session is typically a termination or closing session where referrals and recommendations can be provided. This session supports the child ending therapy as it allows the opportunity to review all the good work done and to say goodbye, which is therapeutic for young children.

Approaches

My therapeutic approach to treating children with complex trauma includes contemporary psychoanalytic theory and attachment theory. Object relations theory is rooted in psychoanalytic theory. The therapeutic relationship provides a framework to examine a patient's object world and their art, a world for both object and subject to participate in (Robbins, 1987; Winnicott, 1971).

Art forms allow the patient and art therapist to participate in a unique relational space that can offer kinesthetic, auditory, tactile, and visual levels of participation. This space with its multisensory characteristics is associated with early caregiver–infant relationships (Robbins, 1987). Therefore, art therapists invite participation in a unique relational space that mirrors and influences attachment experiences.

Attachment theory explores the early attachment relationship between caregiver and infant. Attachment experiences shape how a person regulates internal affective states. Contemporary attachment theories show the right hemisphere of the brain is the center of self-regulation and is shaped by attachment experiences. If attachment is disrupted, an inability to modulate internal affective states occurs, thus increasing the chances of emotional dysregulation. In normal attachment, both caregiver and infant's right hemispheres are interacting when facial mirroring and mutual gaze attunement are experienced, which leads to shared states of arousal and affect, thus shaping how a person regulates their emotions (Schore, 2000).

Case Study

Katherine's parents divorced when she was four years old, and parental conflict was ongoing. At age six, Katherine witnessed an incident of violent, physical injury as it occurred to her mother by her mother's boyfriend. Her mother required hospitalization for the incident and was reported to have restricted custody following. Her mother's whereabouts were unknown for the first two years of Katherine's treatment. Near the end of Katherine's sessions, the mother engaged in her daughter's treatment as her whereabouts became known and she entered a local treatment center for alcohol and drug rehabilitation.

Katherine was reported to experience early difficulties in infant–mother bonding. She was reported to have interpersonal conflicts with her family at home and peers at school. Katherine's family at home was composed of her biological father, his girlfriend, and their six children from separate marriages aged three to 19. Her family lived in a rural setting about an hour outside the capital city. Katherine's family moved often from one rural location to the next. As a result, Katherine was uprooted to attend five different schools over the span of the four years we worked together. She described difficulties in her relationships and reported not having many friends.

Katherine was seven years old at the time of our first meeting. She engaged in treatment for four years. Katherine presented with complex trauma, dysregulated mood, and disruptions in attachment in her relationships and to places. I planned to help Katherine regulate her emotions and invite a narrative for her experiences by offering a range of art media to regulate and gain mastery within a supportive therapeutic relationship.

Intake Session(s)

Katherine was provided with an open directive, a range of art media to assess themes and her capacity to self-regulate. She appeared frightened, as she watched me wide-eyed. I implicitly tuned in to her distress, as I worked towards an attuned connection to Katherine by neutralizing her strong emotions, reflecting a calm expression and comforting tone.

Katherine chose to work with clay, and I asked her if she knew what she might make. She shrugged, not saying a word as she rolled out the media on the table. She formed a bird that was injured and needed "surgery" (Figure 2.1). Her visual communication and observed

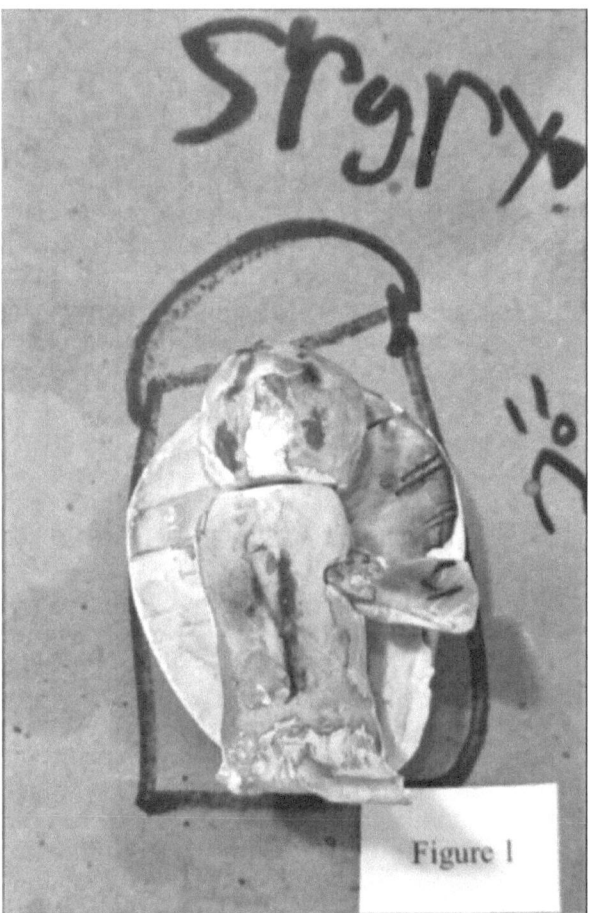

Figure 2.1 The Injured Bird

affective state reflected the report of the patient's witness to a traumatic event. The patient's presentation changed following our first meeting.

Early Sessions

During the first year of weekly art therapy, Katherine showed much emotional dysregulation. She did not verbally communicate and only communicated her affective states of arousal as she painted the walls of my office, the art table, plants, furniture, and once tried to paint me. During this early time together, I would feel so overwhelmed and helpless at the mess she showed me that I thought I might not be able to continue our work together. While in my office writing this paper, I could see paint marks that remained on my office wall from Katherine. I smiled as it reminded me of our early time together and how much she had grown.

Early art therapy sessions helped Katherine to regulate her anxiety by offering uncontrollable media within a supportive therapeutic relationship. Wielding a paintbrush and a sly smile, Katherine started to paint on the table and this time I offered her a large 18 × 24-inch paper to provide containment. Her first attempts took one step forward and two steps back as paint flew onto the paper and other times onto the wall and furniture. I attended to her intense state of emotional dysregulation as I reflected how much there was to share with me that it seemed difficult to fit onto the piece of paper.

Figure 2.2 shows a large fish in a dark environment. The fish appears wide-eyed and alone. I wondered aloud what the place was like for the fish or if her painting might have a story. Katherine's eyes widened, like the fish, as she shared how scary the place was for the fish. The fish was no longer alone as we stared into the dark environment and witnessed how scary a place that was for a fish. As I sat with Katherine, she did not look at me, only at her painting. I let her know that I could see how scary a place it was for the fish and if she ever wanted to let me know what the fish found so scary, I would want to know.

Katherine was now showing an increase in emotional regulation as she put words to her overwhelming feelings. In Figure 2.3, titled *Lost Goose* she depicted a mother duck who looks down upon a sad baby goose. The baby goose looks up towards the mother duck tearfully. Katherine appeared sad and I told her I could see the goose felt so sad about its mother and wondered aloud if this is why the goose was crying.

I encouraged Katherine to say more about the story of the baby goose and the mother duck. I asked Katherine if there was a story to her drawing and she wrote, "here is a goose, a sad goose, its mom did not want her". As I read the story aloud to her, she quickly scribbled out the word "want" and added "find her yet". The story of her drawing now read

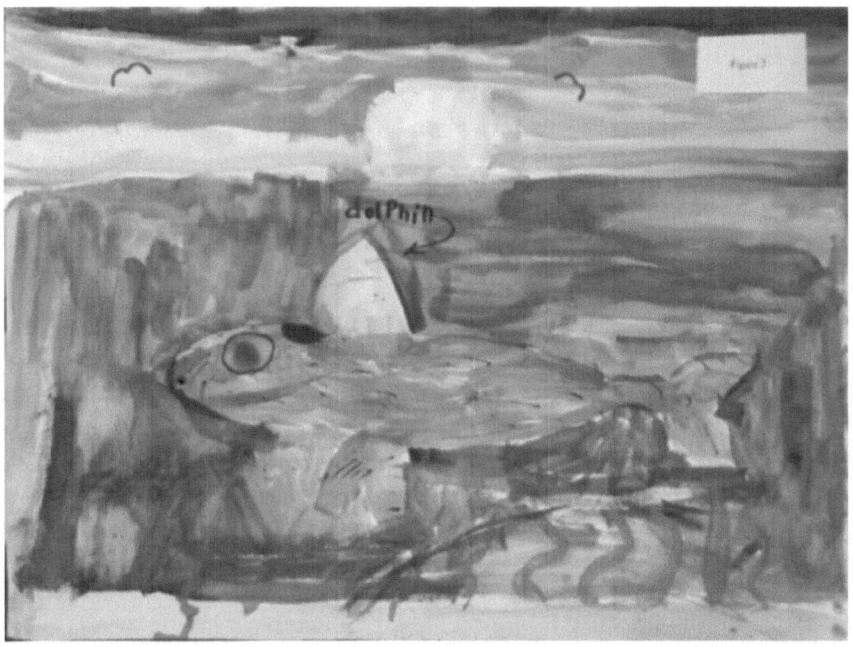

Figure 2.2 The Large Fish

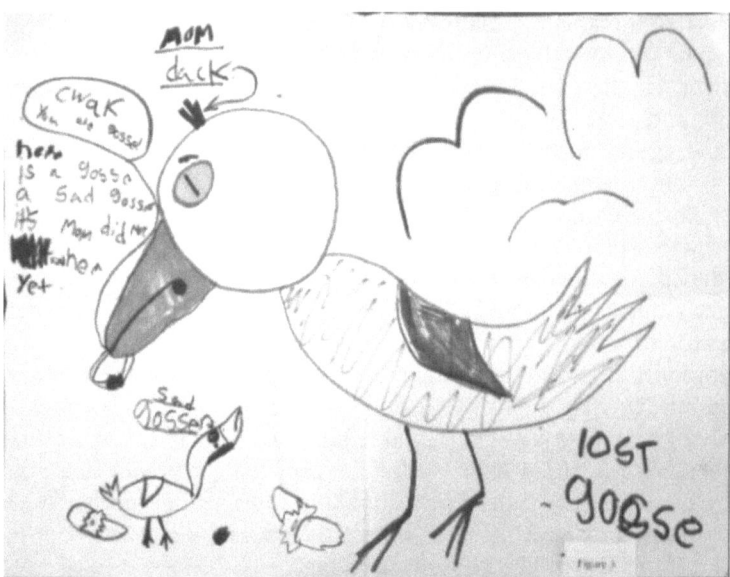

Figure 2.3 Lost Goose

"here is a goose, a sad goose, its mom did not find her yet". Katherine could not acknowledge that a mother might not want its baby so she created a narrative that was protective and hopeful.

Figure 2.3 shows Katherine's use of the defense mechanism of displacement to redirect her scared and sad feelings, by representing something threatening in a less threatening object. Defense mechanisms are protective and can shield a developing person from problems that arise from early relational wounds (Robbins, 1987). Katherine's dealing with the loss of her mother was portrayed in a story of the mismatch of a mother duck and a sad baby goose that was unwanted. This demonstrates the use of displacement and use of narrative to neutralize overwhelming feelings of sadness (Shore, 2013).

Later Sessions

Later in art therapy sessions, Katherine showed interest in the sandtray. She showed progress as her verbal communication increased and her emotional dysregulation decreased. Her father reported Katherine showing improvement in emotional regulation both at home and at school. I continued to recommend individual sessions for Katherine, to which her father agreed. For the first two years of treatment, I had no communication with Katherine's mother, then the mother showed up to one of Katherine's sessions unannounced.

Katherine's mother let me know she would be joining her daughter's session that day and I, surprised, encouraged the mother to give her daughter a sense of autonomy over her sessions by not joining that day. The mother joined the session against my advice and used the time to provide an account of her trauma. I found myself intolerant of her mother's behaviors and wanted to cast her out of the session. I patiently provided redirection throughout the session.

Katherine showed a dysregulated self-state as she again painted on the table, the walls and her mother. Katherine giggled as she sat in her mother's lap, painting her hands. I commented on how close they appeared and then her mother showed photos of a young Katherine. Her mother then scrolled to a photograph of her own badly bruised body from the earlier incident of physical abuse that required surgery. Katherine appeared frozen as her mother began to share the traumatic images and unbearable emotions of that day.

I had worked with Katherine for two years before her mother's whereabouts were known. Her mother was engaged in her own therapy and visited Katherine during the weekends. Now with her mother's support, I elected to continue to support Katherine and her sense of autonomy by continuing to have independent sessions without her parents.

Katherine arrived at an upcoming session and let me know that she wanted to try the sandtray. She said that she would be making movie scenes and reassured me that these movies had no connection with real events. I told her that I believed her and wanted to watch one of her movies. Her cast for her first movie was a family with a young child. First the mother, then the father and then the child entered the scene, falling from the sky above. Katherine appeared frightened each time the child fell uncontrollably into each new scene. I shared it seemed frightening for the child to have the feeling of not knowing where she would land next.

During the making of Katherine's movie, the family's cat entered the scene. I started to get to know the cat's personality, quick to pounce on family members, often starting fights, and repeatedly was the outcast of the family. During the making of a sandtray scene, the cat went missing. I found the cat was missing from my office the following session.

In subsequent sessions, Katherine created missing posters for the cat. I asked her if she thought the cat had been stolen. She presented with restricted affect as she asked if I knew who had stolen the cat. I maintained curiosity about what happened to the cat and shared how awful it was that the cat had gone missing from her family.

Katherine brought the cat figurine from the sandtray collection into a session near the end of our time together. She took the cat figurine out of her pocket and handed it to me. "Oh, you found the cat?" I said with warmth and curiosity, and let her know I was so very glad the cat had been reunited with her family.

Katherine's mother was now reunited with Katherine and her family. Her parents were reported to have shared custody. Katherine would soon move to live with her mother who was two hours away from my office. I recommended her parents schedule closing sessions with me, and for Katherine to continue work with a child therapist. I provided a referral for a child therapist who was in close proximity to her mother. Four 60-minute closing sessions were provided so that Katherine was able to say goodbye and review all the good work she had done over the years.

Outcomes

Long-term work with Katherine over the course of four years allowed for a reparative relationship that supported her to regulate her emotions. She showed an increase in emotional regulation as she put words to her overwhelming feelings and made use of art as a container for her intense emotions. Her use of defense mechanisms shielded her from the relational wound of her mother's abandonment. The outcome of our relational work together showed the patient used a range of art media that fostered self-regulation and developed a capacity to process and put words to overwhelming feelings that gradually improved within a supportive therapeutic relationship.

Concluding Statements

Children with complex trauma have a powerful impact on those who work with them. My early sessions with Katherine provoked strong emotions and feelings of helplessness. These emotions were meaningful to tune into, as they provided a sense of what it might feel like to be Katherine.

The emotionally attuned therapeutic relationship with its multisensory matrix of art media offered characteristics associated with early affective, non-verbal functions. The therapeutic relationship Katherine and I shared did not alone accomplish the repair of disruptions in attachment. The affective exchanges and shared states constituted an emotional feedback system between Katherine and me that fostered an increase in self-regulation and positively influenced her attachment relationships.

NARRATIVES EXPLORING ANXIOUS REACTIONS

PEG DUNN-SNOW

Setting and Approaches

As mentioned in Chapter 1, Children's Corner: Art Therapy for Children is an art therapy practice that serves children between 5 and 12 years of age through varies treatment approaches.

Case Study

Susan was an only child, living with both of her parents. She was ten years old and was attending the fourth grade in a private parochial school system. A little more than a year ago, her father's best friend, Uncle Bob, was hospitalized and within a few days, while still in the hospital, he died. Unknown to Susan, her uncle had been battling cancer for several years, so it came as a shock to her when he seemingly died suddenly. The day that he died was identified by both Susan and her parents as a traumatic event for all of them as Bob and his wife were neighbors and the families saw each other weekly. Together, they went on vacations and celebrated the holidays and other special family events. Since Bob's death, Susan's parents became concerned about the changes in behaviors they saw in their daughter. She was no longer the happy, confident girl they knew but instead she was withdrawn and anxious and recently these behaviors had gotten worse.

Intake Session

Family Information and Preliminary Diagnosis

Susan was first seen in March of the school year. During the intake session, a preliminary diagnostic impression of anxiety disorder, unspecified, was made based on the following information. In this session, Susan's mother reported that Susan had become anxious, agitated, tearful, and sometimes angry. However, when the parents would ask Susan about her behaviors, Susan could not give them an explanation. When the discussion of the death of Susan's uncle became the topic of discussion, Susan's mother began to cry and Susan showed signs of becoming agitated. Susan reported she was upset because her mom was upset and crying and not because her uncle had died. Also discussed during the intake session was Susan's anxiety about her dad leaving the house, which was evidenced by her calling him frequently when he was away and asking him when he was coming home. It was also reported Susan became angry when her dad did not arrive home at the time he had planned to when he left the house. During this session, Susan also identified two other traumatic events that had taken place in her life. When she was eight years old, she had a scary dental visit, and when she was five years old, her paternal grandmother died.

Assessments and Treatment Plan

With information given in the intake session, it was determined that Susan's initial therapy would be trauma-based, and the Instinctual Trauma Response (ITR) would be used (Tinnin & Gantt, 2013). This protocol is a combination of art therapy, narrative therapy, and parts work as described in writings about the Internal Family Systems (IFS) approach to therapy (Schwarz, 1995; Spiegel, 2017).

Trauma-Focused Therapy

The First Therapy Session

It was two weeks later before Susan attended her first therapy session. Before the session, her mom contacted me and told me Susan's dad wanted to come to meet me and participate at the end of the first therapy session. During the session with Susan, after we discussed the three scary events she identified in intake session, Susan chose to create a graphic narrative about the day Uncle Bob died.

The protocol began asking Susan to draw one of her safe places as a grounding activity before she began her graphic narrative. Next, she was asked to draw a series of sequential pictures of the event, as she remembered them, and then tell a story about each drawing. The story was directed through a series of questions asking Susan to answer in the third person and include her thoughts, feelings, and what her body was doing as part of her memory of the event. At the end of the session, I read Susan's story to her. It was with her drawings and story that Susan identified her responses to the death and loss of her Uncle Bob and what followed afterwards. What is most important in addressing trauma is helping the client understand his or her responses to the traumatic event versus the trauma itself (Porges, 2011).

When both parents were invited into the last part of this session, Susan discussed her graphic narrative with them. I suggested that Susan, after experiencing her uncle leaving his home, going to the hospital, and then never coming back home, might be one of the reasons she had become fearful about her dad leaving the house without her. Was she thinking he could leave the house, go somewhere, and never come home too? When Susan was asked that question, she shrugged and said, "I don't know, maybe". Neither parent agreed or disagreed with this idea and contributed very little to this discussion. Susan was then asked if she was worried about anything else going on at home. Much to her parents' surprise, Susan said she was also worried about how often she would see them fighting. Both parents seemed not only surprised but also embarrassed by their daughter's disclosure, and seemed to dismiss it by not contributing to the discussion about this topic either. That was also the last time Susan's father came to a session.

The Second Therapy Session

The second therapy session took place a week later. Susan reviewed her drawings and story to determine if it was finished. She decided her graphic narrative was incomplete and added more drawings and text to her story. At the end of this session, we reviewed her additions with her mother. I told Susan I would type up her finished story and bring her a copy to take home during our next session. I told both Susan and her mom I wanted to begin parts work with Susan during the next session and continue to discuss Susan's use of her avoidance part featured in her narrative about the death of her uncle. It was important to discover whether this part developed any false beliefs during that trauma event that are still influencing Susan's behaviors in the present (i.e., her strong fears of being separated from her dad based on her uncle).

Schwartz (1995) developed the IFS theoretical approach to psychotherapy and identified a family of personality parts within everyone, including young, wounded parts that hold painful memories and protective parts that try to shield a person from their painful experiences. These parts fight with each other and with the person's core parts, a concept that makes up the confident, compassionate, whole person who lives in all of us. IFS focuses on healing the wounded parts by correcting the false beliefs they have come to believe as truths about themselves and others. The IFS approach also focuses on convincing protector parts that the person's core parts can cope with challenges presented by past life events. When successful, relationships amongst the parts shift the balance of power over to the core self.

The Third Therapy Session

Four weeks went by before Susan attended her third art therapy session. This session began with a review of her completed narrative, and afterwards Susan was given a copy of her story and drawings to take home with her to keep and reread (Davis, 2019).

After four weeks, Susan was no longer interested in continuing a discussion about her uncle. Her comment, when asked about her thoughts, feelings, and behaviors about dad when he would leave the house was, "It's getting better". When asked what was getting better, Susan was unable to reply, or perhaps she was avoiding the subject. If Susan was avoiding the topic, it was similar to how she initially dealt with her uncle's death as recalled in her graphic narrative. "… Susan, age nine, would take care of herself '[by] trying to let go of her Uncle Bob's memory and thinking about the next great thing that would happen …'".

With almost 40 minutes left in this third session, it became clear that Susan wanted to talk about something else that happened to her in school since the last time we saw each other. For the remainder of this session, she talked about being bullied daily at school by one of her classmates. When asked if she had told her parents, Susan shook her head no. When asked why she had not confided in her parents, she said because the classmate is also their neighbor, and "we go on vacations together" and "Valerie treats me differently when we are away from school". I suggested to Susan that when her mother joined us during this session that she tell her she is being bullied at school. When Susan's mother was told what was going on, her reaction again was one of surprise. I suggested having a discussion with Susan, Valerie, and their mothers to try and resolve this conflict before it could escalate. In preparation for Susan's session next week, parts work was again discussed with Susan and her mother that could address Susan's coping strategies as revealed in her graphic narrative. There was also a discussion about helping Susan identify her experiences of success through some type of self-portrait that could address her loss of confidence that her parents have observed and were concerned about.

Susan's Story

Safe Place: Susan, age ten, has a safe place. Her safe place is her room at home. Susan, age ten, feels safe in her room and thinks about getting good grades at school. Her body is relaxed when she is in her safe place as she lies on her bed reading a book.

The Story of How Bob Died

Susan, age nine, was out to dinner with her family and Bob's family. She was thinking about what she wanted to eat and was feeling hungry. Her body was sitting at the table.

Next, Bob is in the hospital with his wife Lena and he has died. Bob had cancer for many years. After school that day, Susan, age nine, was in her parents' bedroom lying on the bed when they told her that Bob had died. Susan, age nine, was feeling shocked and thinking and wondering how her parents would react to Bob's death.

Later that afternoon, Susan, age nine, was in the car with her mother getting ready to go to her karate lesson. Her mother began to cry and could not drive the car so Susan, age nine, could not go that day. Sitting in the car with her mom, Susan, age nine, was feeling mad because she could not go to class but continued to be concerned about her parents and how they would continue to react to Bob's death.

Susan, age nine, would take care of herself by going to her safe place, her room. She would try to get her body to relax. She felt safe and thought about how much had been going on and tried not to think about it (Figure 2.4).

Susan, age nine, was with her family and Bob's family going to visit a lighthouse to see Bob's stone. Susan, age nine, was feeling happy because she got to go to the top of the lighthouse and the view was amazing. However, Susan, age nine, was also sad because she also had to go see the stone. Susan, age nine, was thinking of a memory she had about Bob and her body was looking all around. They were at the lighthouse for three or four hours.

On another day Susan, age nine, was at home on the couch in the family room (Figure 2.5). "She was trying to let go of Uncle Bob's memory and trying to think about the next great thing that would happen". Susan, age nine, was feeling relaxed while lying on the couch.

Today, Susan is ten years-old and goes to karate classes two times a week. When she is at karate, she does a lot of exercises as she thinks about trying to stay focused. She is feeling tired after her classes.

The story entitled *The Story of How Bob Died* had a beginning, a middle, and an end and it happened a year ago and it is over. THE END

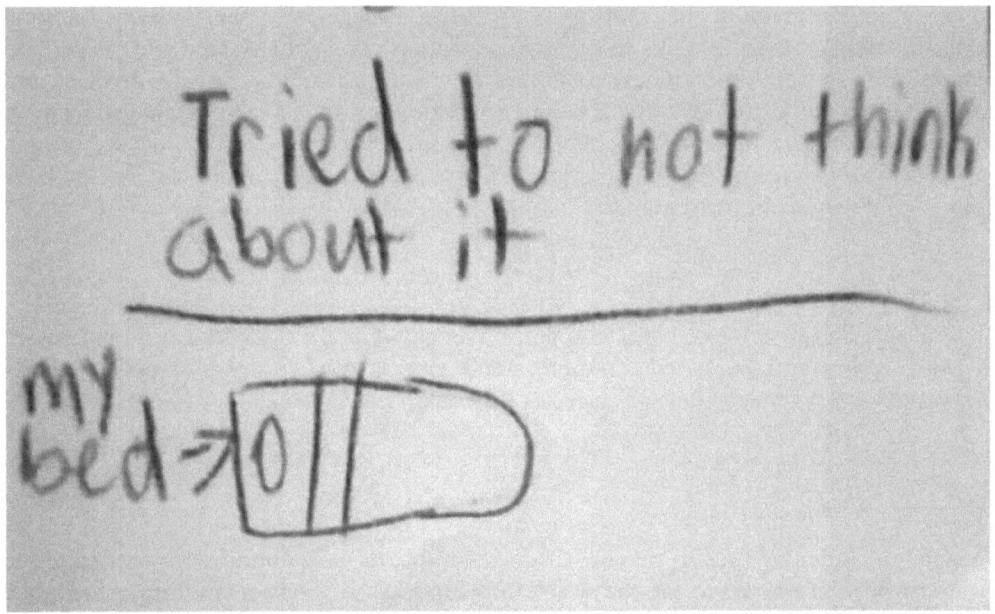

Figure 2.4 Trying Not to Think about Uncle Bob

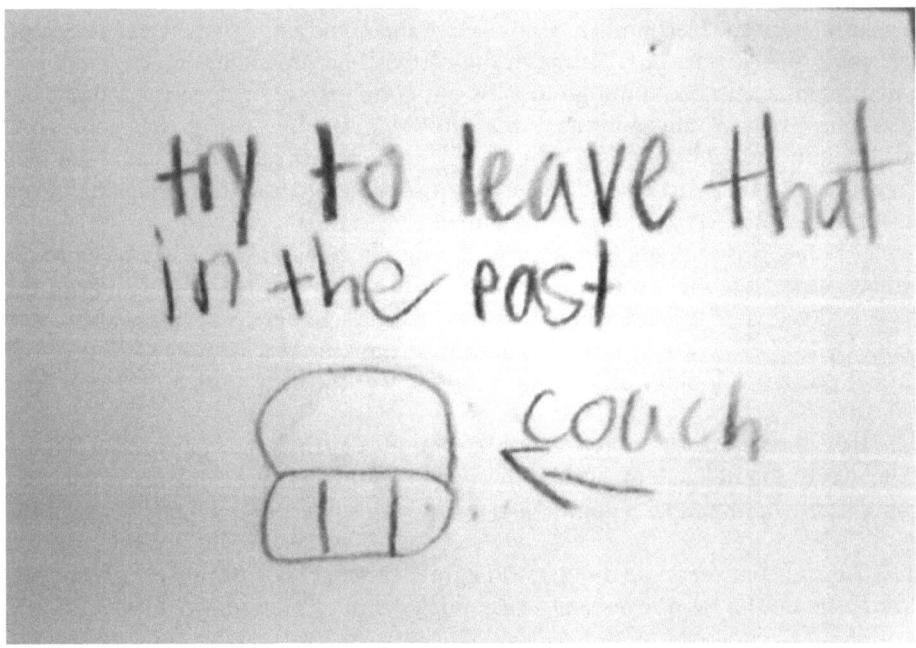

Figure 2.5 Leaving Thoughts in the Past

The Fourth Session Became the Termination Session

Unfortunately, another five weeks went by before Susan came back for her next therapy session. This fourth session also turned out to be Susan's termination session. At the beginning of this session, I asked if Susan's mother would participate in the entire session this week in order to review the initial reasons Susan's parents wanted therapy for their daughter and whether new goals and objectives should be identified at this time. I also wanted to find out from both Susan and her mother the status of the five issues that Susan had discussed previously in her therapy sessions. The five issues included the death of Uncle Bob, Susan's anxiety about dad leaving the house after Uncle Bob death, the parents' frequent fights that Susan was witnessing at home, the bullying at school from one of Susan's classmates, and Susan's diminishing self-confidence as observed and reported by her parents.

It was reported Susan was no longer troubled by her uncle's death and Susan believed her anxiety about her dad leaving was connected to losing her uncle. According to Susan's mother, Susan's anxiety was under control now, especially since her dad was beginning to call when he knew he would be late coming home. The mother took responsibility for Susan's witnessing her parents' fights and she and Susan's father are trying to make sure their fights are done in private with Susan's inability to hear them. The mother also reported that nothing was done about the bullying. Susan was experiencing at school by their neighbor's daughter, Valerie. The mother stated she believed there was a third classmate in the classroom who was stirring up trouble between Susan and Valerie. Susan reported that two days ago, Valerie told her she thought the other classmate was mean. Susan's mother was surprised to hear that Susan again had not confided in her about this exchange with Valerie at school. Susan's mother heard for the first time in this session that the bullying at school appeared to be stopping. The mother never mentioned the issue of Susan's diminished self-confidence. The mother felt that all the issues listed in the summary of the third session above were beginning to be resolved and that Susan was doing much better. She believed Susan could stop therapy at this time. Susan agreed as long as she could come back if she needed more therapy in the future.

Proper Termination

At the end of this fourth session, Susan added her drawing to my goodbye journal, an activity I ask children to do when I have the opportunity to conduct a proper termination with my clients. Susan, her mother, and I also agreed that the door to my art therapy office was always open to them in the future.

Outcomes

Susan was compliant in her art-making and discussions during her brief art therapy experience. It appeared that she benefitted from her time in therapy when she had a chance to understand that her anxiety about her dad leaving the house without her was directly connected to her perception of how she lost her uncle (i.e., Uncle Bob left his home and a few days later he was gone and never came home). However, Susan's graphic narrative illustrated that she frequently used avoidance as a coping mechanism and was reluctant to confide in her parents when she was conflicted about other issues, like being bullied at school and witnessing their fights. One of the reasons Susan was brought to therapy initially was because she could not or would not explain her behaviors, which her parents found troubling. Due to the inconsistent therapy schedule and the short time Susan's attended therapy sessions, there was no time to discuss healthier coping strategies with Susan nor was there any opportunity to address Susan's diminished self-confidence, the bullying at school, or the witnessing of her parents' ongoing conflicts at home.

Developmental Concerns

I also wondered if Susan's language development was a factor in her inability to express herself verbally to her parents. Again, there was no time to determine if Susan could benefit from attending Speech and Language sessions to improve her vocabulary and language skills.

Conclusions

Susan was a bright but guarded young girl who reportedly was academically successful in school. Susan's cognitive skills appeared to match her chronological age but it appeared that her social and emotional skills and possibly her language skills were not age appropriate. When she created her graphic narrative about the death of her Uncle Bob, it was evident that her primary coping strategy was avoidance.

It appeared that Susan learned to use avoidance as a primary coping mechanism from her parents. Her father only came to Susan's first therapy session, during which Susan brought up not only her fears of when he was absent from the home without her but also about the frequent fights she had been witnessing between her parents on a weekly and sometimes daily basis.   During her third session, Susan told her mother about being bullied by a classmate which seemed to make the mother uncomfortable when she heard this news. The mother explained the classmate who was bullying Susan was actually the daughter of a neighbor. The families were very friendly and spent time together on a weekly basis. Susan's mother admitted that Valerie does treat her differently at home when they are away from school.

In Susan's fourth and last session, Susan's mother reported she had done nothing about the bullying and did not address the problem with her neighbor. The mother believed the problem was caused by another girl in the class who was causing trouble between Susan and Valerie. Susan's mother believed the girls would sort out their problem between themselves. The mother did admit that the parental fights at home should not be witnessed by Susan and she and her husband would try harder to keep their fights private. Not bringing Susan to therapy on a consistent schedule also appeared to be an avoidance behavior by the parents.

I believe Susan does not feel safe confiding in either of her parents about her thoughts, feelings, and anxious behaviors. Until this family can improve their communication with one another and until the parents can be more present to their daughter's emotional needs, Susan will continue to react anxiously to situations that trouble her. Susan may also have difficulties developing trusting relationships with others. This family would benefit from family therapy in the future to address these issues.

DISTANCE AND PROXIMITY IN ADOLESCENCE: A RELATIONAL VIEW OF THE USE OF THE ART THERAPY SPACE WITH TWO ADOLESCENT CASE STUDIES

MIA DE BÉTHUNE

Setting

These two case studies took place in a private practice studio in a suburban setting in the Northeastern United States just above a major metropolitan area. The studio was spacious with two large tables covered in craft paper, making them a clean and available area for any type of art activity. The studio was stocked with all manner of art materials from a variety of papers, paints, drawing media, and markers to various types of modeling clay to woodworking tools and fabrics. I, the art therapist, maintained an area to one side as my own personal workspace and the walls had cork boards to accommodate large drawing and viewing of artwork from a distance. The two clients were an early adolescent girl and a middle adolescent boy. Ten-year-old Mina displayed anxiety and aggression and was seen with her mother at first. Parallel sessions were also held with both parents during the first six months. Eventually, she came on her own for six years before sessions moved online during the pandemic and the final two years of her treatment. Fourteen-year-old Carey was depressed and selectively mute. He was seen individually at first with parallel sessions for his parents. Eventually, family sessions were used to enhance communication toward the end of treatment.

Approaches

Both case studies used a relational lens to examine the development and attachment style of early, middle, and late adolescence for these two youths as seen through their use of space within the art therapy studio. Space was considered in its physical, embodied, and symbolic aspects through images and objects created by Mina and Carey, who displayed varying tendencies based on their shifting needs and issues. Shifts in distance and proximity with me, the art therapist, seemed indicative of development as Mina grew from a clingy and physically demanding young child to an older adolescent with stronger coping skills and the ability to create her own space within the therapeutic alliance. Symbols created by Carey seemed to represent his negotiation of the therapeutic space and alliance with me as he began reaching beyond carefully defended boundaries. Shifts in the distance he maintained from me seemed to indicate his developmental needs, as he went from barricading me over the course of many months to inviting me to share his space and accept encouragement to develop his voice.

Adolescents learn to become independent through gradual disengagement from the support of parents and others whom they depend upon in childhood (Steinberg, 2014). Disengagement is accomplished through experimentation with shifts in the distance or proximity with important persons in life. The required shift from the protective sphere of parents to the social sphere of peers is often marked by ambivalence, particularly toward parents who must be left behind. These swings between closeness and distance, if recognized as a step towards independence, can open avenues of communication that aid a teen's natural course of development. The art therapy studio is a perfect setting for this to occur.

Review of Literature

Attachment and Mentalization in Adolescents

Adolescence marks a time when attachment bonds are tested because of the dramatic physical, neurological, and psychological changes that occur during puberty (Steinberg, 2014). "Identity formation, peer relationships, body relationships", and the need to become independent make "the attachment system" more relevant in adolescence (Steele et al., 2015, p. 16). Teens will test the strength of attachment relationships (Steele et al., 2015), and yet those who have disorganized or insecure attachment ties may find their ability to form new relationships compromised. This inability may be due to poor affect regulation and lack of verbal skills. Additionally, their sense of physical boundaries and self may be fragmented and easily threatened (Carlson et al., 2009; Steele et al., 2015). These deficits make the transition from family bonds to new bonds with peers more difficult. The capacity for reflective functioning (RF) is an important aspect of attachment bonding, which helps adolescents create meaning in their lives by understanding the reality of other people's thoughts in relation to their own. RF, or the ability to think about mental states, "is crucial to the development of the self" (Steele et al., 2015, p. 22). Generally, RF develops in relation to a primary caregiver through satisfactory attunement. RF or "mentalisation" (Bevington et al., 2012, p. 2) provides the security of understanding another person's thoughts and actions while they also understand yours.

Deficits of Attachment and Mentalization

Adolescents with emotional problems of depression, aggression, dissociation, or post-traumatic stress disorder (PTSD) have been shown in studies of mother–infant attachment bonds to have parents who "consistently show a lack of attunement and fail to pick up on their infants' signals" (Steele et al., 2015, p. 18). Lack of attunement with an infant can lead to insecurity and conflicted interpersonal skills in adolescents (Steele et al., 2015). These youths also tend to have a limited ability to understand or express their own emotional states and may instead act out emotions through physical means, including self-harm. Lyons-Ruth et al. (2013) showed a direct correlation between "maternal withdrawal to infant's attempts for emotional proximity and self-injury" (Steele et al., 2015, p. 25). Though they may no longer want hugs and physical contact from their parents, they still need and crave "emotional proximity to and *perception* of being accepted and protected" (Steele et al., 2015, p. 26).

Having an adult understand what their behavior means can help a child become a well-integrated adult who understands themselves and their emotions (Steele et al., 2015). When the ability for emotional regulation "fails to keep up with cognitive or sexual maturation" (Dil et al., 2016, p. 84), depression can occur. Depressed adolescents suffer from feelings of confusion and "find developmental tasks overwhelming" (Dil et al., 2016, p. 85). Resultant feelings of shame (Dil et al., 2016) may become maladaptive, causing the teen to turn inward, protecting a fragile self and unable to form relationships with peers. Their understanding of self may be incoherent (Steele et al., 2015, p. 19; Beebe et al., 2012; Beebe & Steele, 2013) and lead to poor interpersonal skills.

Children who have sensory differences, exhibit attention deficit disorders, or struggle with learning disabilities are often among those who show acting-out behaviors and maybe even more at risk (Peleikis et al., 2022). They can develop "narcissistic depression" (Dil et al., 2016, p. 85) because they often feel stigmatized and alone. Gurian (2017) described male anhedonia in boys who were not emotionally nurtured, which resulted in depression, poor school performance, lack of verbal expression, and addiction to video and computer stimulation, including pornography.

Use of the Art Therapy Space in Treatment

Early attachment relations can be projected onto the art therapy space through the art material and the relationship with the therapist. Creative art therapies stress empathy and "a receptive mirroring stance toward the client" (Johnson, 1989, p. 89) by creating a sense of holding and employing all the senses in an attuned manner. The tendency to approach or withdraw, seek proximity or create distance from others is rooted in past experiences of reward or punishment with regard to intimacy (Dosmantes, 1992). Thus, the art therapist is drawn into the adolescent's internal world of attachment ties (Hilbuch et al., 2016) and can help teens develop a deeper understanding of self through the use of space, materials, and the therapeutic relationship.

Mina: Anxiety and Aggression in Early Adolescence

Mina was a small, ten-year-old preadolescent girl with long, black hair and an expressive face with large aquamarine eyes. She first came to art therapy because she had been biting and hitting other children in elementary school. She was of Polish, Acadian, and Native American heritage and from a middle-class family. Neurologically sensitive as an infant, she was an unplanned pregnancy for her young professional parents. She was often handed around backstage when her mother, a dancer, was performing. Mina's previous therapist had moved to another state and her mother sought me as an art therapist because Mina loved to paint. Upon meeting her parents, who both worked in the theater world, they disclosed that each had lost a brother within the past ten years. Mina's mother, especially, continued to struggle with her grief.

Intake Session

In the first session, Mina seemed shy and eager to please and requested her mother stay in the room. She presented me with a picture of her dog, a pit-bull, of which she was both fond and afraid. I noticed quickly that she reverted to baby talk, preverbal noises, and facial gestures when frustrated or anxious. If I asked any direct questions about her thoughts and feelings, Mina responded by hissing or even growling, like an angry cat. There were school reports of her physical aggression when she could not communicate her needs, and it was immediately apparent that she was also extremely sensitive to light, sound, and tempera-ture. The ticking of the watch on my wrist was a loud pounding noise to her ears. She had received occupational therapy in preschool for sensory processing but was denied services in elementary school because she did not meet the severity threshold for Attention Deficit Hyperactivity Disorder (ADHD) or anxiety disorder.

Assessment and Early Treatment

Mina described her need to come to therapy as "my therapist left" and "my mother says I'm destructive". Initially, she completed several art therapy assessments (The Kramer Assessment; Kramer & Scheur, 1983; The Kinetic Family Drawing; Hardin & Peterson, 1997; Formal Elements Art Therapy Scale; Gantt & Tabone, 1997) that revealed anxiety and depression, but also an exceptional ability for visual-spatial skills. As her mother was a professional dance teacher, it was not surprising to learn that Mina was a skilled ballerina who had been dancing from the age of three.

Mina brought an infant-self into therapy with the baby talk, as well as a need for physical intimacy through proximity (a need for touch) and aggressive actions toward me as the therapist. The art therapy space greatly enhanced the opportunity for this physicality to be expressed and explored, so that eventually she was able to create more secure personal boundaries as she matured. Throughout treatment, Mina consistently engaged in symbolic play through image-making, puppets, doll-making, and games that had themes of aggression and anger. These often included a mother figure who was either angry, vulnerable, or sad.

I frequently observed her internal mother-voice self-criticism, and so parallel to my work with Mina, I coached both her mother and father in parenting skills and boundary setting. I especially worked to boost her mother's confidence in her ability to be a parent as well as to explore her own feelings of grief about Mina's uncle. Gradually, I heard more expressions of compassion and pleasure toward Mina. This seemed parallel to a growing ability for more sophisticated, age-appropriate problem-solving behavior. The skills appeared especially around creating three-dimensional projects she called "monsters" which were made by scrounging through my recycle bins (Figure 2.6).

Expansion into the Studio

Although initially timid within the therapy space, Mina soon exhibited an expanded self and a frenetic need for movement within the entire room. Visually, this took the form of her need to cover any clean space on the two work tables in the studio with her own marks using paint or markers (Figure 2.7). She would often exclaim, "This is mine!" and seemed to assert her need to be seen. This expanded energy also took the form of highly physical games of paddle tennis over the work tables in which it seemed important to not only win but also to "slaughter" me as her opponent, or punching battles with puppets where my puppet was the target. Both seemed a healthy development in terms of her ability to express more open feelings of anger and aggression toward me without having to please me all the time.

As I set limits around physical aggression toward me, Mina began to express herself more verbally. Her calling me "slow" or "bad" seemed a projection of bad feelings about herself that we then explored. I was often exhausted by both her physical and verbal aggression and began to use small self-disclosures related to this activity. Mina seemed able to tolerate this and to genuinely hear me, thus developing a relational capacity for empathy; an ability to "see" the other. Often after the aggressive play, she would settle down to create another "monster". This series of small creatures seemed to reflect her current wants and needs but also seemed a way to rework her own identity as a destructive child.

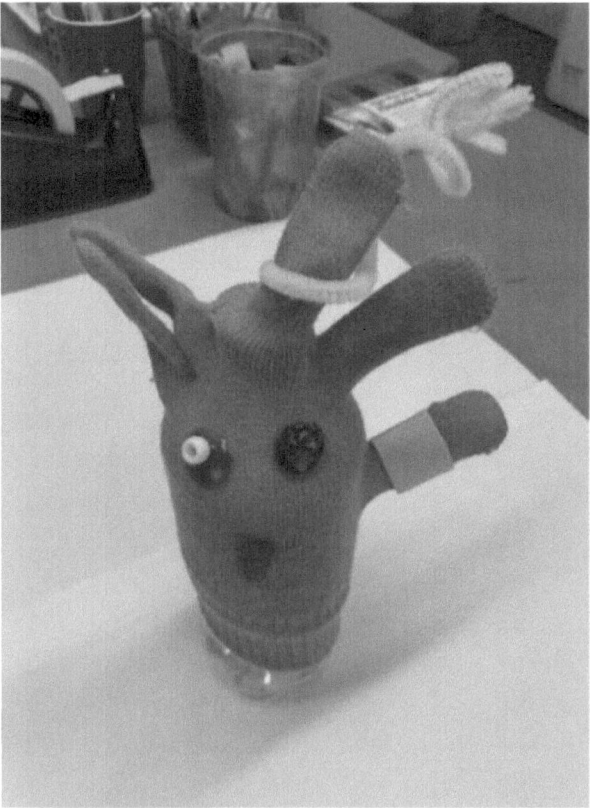

Figure 2.6 Mina's Monster

Growth and Progress

Mina's need to regress and become "baby-like" diminished over our first few years together. She began to tolerate it when I pointed out her baby speech and wondered about her need for it. I also suggested that Mina make a dictionary of her own "Mina Speech" – a project she took up with great enthusiasm. The focus of therapy then shifted toward discussing more anxiety-provoking material such as the death of her uncles, friendships in middle school, and schoolwork. Mina no longer responded to questions by hissing but instead said, "awkward" or repeated the word "cupcake" several times. When it came to school work, Mina would shrug and say, "I hate reading" or "I just don't care".

As Mina's schoolwork became more of a focus in therapy, I suggested to her parents that she have a psychological evaluation. I prepared Mina for this by explaining why she needed the testing and she seemed able to hear that she might need support to "do better". Both parents had become more mindful of their interactions with her, particularly around the support of homework. She was finally given a diagnosis of both anxiety disorder and ADHD and improved rapidly once school accommodations were implemented. These included modified homework, a front seat in the classroom, and lengthened test times. Mina

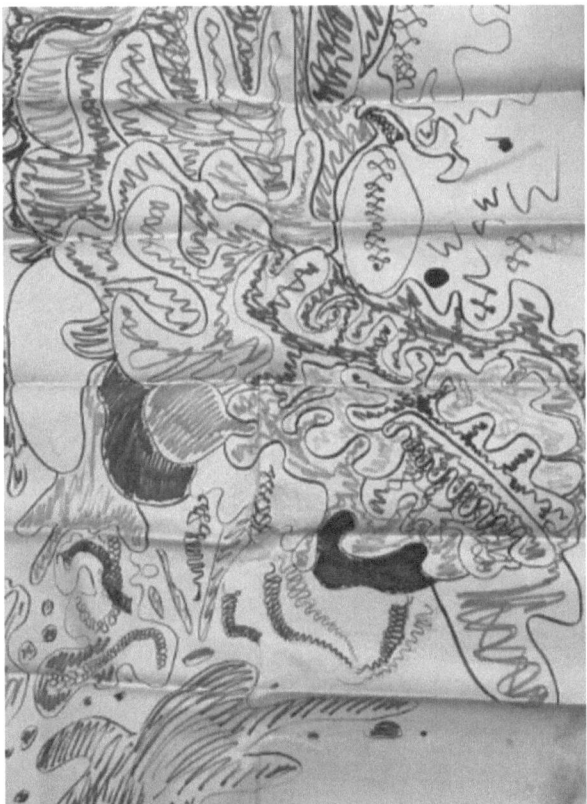

Figure 2.7 Mina's Drawing on Tables

began to succeed in some classes and reports indicated that she was more motivated, and she was completing homework on her own initiative. Sometimes she even brought work into therapy. There were no more incidents of classroom aggression and Mina began to describe friends that she was sitting with in the cafeteria.

Creating Boundaries Within and Without

Through the support of her teachers, her parents, and myself, Mina made gradual but steady improvements in feelings of competence, self-esteem, control of impulsivity, and self-reflection. Support from her parents seemed to make Mina a more confident and happy child. Within the art therapy room, Mina was more self-directed and able to engage in a give-and-take with me as her therapist. Of course, this was not the end of the story. I continued to work with Mina as she graduated to toe-shoes and excelled as a dancer even as she faced the vicissitudes of middle and high school. One final chapter relays the shift toward a more distant independence that occurred for her within the therapeutic space.

Later Sessions

By the age of 14, Mina was well entrenched with a group of middle school friends who were into Japanese Anime and popular music. She experimented with having crushes on both boys and girls and eventually had a boyfriend. She no longer made much art in therapy, nor would she talk to me, as is typical of middle adolescents, but she never missed a session and showed up every week. Her physical appearance began to include darkened eyeliner, ripped jeans, and brilliant color of every possible shade in her long hair. The color changed weekly. Though she would not talk about her friends or boyfriend, I had learned to ask oblique questions and just remain present. Generally, as she was leaving, she would drop small clues as to her inner life (e.g., "J and I had a fight and got kicked out of French"). Her most consistent behavior was to drop her heavy backpack on the floor, sigh, and then lay most of her body on the same work tables that we had once played paddle ball over and that she had covered with paint. She often lay there for a long while as if retreating into a sanctuary.

In the fall of her 15th year, her mother became panicked because Mina was cutting herself. Because of our rapport, I was able to speak very frankly about this, and she listened, scowled, and did not speak, but paid attention. I was able to determine that she had been sexually involved with her boyfriend and was frightened. The old non-verbal and anxious Mina had returned. While I normalized sexual experience and described how frightening it could be, Mina and I began working with Origami paper. She folded an exquisite three-cornered box. When I speculated that it would make a wonderful hideout, Mina's eyes lit up. I suggested that she could construct a box big enough to get inside and she became as excited as she'd been when creating her monsters. Over the course of several weeks, we constructed her box together (Figure 2.8). When it was finished, she went inside and spent the rest of the session silent, sending only a small slip of paper out the top with the word "hello". This was the last project Mina created with me.

Outcomes

During the COVID-19 pandemic, she was doing well in an alternative high school and I didn't see her for several months until she agreed to meet online. Something about the security of her room (another little box) and the distance created by Zoom seemed to allow her to open up and become chatty. Sometimes she shared with me clay or painting projects she was doing for school and very often we just sat in silence or talked about her favorite Anime shows. We met consistently online once a week until she graduated a year later.

Discussion

From her initial session in art therapy, Mina presented as a child who might be described as having an "incoherent internal working model" of self (Steele et al., 2015, p. 19). Her parents, still focused on their careers in their early twenties, were not prepared for an infant or the mirroring required to care for one (Lyons-Ruth et al., 2013). Her mother, especially, was anxious in relation to caring for a baby that was highly sensitive (Peleikis et al., 2022). Overwhelmed and confused by Mina's demands, she projected onto her the identity of a destructive child. Given the regressive behavior Mina presented with – baby talk, biting, and physical aggression – it seemed likely she had missed out on some of the benefits of

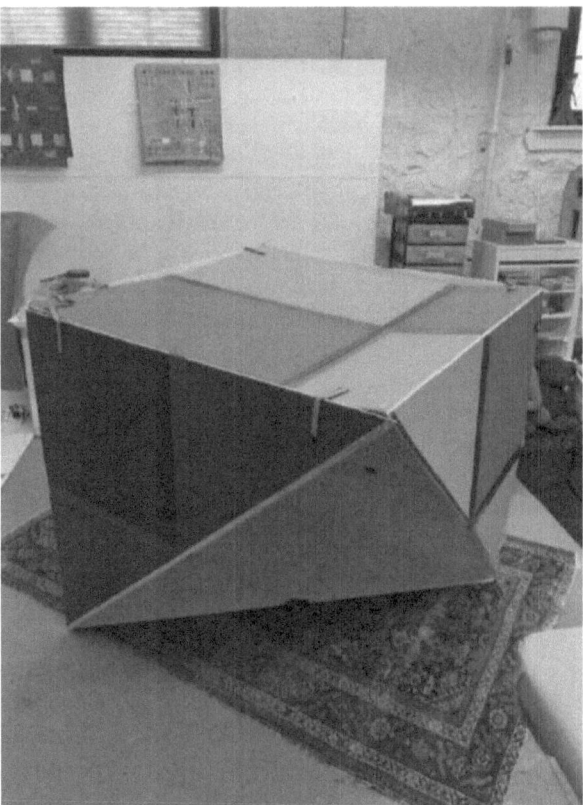

Figure 2.8 Mina's Box Hideaway

secure attachment bonding in infancy (Beebe & Steele, 2013) and was acting out her needs through a primitive form of communication.

Using the space within the art therapy studio (Hilbuch et al., 2016), we began to renegotiate Mina's ability to have her needs met. Mina's initial need for close proximity and touch from me, as well as her physical aggression, may well have represented a fragmented and poorly regulated nervous system (Carlson et al., 2009; Steele et al., 2015). I began negotiations by first accepting and then setting limits on this behavior thus, helping Mina to self-regulate just as a mother teaches her infant (Beebe & Steele, 2013). Mentalization and RF played a significant role, initially in my attuning physically to Mina (Bevington et al., 2012), and eventually in my verbal wondering about her baby talk. But mentalization and RF also occurred through artmaking. Though Mina was verbally regressed, she excelled in symbolic representation. I would wonder what her pictures were about and, thus, began to help give meaning to her actions. In this way, art therapy and the open space of the art studio were a perfect match for this young girl who could express herself by making things and, as a trained dancer, moving her body in relation to me a new attachment figure in her life.

Mina's creation of "monsters" was particularly ingenious as she could take a broken pen and turn it into another character who could tell part of her story. In a family where there had been significant losses, Mina carried the heavy burden of her parents' grief. She turned everything from soda cans to empty iPhone boxes into characters that went home in her backpack encouraging her mother's despair that she would become a hoarder. She gave them names, assigned them personalities, and held funerals for them. In this way, she appeared to be using them as both attachment objects that linked her home life to her progress in the studio, as well as a way to work through feelings she could never fully explore verbally. Additionally, they seemed objects of identification that allowed her to recreate herself as not just "destructive" and helped her to move developmentally into the age-appropriate identity-seeking of middle adolescence (Steinberg, 2014). Her later behavior, typical of adolescence, showed an embodied sense of shifting identity with changing hair color and sexual experimentation. The safety to just "be" and throw herself down on the studio tables seemed to indicate a holding container (Dosmantes, 1992) she could trust. Her final act of creating a discreet area within which she could retreat speaks to a more differentiated self that no longer had the primitive need to consume the space or my awareness. She appeared to use my empathic holding (Dosmantes, 1992) to retreat into calm self-reflection and regulation as evidenced by her allowing me to help her out of a spiral of self-harm. It was a privilege to witness and accompany her over many years as she occupied and used space within the art therapy studio to experience a broadened sense of self and her abilities.

Carey: Depression and Selective Mutism in Middle Adolescence

Carey was a 14-year-old selectively mute boy with a stocky build and bright blue eyes, who created weapons out of wood as a way to ward off any threat I might present to his fragile identity. He was white, of Northern European descent, and from a middle-class family. His mother breastfed each of her three boys until they were four years old and then turned her attention to the next infant. The four-year-old toddler, Carey, her middle child did not react well to abandonment and stopped talking. When challenged to express himself at 14 years of age in art therapy, he had difficulty forming words and seemed more comfortable expressing himself visually. When he did speak, his language was stilted and he was resistant to talking. Carey had been seen by an art therapist as a toddler. He had been prone to tantrums and playing with feces. His parents described how his older brother Jason, four years older, would speak for him to get his needs met. As a teenager, Carey's parents felt he wasn't trying hard enough in school and was too wrapped up in computer games. Their main concern was that he had no interior life because he would not talk to them and had trouble articulating thoughts. After his first art therapist, he worked with a drama therapist for many years. Prior to his work with me, this drama therapist and Carey were at an impasse because Carey would not speak.

Intake Session

Carey presented to me as shut down with flat affect, a constricted body, and little eye contact. He was, however, willing to draw and I engaged him in several art therapy assessment tools (Kramer Assessment; Kramer & Scheur, 1983; Human Figure; Hardin & Peterson,

1997; Bird's Nest Drawing; Kaiser & Deaver, 2009) to determine ego strengths, coping mechanisms, and his relationship with his family. His drawings showed a young man with considerable visual skills that did not carry over to work in paint or clay. This seemed to indicate a disparity between cognitive and emotional development. His first pencil drawings were of knights wearing highly detailed armor perhaps indicating a need for protection from the world (Figure 2.9). Assessments related to family indicated support, but a lack of personal space or agency. His mother described their home as small with little privacy and the boys all sharing a room. His clay and paint works were simple and depicted machine-like objects that seemed to show a need for distance from difficult, perhaps primitive emotions. I was able to assure his parents that Carey did indeed have a rich interior life, but one that was well guarded.

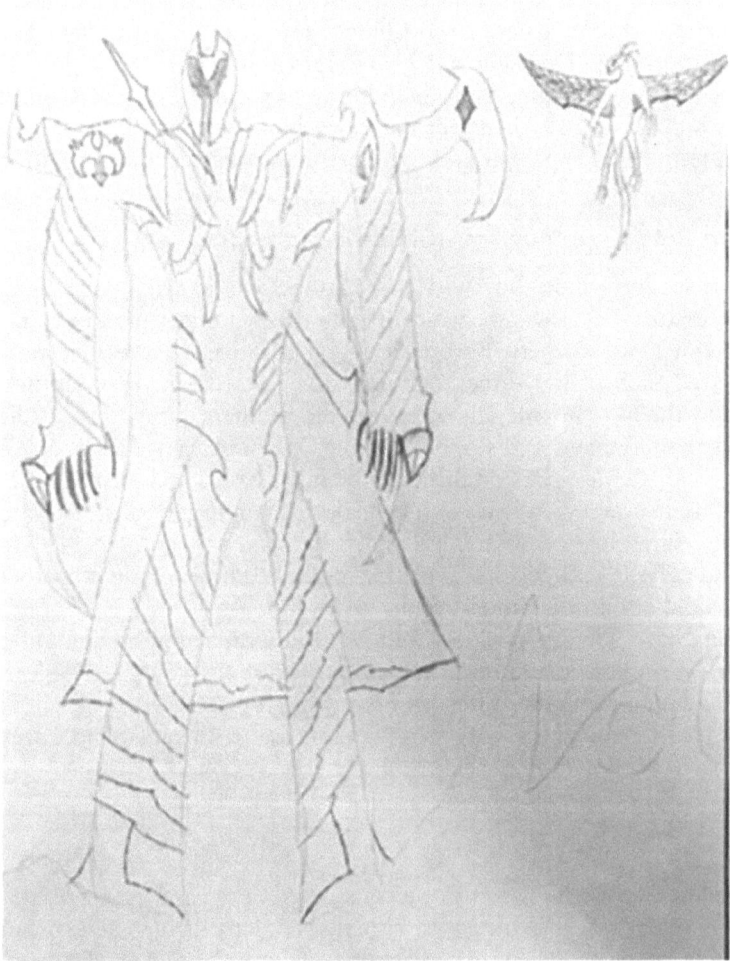

Figure 2.9 Carey's Armored Knight

Early Sessions

When I asked Carey about his previous therapist, problems in school, or life at home, he shrugged and said, "I don't know". It seemed easier for him to discuss his drawings – an imaginary world of knights, dragons, and robots. When questioned about his work, it took him several minutes to formulate a response and I learned to wait. When I said, "I know it's difficult for you to find words and it can take time for you to answer. I'm okay with that", Carey seemed to relax and tolerate my questions. He then seemed eager for sessions so he could make new drawings that I would ask him about. Over the course of three weeks, the knights became less armored and a human face appeared.

Carey's mother Sue brought him to therapy once a week without fail. Sue and his ten-year-old brother John always waited in the reception area. After the session, she would ask Carey about it, offering him little privacy. Parallel work occurred with his parents once a month, mostly with Sue, as his father Dan worked full time. Both she and Dan shared family histories of alcoholism and mental illness. Sue revealed anger and depression. She was quick in both her movements and her judgments about others, especially her husband and sons. She seemed to focus a lot of anger on Carey whom she saw as purposely underachieving. She described him as reminding her of a sibling who was mentally ill and it seemed difficult for her to have any empathy toward him. She also expressed dissatisfaction having given up her own career to raise three boys in a tiny home without privacy. She was, however, devoted to volunteering at school and church, almost to the exclusion of her own needs. When Sue and Dan were both present in sessions, he let her do the talking and described Carey as being a lot like himself.

Rupture, Distance, and the Slow Process of Repair

After two months of art therapy, I suggested to Sue that Carey might have a language disorder. She was resistant to this idea because they had just paid for John to be tested and were adjusting to his diagnosis on the autism spectrum. I suggested we could return to the idea at another point and not mention it to Carey, but she did so anyway. When he came into therapy the following week, he made no eye contact and turned his whole body away from me with arms folded. He drew a picture of swords that day (Figure 2.10) and I commented at the end of the session that perhaps he was angry at me for speaking to his mother about him.

In our next parent session, Sue confirmed that she had told him that I thought he had a language disorder and said he had denied having anything of the sort. Thus, began a six-month period during which Carey withdrew from me and began making weapons and eventually swords out of balsa wood. All of these I observed and commented on. He seemed to have begun defining the therapeutic space in a way that was useful to him, which included defining his relationship with me.

Over the course of that year, I began to see a pattern. Initially, sword-making involved aggressive action with a knife followed by sandpaper to refine the object. During this process, he spoke to himself as if defining his idea. Though I stayed close by to ensure he didn't get hurt and even vocalized concern at times, he maintained a safe distance from me across the two large tables in my studio. My laptop computer was set up between us playing his Spotify list and creating both a physical and an aural barrier – a space within the therapy space. It became a ritual for him to ask my permission to turn it on. Of necessity, he began

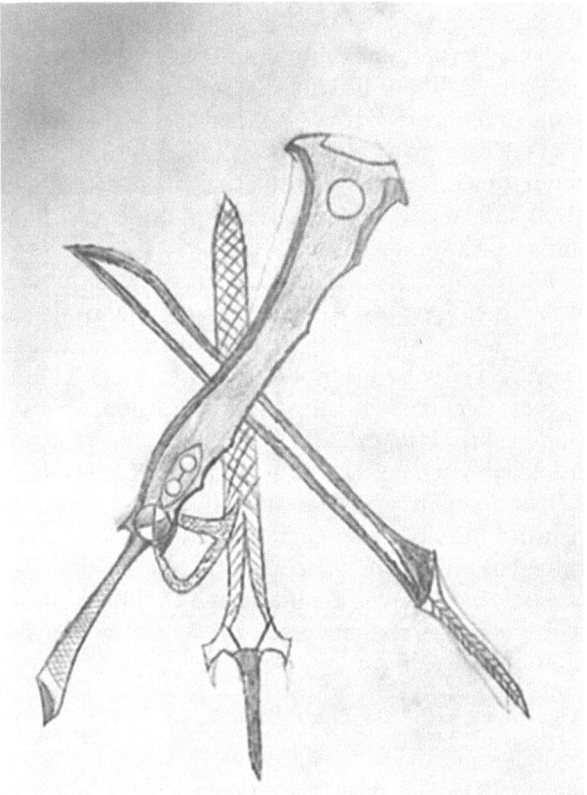

Figure 2.10 Carey's Weapons

to rely on me for various tools and supplies as well, which caused him to engage verbally. Then he would withdraw across the room again. However, his physical comfort with moving about my studio and experimenting with materials grew over time. I confined my comments to the aesthetic enjoyment of the weapons he crafted and his increasing skills. If I made any comments about their meaning or his occasional wielding of them, as if a character in one of his video games, Carey would shut down and become once more mechanical and emotionally flat.

I noticed too, that after his mother had come in for a session, his body language would be constricted and he would not make eye contact. I began to wonder aloud if her visits made him angry. Eventually, Carey acknowledged this and began wanting to know what we said about him. I was happy to share. Over time his body positioning in the session seemed to turn in my direction. His verbalizations seemed more intended to draw me in (e.g., "I wonder how I should do this?"). He also seemed more able to tolerate my comments about his work and my questions about their meaning.

Later Sessions

Over nine months, Carey made a lot of progress, but his attendance decreased to twice a month because of sports and volunteer work. Every time he came in, I had to work to re-establish the delicate thread that connected us. Sue had prioritized other activities over therapy and seemed threatened by his developing attachment to me. Dan, however, had increased his involvement with Carey because of the woodworking and facilitated the use of his basement workshop. Both parents remained concerned about his computer video game consumption and his mediocre grades. I revisited the idea of having him tested and this time they agreed.

I presented the idea of testing to Carey as a way to "learn how you learn", which appealed to him and seemed to take pressure off his relationship with his parents who considered him lazy. Testing revealed that Carey did not have a language disorder and was in fact superior in some aspects of cognition. This greatly increased his self-esteem. He did, however, have executive functioning deficits which affected attention and organization. Over the next year, his mother devoted herself to helping him with organizational strategies, his psychiatrist prescribed a stimulant for Attention Deficit Disorder and attendance in art therapy became consistent as Carey's grades steadily began to improve.

That fall, Carey discovered I had masks on my supply shelf. He seemed ready to begin not only looking at his own identity but revealing it to me. He painted a series of masks and canvases, which seemed clear self-representations. Parallel to these symbols came the ability to describe his work in more emotional terms. One abstract image of a purple face he labeled as "ambiguous", which I pointed out was a perfect description of how many people his age might feel. Another image from that period showed an emerging self in the form of a rising dragon like a phoenix (Figure 2.11).

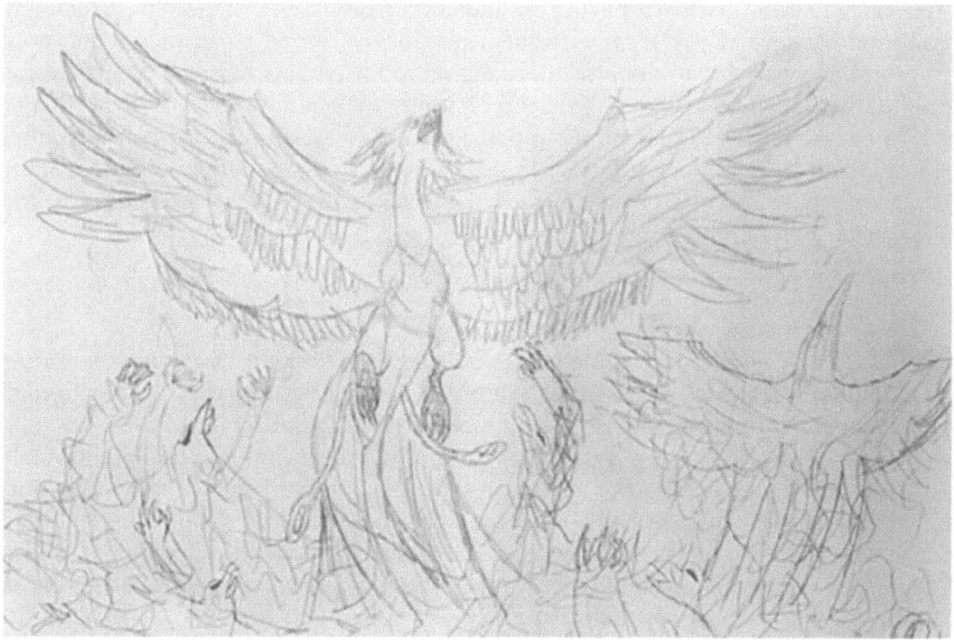

Figure 2.11 Carey's Rising Dragon

Growing Trust and Proximity

Over the course of his 16th year, Carey continued to invite me into his world, told me about his favorite Anime shows, and began planning comic-con costumes. These activities involved my sitting side by side with him at the computer rather than on the other side of the table. He confided that computers were his safe space despite battles at home with his parents about their use. In the studio, I allowed him to use my computer and he became more comfortable sharing his concerns verbally. Two projects from this period seemed to symbolize the intimacy that had grown in our therapeutic dyad. Carey created a dragon's egg out of Styrofoam and relied on me to supply thumbtacks to make its scales. He also sought my help in creating an armored wrist cuff as part of a costume and this required close contact as I applied plaster gauze to his arm.

Outcomes

During his 17th year, Carey confided that he liked a girl. This became apparent through an image of a heart surrounded by question marks. We explored the possibilities of being accepted or rejected, or being just friends and how he might feel about each. When Carey was rejected, he declined to discuss it and instead launched into an elaborate scheme to build his own computer over the summer. His parents did not agree and doubted he would ever leave home and apply to college. I proposed family therapy and Carey agreed. Over the course of three or four sessions, he was able to express pent-up rage at his parents and they were able to communicate their frustrations with him. Both parties negotiated compromises around computer use and impending college applications. In his senior year, Carey appeared more verbal, open, and positive as he sought my advice about college choices.

At this time, he also disclosed having an addiction to online pornography, which had been going on for several years. He attributed his positive mood to an online anti-porn support group. He was able to disclose his addiction to his parents during a family session in which he was articulate and able to defend himself. Our relationship, however, became strained, as he also defended his online support group over actual therapy. Not long after that, Carey asked to terminate with me. In a parting session, the family appeared more related. Carey was 18, on the threshold of leaving home, and no longer needed me to feel connected to his own family.

Discussion

Carey could be described as an adolescent who had experienced misattuned parenting from early childhood (Steele et al., 2015). As a result, his abilities for reflective functioning and interpersonal relating were compromised as were his academic abilities and emotional expressiveness. This made Carey a depressed, socially anxious, angry, and emotionally delayed youth (Dil et al., 2016). His addiction to both computers and subsequently pornography fits well with Gurian's (2017) pattern of male anhedonia. Art therapy seemed a perfect match for his developmental stage as an adolescent who lacked language and needed the physical space and symbolic language of art to communicate his complex interior world. Carey's use of the art therapy space was particularly moving as he initially used not just images of armored knights but also the physical length of my art tables and the aural shield of Spotify music to keep me at a distance. With his mother's intrusive anger towards him, it made sense that he should defend himself against me. My use of gentle speculative language with Carey about his art images and his inability to speak quickly seemed to provide reflective functioning (Steele et al., 2015) as well as the narcissistic mirroring (Dil et al., 2016) he missed as a toddler. This mirroring through observation and titrated verbal reflection continued through his year of weapon-making and culminated in the revelation of his being tested and revealing intellectual strengths. Carey's evolution as documented through his artwork went from a depersonalized and armored knight with a tiny dragon (Figure 2.9) over its shoulder to a rising, wild dragon headed into the sky (Figure 2.11) as if freed from the shackles of depression and anxiety. He appeared to use objects created in my presence to define his identity and to develop his own voice.

Conclusions

Both Mina and Carey appeared to benefit from the unique space offered by an art therapy studio setting. This studio provided an attachment perspective where their particular developmental needs could be acted out, mirrored, and explored through the use of movement, symbol making, and, most importantly, distance and proximity seeking. In the ultimate goal of achieving selfhood and independence through their adolescence, these two developing young adults appeared to use an active creation of space within the space of the art therapy studio, that supported their needs and search for meaning about themselves in relation to the other. Art therapists can pay close attention to strivings for distance or proximity within this age group to help their adolescent clients articulate confusing feelings that can arise when maturation pushes them toward adulthood.

NEGOTIATING GRIEF WITHIN CULTURES

DIXIE MOORE

Setting

My open studio model offers both individual and group sessions. I also see clients at a grief center and sometimes those clients switch to my private practice. Many materials are available for clients. Media is selected according to the client's needs upon arrival. I provide a variety of 2D and 3D media choices and guide clients accordingly. Some clients work with me in the studio for years.

Approaches

I am an art therapist as well as a certified trauma specialist, so I incorporate neuroscience and creative arts (visual art and dance) in my sessions along with yoga therapy. I am trained in Eye Movement Desensitization and Reprocessing (EMDR; Shapiro, 2014), Somatic Experiencing (Levine, 2010), Polyvagal Theory (Porges, 2011), and Internal Family Systems (IFS; Schwartz, 1995).

I work with all ages. Some of my clients are four years old and some are 59. The majority I see are young adults. What I have observed is that trauma affects all of us the same, no matter what developmental stage. Essentially our bodies keep track of each event because it becomes a physiological experience. It is important to understand that grief and trauma treatment can be supported by specialized trauma approaches for transformation and healing. From a perspective of trauma integration, I aspire to work addressing the physical, mental, and emotional responses. I agree with the tenet that the physical and mental bodies are not separate, but instead are viewed as one.

Safety is my primary target when working with new clients. My next goal is to help them understand neuroplasticity and how it can work for them instead of against them. By using a three-tier approach, bottom-up, top-down and horizontal, clients become aware and develop life skills.

Once clients feel safe to be in their body, I start with bottom-up techniques where we work through the body and begin to deactivate the amygdala (fear center) and regulate the insula (interoception; Porges, 2011). Incorporating a polyvagal-informed approach helps clients feel safe. I teach them how to map and befriend their autonomic nervous system. This bottom-up approach takes anywhere from six months to a year depending on the level of trauma and grief the client has experienced. Media choice plays a big role in my sessions. Although I practice an open studio model, I guide my clients to possible media that can better inform them where they may be experiencing grief and trauma in their bodies that day. I combine both the Expressive Therapies Continuum (ETC; Hinz, 2019) with the Polyvagal Theory allowing for clients to experience the present moment. If I see a client may need a deeper dive into another trauma-informed approach, I refer them to other clinicians that are certified in specific trauma therapies.

Client

Jean-Marie's heritage is Houma (Indigenous) and Cajun. It is important to note, South Louisiana has a unique cultural identity. We are made up of a combination of Louisiana Creole, Cajun, West African and Indigenous. Cajun and Louisiana Creole have their own distinct French languages. For example, Louisiana Creole language is different from Haitian Creole. And we come in all skin colors depending on how much Indigenous (N8V) and/ or West African ethnicity is in our bloodline. We have several Indigenous nations in South Louisiana that others have never heard of or been educated about in the United States.

I first started seeing Jean-Marie at age 12 after one of her parents died from cancer. The cancer illness was long and began when Jean-Marie was only five years old. She was experiencing hyperarousal, panic attacks, disordered eating, and was cutting. At one point prior to our work together, Jean-Marie had been admitted to Children's Hospital for attempting suicide. The living parent was desperate for help and was referred to me by a colleague who knew I would have a cultural connection to the family. Jean-Marie is the only child and disconnected from cousins that live here because of the living parent's *uncomfortableness* with their culture and religious practices. The living parent was raised evangelical, but the deceased parent's family practices both Catholicism & Indigenous Spirituality traditions. Religious trauma and cultural trauma were evident during the first intake with parent and client. The living parent was clearly grieving and suffering from generational trauma of their own.

Intake Session

The living parent is from a rural town in central Louisiana and disconnected from the culture in South Louisiana. The living parent is Cajun French but disconnected from their roots because they were raised in a conservative evangelical home. The parent that died was an artist and cultural bearer and deeply connected to their Houma and Cajun cultural identity. The living parent was grieving and felt isolated and alone. The parent ended communication with their own family 12 years ago. Jean-Marie was guarded during our initial session, likely due to her sensitivity and protectiveness of the living parent's separation from family.

Jean-Marie was seeing a psychiatrist at Children's Hospital when we first started services. The client was prescribed anti-anxiety medication after her hospitalization. The initial diagnosis was Adjustment Disorder. Jean-Marie spent two years in cognitive-behavioral therapy before starting with me.

Early Sessions

Non-Art Therapy Assessments

I first administered the Trauma Screening Questionnaire (TSQ; Brewin et al., 2002), a dissociation scale survey to which Jean-Maire scored high. I staggered the following assessments to follow up on the findings of the TSQ. I used the Trauma Checklist Assessment (Elliot & Briere, 1992), the Adverse Childhood Experiences (ACEs; Felitti et al., 1998), and a Body Perception Questionnaire Awareness (Porges, 1993).

Art Therapy Assessments

To assess Jean-Marie's stress levels and coping skills, I administered the Draw a Person in the Rain (Willis et al., 2010). During the second session, I administered a modified Bird's Nest Sculpture assessment with the living parent to help understand family roles and attachment between the parent and Jean-Marie. (I created this from the original Bird's Nest Drawing Assessment; Kaiser & Deaver, 2009).

Treatment Plan

To address the findings of the assessments, we created a treatment plan including long-term goals and short-term objectives. The long-term goals included development of: regulation skills that would help Jean-Marie move through heightened autonomic nervous system responses instead of getting stuck in fight or flight; achieve anchoring tools based on Polyvagal Theory to map her autonomic nervous system through yoga, art, and breathwork; and recognize triggers and apply coping strategies before the nervous system collapses into dangerous or life-threatening responses.

The short-term objectives included learning to anchor through a series of vagus nerve reset exercises; participating in a trauma-sensitive group for additional support; keeping an altered-book feelings journal to help identify emotions while keeping them contained until the next session; and developing an emotional vocabulary through art and movement.

Sessions

I began seeing Jean-Marie eight years ago, beginning at the end of middle school through high school and now into college. We initially did weekly sessions for four years, then twice a month for a year and a half. When the pandemic hit, some regression occurred. I saw her weekly until 2021. After that we saw each other every three to four weeks. The parent did make Jean-Marie's healing path very difficult at times. The parent never went to any type of therapy for their own healing. Sadly, this is true for many of my younger clients. I always express to parents or guardians that a dysregulated adult cannot regulate a child. Fortunately, through specific trauma modalities like EMDR, Polyvagal Theory, and IFS, we were able to create a clear path of integrating the trauma for Jean-Marie. She developed tools rooted in the neurobiology of trauma, which were essential to move through this healing journey.

When a person experiences a trauma that significantly interrupts and disconnects them from daily living, they usually stay at that developmental age of when the incident occurred (van der Kolk, 2015). Trauma disconnects the psyche from community and interrupts time and memory. This was quite evident in Jean-Marie's artwork as well. The deceased parent got sick when Jean-Marie was five. There were quite a few sessions when I met Jean-Marie's five-year-old part through artwork and baby talk. I incorporated the IFS approach and we identified that part and began to integrate it and any other parts that would arise through our journey. Unfortunately, we do not have a lot of earlier artwork where we saw the five-year-old part emerge. Jean-Marie would make scribble drawings in some sessions and talked about drawings with the deceased parent in a baby voice. It was an interesting process to observe and see how the IFS trauma approach worked well with art therapy.

I rarely use directives because I want my clients to develop trust in their own nervous system. I simply guide them to media that I believe will help them *see* themselves. What I have noticed in my 10 years of doing grief and trauma work is that clients first gravitate to clay. Usually, during the first three to four sessions, they work with clay and most of them make vessels. I find this fascinating because art therapy is essentially about metaphors and is symbolic in practice. Both clients and I see these vessels as support. The vessels became something to hold their grief, their fears, and their disconnection from others. Jean-Marie gravitated to collage, then oil pastels, and onto watercolors, eventually using all three depending on her emotional affect that day.

When we switched to online sessions, Jean-Marie was able to create a space in the house that was private and safe. Because her deceased parent was an artist, Jean-Marie used her parent's watercolors and pastels, which created a special connection. Since the pandemic, Jean-Marie hasn't always seen me in-person but when she does, she continues to select pastels and watercolors.

Jean-Marie's healing journey has been remarkable to witness. Our earlier sessions were difficult but with both individual and group work she began to trust herself and find her voice. We reflected on her past artwork and had some profound *ah-ha* moments, including addressing generational trauma and historical grief and loss by creating altars for birthdays and death days. We explored the nuanced relationship between the living parent and Jean-Marie through layering of collages. At one point she repetitively cut the heads from pictures of people in magazines and collaged them on various objects. She then began to feel comfortable in her body (Figure 2.12). Jean-Marie no longer would get stuck in her head with intrusive thoughts that would interrupt the process.

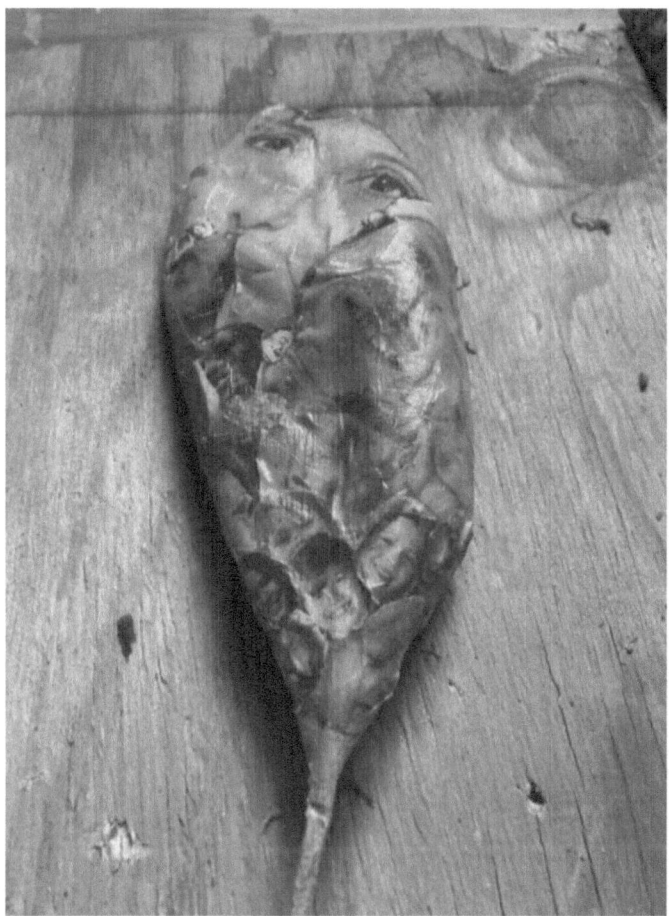

Figure 2.12 Collage on Leaf with only Heads Jean-Marie Cut Out

Jean-Marie's later work also emphasized collage. One directive asked her to map her nervous system and experience her internal surveillance system. Its intent was to explore her internal compass meditating in each direction. The process started with movement, then art-making, and later included yoga and breathwork (Figure 2.13).

Outcomes and Conclusions

I continued to see Jean-Marie through her university experience. Jean-Marie has grown emotionally and spiritually and has discovered who she is and embraces her current identity.

She is currently an undergraduate student majoring in a creative arts therapy profession. We are doing a deeper dive into the Polyvagal Theory and learning how she can incorporate her modality into this theory. Jean-Marie's living parent has not changed much but

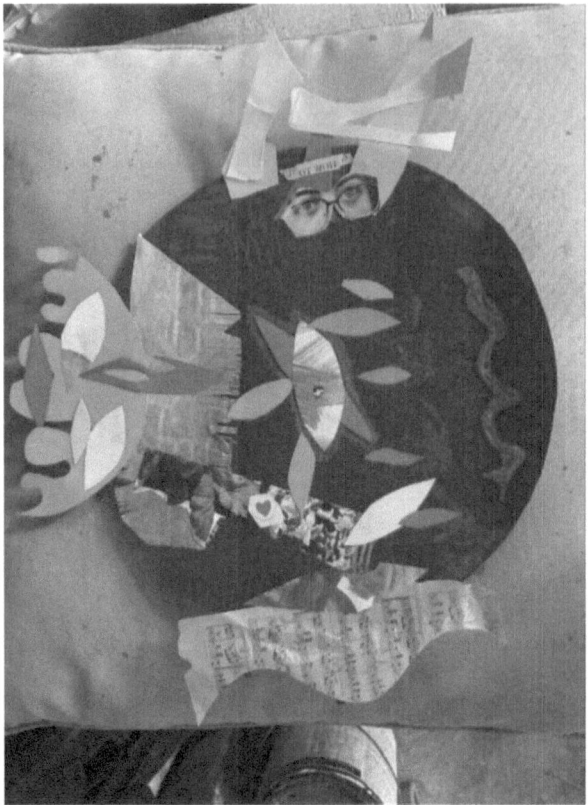

Figure 2.13 Jean-Marie's Latest Collage

Jean-Marie has progressed. She stopped taking medication for anxiety four years ago. She had been able to move through many difficult situations and stay regulated. As a senior in the fall she lived in an apartment with two other roommates.

FINDING AN ADOLESCENT IDENTITY

JILL MCNUTT

Setting

Maranda was in the seventh grade when she was referred to an in-school counseling center where I served as an art therapist. Maranda was the oldest of two children and lived with her single mother in an apartment within walking distance from the school. The organization I worked for was a non-profit agency specializing in runaway, homeless, and at-risk youth. My office in this middle school was a small room toward the center of a long hallway. I imagined it used to be a walk-in closet. There was enough room for a small desk with a chair and another chair positioned at the side of the desk. The room had no windows and between classes when there were students in the hallways changing classes, there was no privacy in coming and going.

The guidance counselor who referred Maranda indicated that she had low self-esteem, depression, and anxiety. In tandem with intake and assessment protocols, I typically use response art. My response art about Maranda usually contained a shadowed young girl with a hovering rain cloud. Each time she walked into my office, the air felt chilly, and she typically had her hoodie pulled closed revealing not much more than her nose. She immediately sat in the chair with her shoulders curled in and neck pushed toward her knees. She responded when I spoke, but in a very soft voice that I had to lean into to hear. We completed the intake paperwork including demographics, her thoughts on why she was referred, limits of confidentiality, and a consent for treatment form. Her reasoning for why she was referred was that she wanted to fit in.

Approaches

Adolescence development, as framed by Erikson's psychosocial stages, centers around the conflict of identity versus role confusion. This stage navigates the complexities of identity formation and strives to establish a cohesive idea of self (Erikson, 1967). During these years, adolescents shift priorities from parents and adults to peers (Riley, 1999). Because of the lessening trust of adults during this developmental stage, it is important during the teen years to provide consistent positive regard and non-judgmental support to clients consistent with Roger's person-centered care (Rogers, 1951). Offering adolescents the supportive atmosphere to explore identities, emotions, and concerns provides validation. Goals of therapeutic interventions during these years include resolution of identity conflicts and fostering a healthy sense of self.

First Session

At this point in my career, I used collage as an introductory meeting exercise. Collage is an accessible medium that reduces initial hesitation in art-making, and provides valuable discussion points around the broad range of images that often make up the artwork (Raffaelli & Hartzell, 2016). I invited Maranda to skim through a small pile of magazines and tear out images that spoke to her. She selected four images: one was a flock of geese, two were flowers, and the fourth was an image of the Taj Mahal in India. I then asked her if she had reflections on any of these images, to which she shrugged her shoulders. I offered her paper, scissors, and a glue stick to create a collage. She quickly glued the four images in random order onto the white paper in such a way that none were touching the others. After she finished her collage, I again asked for any reflections. She offered a slight smile but remained silent.

I was not long out of my education at this point and had a minor in art history, so I often shared points about artists and artworks that I thought were pertinent to my clients. In Maranda's case, I pointed out that the Taj Mahal was a mausoleum and was built as an elaborate tomb to honor the life of a beloved wife. Maranda looked up at me with a surprised look, curled back up into her chair, and looked at the collage. When the class bell rang, she collected the collage, folded it in half, stuffed it into her backpack, and left the office.

Maranda did not return to her session the next week or the week after. The guidance counselor contacted me the following week. She explained that Maranda told her about our session and her anxiety was heightened when I explained the meaning of the Taj Mahal. In my wanting to spread knowledge and break the silent space, I had inadvertently turned away my client. This was a real-life lesson in keeping sessions focused on the client and the client's art. The counselor was able to convince Maranda to come back to art therapy.

Maranda came for her scheduled session the next week. Her 13th birthday was the day after our second meeting. She had no plans for a party and thought that her mother would plan dinner for her and her little brother with a cake. Maranda was concerned about the cake as it wasn't "acceptable for girls to eat sweets". Maranda was, at best, 5'2" tall and had a small frame. She made efforts to fit in by doing what she assumed other girls in school were doing. She had difficulty naming things that she liked and instead reported what was popular.

As our relationship grew, it became apparent that Maranda based her own value on what she thought her peers would want in a friend. She was building her image to please others. This was consistent with Bandura's (1979) social learning theory that posits that individuals learn behaviors through observation, modeling, and reinforcement. I was concerned that Maranda may be influenced by external factors including peers and media. I wanted to explore her self-perception in relationship to her peers. During one of our earlier sessions, I asked Maranda to draw a series of trees, at least five. Using colored markers, she drew five trees of varying styles, shapes, and sizes (Figure 2.14). There was an evergreen tree on a hill drawn closest to the viewer, three trees were on a central hill, and a weeping willow existed on a hill toward the background of the image. I asked Maranda, "If you were a tree,

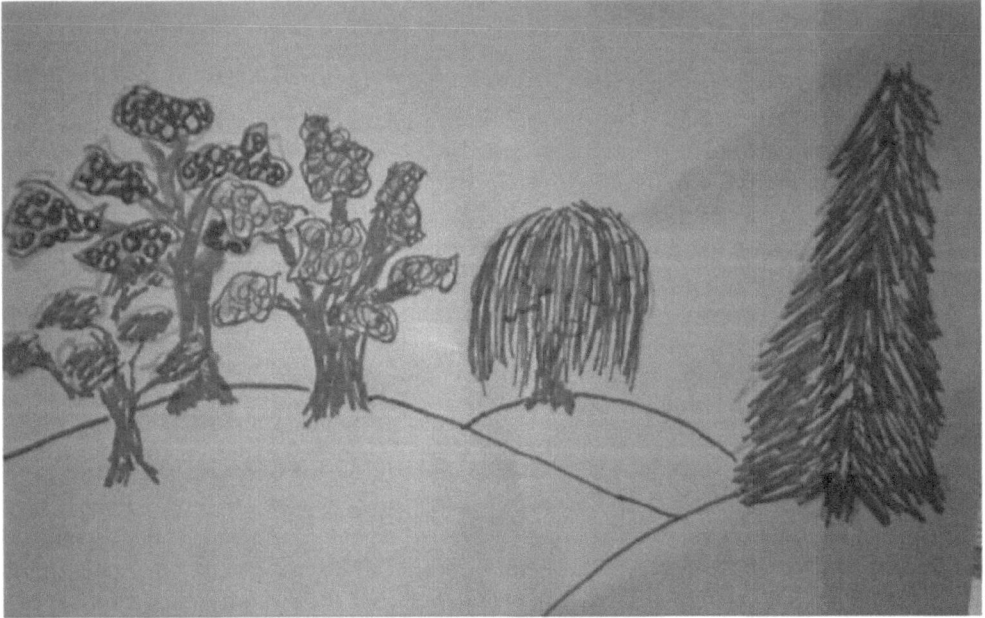

Figure 2.14 Five Trees

what kind of a tree would you be?" She responded by pointing to the tree on the left. This tree echoes the two trees closest to it, with a smaller size and muted color.

Self-esteem and self-efficacy became the central goals of our work together. I wanted Maranda to explore her own interests and trust herself enough to make decisions for her own well-being. I encouraged her to work with masks and self-portraits but she declined both. Maranda did agree to decorate an old wooden cigar box. She used magazine collage and found objects, placing things that she kept to herself on the inside and things she showed to others on the outside. Maranda was very closed about sharing what was being put inside the box or why things were put there. The outside of the box displayed images from playing on the beach, silk flowers, and a few images of women's clothing. Maranda found a string of artificial pearls in the found objects box and quickly tied the pearls around the box in such a way as to inhibit anyone, including me, from opening it to find out what was inside. She opted to leave the box with me when she was finished. Each week when Maranda came into the office she saw her box placed on the top shelf, just where she wanted it.

Maranda never told me what was in the box but she did offer a soft smile when she remembered. Our discussions started to include things that Maranda enjoyed. She liked sharing makeup with her mother, painting her nails, which were often worn and chipped, and wearing plastic jewelry. She liked going to popular movies and playing video games, although her mother would not allow her to have a video game at home. As Maranda started to open up I asked her if she would create another collage that represented her past, her present, and her future. The directions I provided asked her to sort through magazines, cutting out images that would fit in her past, present, and future. Maranda sorted them as she removed the images. The past images included a family, images of comfort at home like fireplaces and holiday decorations. The present displayed advertisements for makeup and popular hair styles, and the future depicted a barber's chair, hair brushes, scissors, and a hair dryer. It also had a sitting area with chairs and a coffee table with magazines to view or read.

As Maranda discussed the collage, she remembered how much she enjoyed painting nails and brushing the hair of her mother and her friends. She started talking about make-up and soon after I noticed she was wearing subtle make-up to school. Maranda was starting to develop her own identity (Erikson, 1967) and expressed a desire to become a hair and make-up specialist after high school.

Maranda still cared what her friends thought, but at this point in time, she started to understand that she could also have plans and desires of her own. I brought out the tree drawing she had done earlier in our relationship (Figure 2.14). I initiated a discussion about how she might be represented in more than one of the trees, and invited her to re-create any of them. Maranda agreed and re-created the weeping willow tree (Figure 2.15). She carefully designed the ground on which the tree stood and started to develop the descending leaf structures. As she drew the leaves that would hang in front of the tree, she depicted them as brushed aside, not unlike a stylist might move the hair to expose a person's face. After she exposed the trunk of the tree, she created an elaborate structure in the bark that included a face. This image reminded me of the first time I met her with her hoodie pulled tight with her face hidden.

Maranda came to my office only one time after completing the second drawing of the weeping willow. When she arrived, she was smiling, and shared with me that her mother was going to take her to get her hair cut at the cosmetology school nearby. She was excited to talk to the student who would be cutting her hair for credit. Maranda was enthusiastic about her mother's approval of her current occupational choice in life. After that session, I

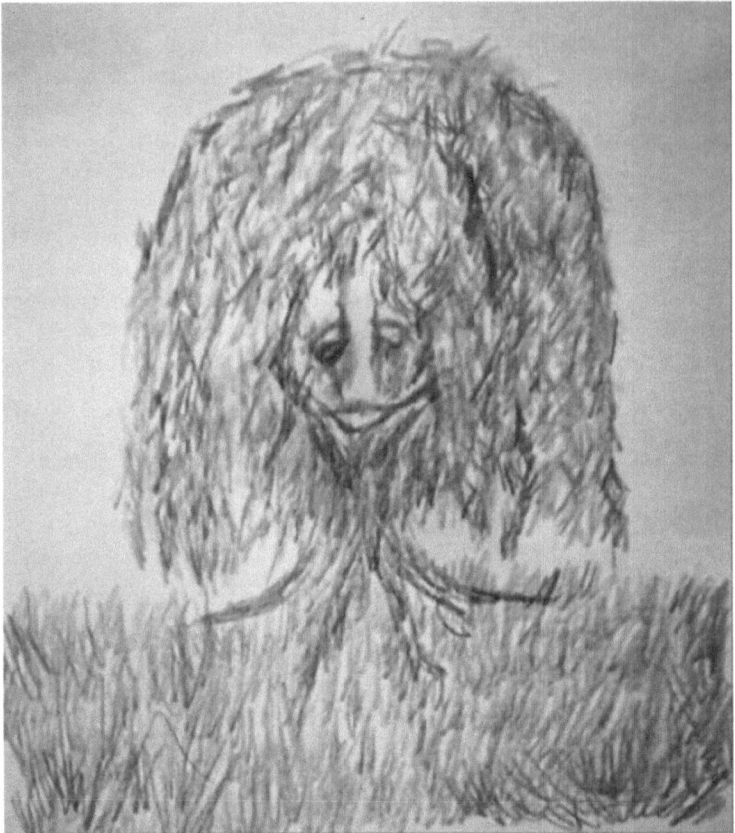

Figure 2.15 Weeping Willow

would only see her in the halls where she would offer me a smile and an acknowldgement using a four-finger wave.

Outcomes

Through our time together, after I pointed out the intention of the Taj Mahal, I provided Maranda a space where she could explore her own identity and express herself without judgment. Providing witness to her process allowed her to find an identity that was not tied to pleasing others. Maranda found a way to serve others and maintain herself. Maranda's artworks helped her to explore herself and her relationships with friends. The box gave her permission to keep some of herself private and to outwardly express what she chose. The collages gave her the opportunity to select images that related to what she wanted and differentiate between her own desires and those of the popular girls at school. Finally, the trees offered her the knowledge that she could carry identities that would fit into various places in the world and interface with various people. Maranda learned that she could be part of a group and still move into a career path of her own choosing.

Conclusion

Throughout art therapy sessions, Maranda exercised creative self-expression, she received positive regard from me and eventually from herself. Throughout her sessions, Maranda developed an appreciation for her own plans and desires and learned a realistic approach to hanging out with friends. She learned that she could be of service to people without having to become the object of their desires. Art therapy helped Maranda to foster a sense of empowerment and self-worth.

FINDING A PLACE TO BELONG IN THE FOSTER SYSTEM

TAMI JOE DELISLE

Art Therapy has a unique power to reach people in the midst of their pain without criticism, condemnation, or judgment, when approached from a perspective of communication. Often clients are referred to our community-based studio to address unspeakable wounds. We are often encouraged to help our clients make art about the difficult experiences as a means to talk through trauma and find a new way out of their impairing memories. However, I find it much more common that we need to allow art to help our clients feel safe enough to trust us.

Community-Based Setting

When Tony was referred to our rural community-based art therapy studio as a part of the county Department of Health and Human Services Comprehensive Community Services, he was at risk of being expelled from school and losing his sixth foster home placement. Early sessions proved difficult as he was unwilling to let his current guardian, a great aunt, leave the space. His wounds were deep and his anger raw. He was easily triggered beyond an effective use of words. He had been left at professional offices in the past and his caregivers never returned. Fear was intense. With his fear came a need for safety. We chose to meet in a small room with dimmable lights. A couch was surrounded by images of trees painted on the wall and a net of soft animals. Across the room, a counter held space for art-making with supplies stored in a cabinet with a few games and sensory toys. This space was comforting and calm to begin to build a felt sense of safety. This space also protected the safety of all people in the room. After a time, Tony would gradually allow his aunt to move further from the room, based on his level of tolerance and trust in me as his art therapist.

A variety of art materials were offered in an attempt to help him move beyond his need for explicit control. First, markers and tracing sheets were used to recreate a favorite video game character, but his need for perfection sabotaged expression. Oil pastel scratch art gave him control without a defined image, but he continued to crave rigidity. His perfectionism worked to almost cloak his authenticity in creating art images. His most utilized media was the classroom-sized chalkboard on the wall. He would diagram a story and quickly erase it, washing the board clean with a spray bottle. While it was reported to me that he liked art, he refused most attempts at creative self-expression.

Tony presented an interesting constellation of challenges for therapy. He arrived with a significant history of trauma. His mother did not survive a car accident caused by his father driving impaired. His father was then deported, leaving Tony in the care of his maternal grandmother at age two. It was later discovered that the grandmother suffered from extreme mental health issues. When it was discovered that she was physically abusing him and neglecting his most basic needs, he was removed to foster care. After years of attachment wounds, he became easily overwhelmed by this new foster family. He coped with the skills modeled to him and acted out with aggression toward the new family. As small children and pets were endangered by his uncontrollable meltdowns, he was again abandoned to a transitional residential center where he was sexually assaulted by a male caregiver. After an extensive search and even more transitions of caregivers, it was found that he most desired to be with his maternal great-grandmother. She was deemed too old to be named guardian, but a great aunt agreed to be his guardian as long as significant support was provided to her. At the age of 12, he was finally diagnosed on the autism spectrum (299.0), in addition to reactive attachment disorder (313.89) and oppositional defiant disorder (313.81; APA, 2022). At 13, Tony came to me feeling broken, worthless, and filled with despair. He feared being left again and fought to manipulate any situation that felt uncertain. He was referred to me to address aggression and anxiety. He needed someone to help him understand that he was loved and safe, even if his brain worked differently.

Tony's fear of abandonment and of men caused difficulties in finding enough support for the family. A male mentor was assigned to help him work on social skills and to provide him with a positive male influence in his life, but he refused his help. He agreed to work with a female mentor who could take him out in the community and practice things like ordering fast food. After he finally became comfortable with her, she had to leave her position. He took great offense and would not agree to another mentor in that role. When his prescribing doctor retired, he was assigned to her replacement, who was male. Instead, a female doctor had to be found to prevent his aggressive meltdowns.

As a part of the comprehensive services, his aunt worked with a parent coach to help her become trauma informed and to apply trauma reactions to her parenting (Levine, 1997). The parent coach helped his aunt see the damage caused by her threatening to send him away if he did not improve his behavior (Perry, 2009). He could not change his reactions without first feeling safe and secure. She needed to avoid shame and blame in order to help this change begin.

Early Sessions

Due to Tony's fear of being left by his aunt, he often demanded that she remain in the session with him. He wanted me to teach her how to help him. Too often, his session started with her reporting all the difficulties of the week. The shame and blame were deep. Together, we were often able to talk through behaviors by first discovering the antecedents, what triggered his overwhelming behavior. His aunt offered her heart and home to this boy, but she had no understanding of autism or the effects of developmental trauma. This led to Tony often believing that she needed therapy more than he did because they were both learning from these conversations. He was referred for individual therapy, and she needed a break from his difficult behaviors. Eventually, he agreed to be left, but "I am not talking to you", was a common refrain and "you can't make me" his body language. I began to introduce him to brainspotting, a form of focused mindfulness connected in theory to Eye Movement Desensitization and Reprocessing (EMDR; Grand, 2013). Brainspotting is a therapy that utilizes eye positions to connect to and process unprocessed trauma or emotional pain in the brain. When clients can hold eye positions connected to specific memories, the brain can release the heavy emotions connected to them. This allowed him space to not engage directly with words (Grand, 2013).

A routine developed. The aunt reported the week's events prior to Tony entering the therapy space. Then, when he entered the session, I asked how he was coping with what happened during the previous week and he would stare at a space, eventually closing his eyes until his time was up. I recognized his need to be seen and I began to draw him. According to Alter-Muri (2010) and Carr (2014) creating portraits of clients provides a form of witness. Never saying a word about the drawings, never asking, and never confronting him. He needed to be seen. I knew the power of the art to hold the space to help him develop a felt sense of safety (Fish, 2012).

Eventually, he felt safe enough to change our routine. Unfortunately, there was inconsistency in his weekly attendance that was overtly experienced. He would be feeling safe and begin to address his anxiety, ask questions for himself, and then he would miss a session. When he returned for therapy, he would again refuse to be seen alone. Subsequent family conflicts would be addressed with his aunt in the room, and the next few sessions he would be unwilling to talk, and I would draw. He would finally admit to feeling better after these sessions. The following sessions he would come prepared with a conflict he needed to understand. Sometimes he would come with a memory he could not make sense of, and we would talk through his perceptions and explore other perspectives. Then he would miss another session and we would be back to needing to build the trust again.

It was very difficult to maintain unconditional positive regard. It was difficult to document or even feel that I was supporting him at all during months of not talking. I reminded myself of the encouragement given to me in my first internship placement with another boy on the spectrum: "He stayed in the room with you, that is success". Tony's aunt would share that she was so appreciative: "Whatever you are doing is working!". I did not feel that I was doing anything. I checked in with his case manager who reported that the school was reporting fewer disruptive behaviors. Tony told his aunt, "She draws me, it is really cool!". The school reported that they knew when he missed a session because he would be very calm after his regular sessions. I reminded myself that healing does not come from the therapist, we just hold the tools for it. We hold the space for healing in attunement.

Later Sessions

A transition occurred for Tony that felt very sudden after years of the above pattern. After significant consideration, and consultation, both with Tony's aunt and case manager, it was decided to ask him to consider allowing an art therapy intern to shadow his sessions. My intern was a male and Tony was very anxious. Their first meeting lasted just a few moments. At the end of the session, Tony volunteered to allow the intern to stay, as long as he did not say anything. The next week was critical. Tony attended an appointment at the county building. While there, his aunt utilized the vending machine and was surprised to discover a dollar coin as part of her change. This excited Tony, he wanted to see the coin, he wanted to have the coin, and could not let go of his desire. His attempt to obtain the coin from his aunt resulted in her arm being badly hurt. Security was called and they encouraged her to file a report to protect her from future accusations. She chose not to, but assured the team that she would have to next time.

The incident became the focus of his next therapy session with me. Tony's aunt took time in our pre-session meeting to describe what happened from her perspective before she left.

He became very upset because he could not understand what he did that was so wrong: "I wanted to see it! Why wouldn't she give it to me?". The effect autism had on his perception made understanding other people's reactions impossible. We engaged in a discussion of personal space, appropriate touch, ownership, and verbal communication, and nothing seemed to help him find the clarity he sought. I decided to switch tactics. "Let's act this out", I said, "I will be your aunt and you be you. Show me what happened". We reenacted the scene from his perspective, then tried to practice a "better way". He still struggled. Then I asked for permission to be him and he could be his aunt. This would give him the opportunity to see the scene from his aunt's perspective. After giggling about being a "girl", he agreed. Only with the witness of the intern was it safe to act out his behaviors, push against his comfort level, and maintain personal safety. With a loud voice, erratic movements, and physical force, I demanded the coin from him. He responded with the same shock and awe as his aunt, without her fear. He looked at me with revelation: "Is that what I do? Is that why people are afraid of me?". He was given a glimpse into his own behaviors that he could not see at the moment. He became a witness to his own impulsive behaviors and understood the words so many adults had been saying to him. The intern and I left the session exhausted, but relieved.

We prepared ourselves for the next session, expecting backlash and an overwhelming nature, stemming from the previous session with a boy who rarely talked, and was sullen and frustrated. Instead, we were met with a boy excited about the art he made in school and a desire to recreate his marker drawing in color. The next five weeks were spent on a marker drawing of a lake surrounded by trees while Tony asked a multitude of questions about his behavior, how to draw better, and how to help people not be afraid of him. His awareness of self opened a window to his personality.

From that point forward, Tony wanted to talk about his limited perception. He came prepared each week with questions, situations, and concerns, "You explain things to me", he said, as he continued to seek out art-making that allowed him control. He began to ask me how to make things look like he wanted them to look. He had begun to develop a "shared will to create" (Vick, 2000, p. 216). For example, when drawing trees I explained it was not wrong because his trees were too close to include branches, they could overlap and intermix with each other. Alongside looking to advance his art-making skills, he also began to ask how he could advance his social skills and get to know people in a "non-stalking" way. Through humor and telling jokes back and forth with each other, Tony began to understand the practice of taking turns in conversation, talking and then giving space for the return. He learned to wait for a response, even if he did not fully listen to it. He began seeking opportunities to interact directly with the intern, the male presence who was not supposed to say anything.

Outcomes

A meeting was held to update treatment goals as his behavior at home and therapy had improved dramatically. His aunt opened the meeting with an observation that things were going very well at home, and she really enjoyed spending time with him now, "except for that hiccup". I asked her nearly under my breath to describe the hiccup, if she felt it was safe. Often, difficult conversations about overwhelming behaviors caused Tony to feel ashamed and he would shut down or become angry and defensive. This time, however, he was able to interrupt the conversation and share his experience:

I felt angry and did what you always tell me. Anger is energy that needs to move and work, so I tried to shovel the snow, but it didn't feel like enough. Everything in life just made me feel angry and I couldn't hold it anymore, so I started to bang the shovel on the snowplow, because it was strong. I didn't want to hurt the car or anyone else, but banging felt good in my body and helped the anger go out…until I broke the shovel and my teacher yelled at me. I did what I was supposed to do to get rid of the anger and it got me in trouble. But I agree, I need to pay for the shovel.

He talked so much in this meeting that we had trouble getting a word in edgewise. He had spent years refusing to accept a mentor in his life for fear of abandonment again and in this session, he requested that the male intern be his new mentor. "I want him. He is funny. I need a 'man wing' to teach me how to be a good date". Fortunately, the administrations involved worked together to make this happen for him. Tony was able to meet with his mentor in his "independent living" program at school and in the community where they continue to build his relationships, social skills, and independence. Art therapy can again focus on processing and understanding the trauma he experienced.

Concluding Statements

Art therapy is often experienced as assisting a client to make art to understand their experiences and emotional reactions. The wonder of art therapy is much deeper than the visual marks made on the paper, it is the emotional marks made in relationships with his aunt, me as the art therapist, men, the school, social services, and the community-at-large. Tony came to me hurt and terrified of relationships. He had deep work to begin to trust me, and accept me. My willingness to engage in radical acceptance of who he was in that time and space and wait patiently for him without judgment, shame, fear, or expectation allowed him to mindfully sit with the things he could not speak about. He found he could trust that I would carry whatever load he had to unburden. He had believed that all these terrible things happened to him because he was unworthy of compassion and I sat with him with an energy of light and love to fill in the empty spaces. This was never expressed in words, but his actions became as gentle as his heart. Instead of approaching the world fearfully, he became able to explore it with curiosity.

There are libraries of books that can describe directives to suggest to our clients, and just as many assessments. The most critically important directive is for the therapist to attune completely to the client to assess where the most connection is needed and let it grow from there. Many sessions I felt I was doing nothing; but feelings deceive us. I was attuned to him, I held the space, I allowed his healing to happen naturally (Moon, 1999). Current research shows that the brain has the capacity to heal itself (Corrigan et al., 2015). When we, as therapists, provide a space of warmth and safety, the brain can rewire positive pathways of thought. Every drawing of him sitting on my couch taught him what it felt like to be cared for and safe (Ickes et al., 2012). He had my undivided attention, even if he asked for nothing.

References

Alter-Muri, S. A. (2010). Beyond the face: Art therapy and self-portraiture. *The Arts in Psychotherapy*, *34*, 331–339.

American Psychiatric Association Publishing. (2022). *Diagnostic and statistical manual of mental disorders: Dsm-5-Tr*. American Psychiatric Association.

Bandura, A. (1979). *Social learning theory*. Prentice Hall.

Barresi, M., & Gilbert, S. (2023). *Developmental biology* (13th ed.). Oxford University Press.

Beebe, B., Lachmann, F. M., Markese, S., Buck, K. A., Bahrick, L. E., Chen, H., & Jaffe, J. (2012). On the origins of disorganized attachment and internal working models: Paper II. An empirical microanalysis of 4-month mother-infant interaction. *Psychoanalytic Dialogues, 22*(3), 352–374.

Beebe, B., & Steele, M. (2013). How does microanalysis of mother–infant communication inform maternal sensitivity and infant attachment? *Attachment & Human Development, 15*(5–6), 583–602.

Bevington, D., Fuggle, P., Fonagy, P., Target, M., & Asen, E. (2012). Adolescent mentalization-based integrative therapy (AMBIT) – a new integrated approach to working with some of the most hard-to-reach adolescents with severe complex mental health needs. *Association for Child and Adolescent Mental Health*. e-Article.

Bowen, M. (1982). *Family therapy in clinical practice*. Jason Aronson Publishers.

Bowlby, J. (1969). *Attachment and loss* (volume 1). Basic Books.

Branje, S., de Moor, E. L., Spitzer, J., & Becht, A. I. (2021). Dynamics of identity development in adolescence: A decade in review. *Journal of Research in Adolescence, 31*(4), 908–927.

Brewin, C. R., Rose, S., Andrews, B., Green, J., Tata, P., McEvedy, C., Turner, S., & Foa, E. B. (2002). Brief screening instrument for post traumatic stress disorder. *British Journal of Psychiatry, 181*, 158–162.

Bronfenbrenner, U. (1979). *The ecology of human development*. Harvard University Press.

Carlson, E. A., Egeland, B., & Sroufe, L. A. (2009). A prospective investigation of the development of borderline personality symptoms. *Development and Psychopathology, 21*(4), 1311–1334.

Carr, S. (2014). Revisioning self-identity: The role of portraits, neuroscience and the art therapist's third hand. *International Journal of Therapy, 19*(2), 54–70.

Corrigan, F., Grand, D., & Raju, R. (2015). Brainspotting: Sustained attention, spinothalamic tracts, thalamocortical processing, and the healing of adaptive orientation truncated by traumatic experience. *Medical Hypotheses, 84*, 384–394.

Davis, N. (2019). *Therapeutic stories to heal and empower*. Therapeutic Stories, Nancy Davis, PhD.

Dil, L., Dekker, J., Van, R., & Schalkwijk, F. (2016). A short-term psychodynamic supportive psychotherapy for adolescents with depressive disorders: A new approach. *Journal of Infant, Child, and Adolescent Psychotherapy, 15*(2), 84–94.

Dosmantes, I. (1992). Spatial patterns associated with the separation-individuation process in adult long-term psychodynamic movement therapy. *The Arts in Psychotherapy, 19*, 3–11.

Dunne, P. (2016). *The narrative therapist and the arts* (2nd ed.). Possibilities Press.

Elliot & Briere. (1992). Trauma Symptom Checklist. PTSD: National Center for PTSD.

Erikson, E. (1967). *Identity and the life cycle*. W.W. Norton & Company.

Felitti, V. J., Anda, R. F., Nordenberg, D., Williamson, D. F., Spitz, A. M., Edwards, V., Koss, M. P., & Marks, J. S. (1998). Relationship of child abuse and household dysfunction to many of the leading causes of death in adults: The Adverse Childhood Experiences (ACE) study. *American Journal of Preventative Medicine, 14*(4), 245–258.

Fish, B. (2012). Response art: The art of the art therapist. *Art Therapy: Journal of the American Art Therapy Association, 29*(3), 138–143.

Fowler, J. W. (1995). *Stages of faith: The psychology of human development and the quest for meaning*. HarperSanFrancisco.

Gantt, L., & Tabone, C. (1997). *Formal elements art therapy scale*. Gargoyle Press.

Gilligan, C. (1982). *In a different voice*. Harvard University Press.

Grand, D. (2013). *Brainspotting: The revolutionary new therapy for rapid and effective change*. Sounds True.

Gurian, M. (2017). *Saving our sons: A new path for raising healthy and resilient boys*. Gurian Institute Press.

Hardin, L., & Peterson, M. E. (1997). *Children in distress: A guide for screening children's art*. Norton.

Hilbuch, A., Snir, S., Regev, D., & Orkibi, H. (2016). The role of art materials in the transferential relationship: Art psychotherapists' perspective. *The Arts in Psychotherapy*, 49, 19–26.

Hinz, L. D. (2019). *Expressive therapies continuum: A framework for using art in therapy* (2nd ed.). Routledge.

Ickes, W., Park, A., & Johnson, A. (2012). Linking identity status to strength of self: Theory and validation. *Self and Identity*, 11, 531–544.

Johnson, D. R. (1989). On the therapeutic action of the creative arts therapies: A psychodynamic model. *The Arts in Psychotherapy*, 25(2), 85–99.

Jordan, J. (2017). *Relational-cultural therapist (Theories of psychotherapy series)* (2nd ed.). American Psychological Association.

Kaiser, D. H., & Deaver, S. (2009). Assessing attachment with the Bird's Nest Drawing: A review of the research. *Art Therapy*, 26(1), 26–33.

Kohlberg, L. (1969). Stage and sequence: The cognitive-developmental approach to socialization. In D. A. Goslin (Ed.). *Handbook of socialization* (pp. 347–480). Ran McNally.

Kramer, E., & Scheur, J. (1983). An art therapy evaluation for children. *American Journal of Art Therapy*, 23, 3–12.

Levine, P. (1997). *Waking the tiger*. North Atlantic Books.

Levine, P. (2010). *In an unspoken voice*. North Atlantic Press.

Lyons-Ruth, K., Bureau, J., Holmes, B., Easterbrooks, A., & Brooks, N. H. (2013). Borderline symptoms and suicidality/self-injury in late adolescence: Prospectively observed relationship correlates in infancy and childhood. *Psychiatry Research*, 206(2–3), 273–281.

Maynard, B. R., Farina, A., Dell, N. A., & Kelly, M. S. (2019). Effects of trauma-informed approaches in schools: A systemic review. *Campbell Systematic Reviews*, 15(1–2), e1018.

Moon, B. (1999). The tears make me paint: The role of responsive art making in adolescent art therapy. *Art Therapy: Journal of the American Art Therapy Association*, 16(2), 78–82.

Peleikis, D. E., Fredriksen, M., & Faraone, S. V. (2022). Childhood trauma in adults with ADHD is associated with comorbid anxiety disorders and functional impairment. *Nordic Journal of Psychiatry*, 76(4), 272–279.

Perry, B. (2009). Examining child maltreatment through a neurodevelopmental lens: Clinical applications of the neurosequential model of therapeutics. *Journal of Loss and Trauma*, 14(4), 240–255.

Piaget, J., & Inhelder, B. (1969). *The psychology of a child*. Routledge.

Pollak, S. D., Cameras, L. A., & Cole, P. M. (2019). Progress in understanding the emergence of human emotion. *Developmental Psychology*, 55(9), 1801–1811.

Porges, S. W. (1993). *Body perception questionnaire*. Laboratory of Developmental Assessment: University of Maryland.

Porges, S. W. (2011). *The polyvagal theory: Neurophysiological foundation of emotions, attachment, communication, and self-regulation*. W.W. Norton & Company.

Raffaelli, T., & Hartzell, E. (2016). A comparison of adults' responses to collage versus drawing in an initial art-making session. *Art Therapy: Journal of the American Art Therapy Association*, 33(1), 21–26.

Riley, S. (1999). *Contemporary art therapy with adolescents*. Jessica Kingsley.

Robbins, A. (1987). *The artist as therapist*. Human Sciences Press, Inc.

Rogers, C. (1951). *Client-centered therapy: Its current practice, implications, and theory*. Houghton-Mifflin.

Schwartz, R. C. (1995). *Internal family systems therapy*. Guildford Press.

Schore, A. N. (2000). Attachment and regulation of the right brain. *Attachment & Human Development*, 2, 22–41.

Shapiro, F. (2014). The role of eye movement desensitization and reprocessing (EMDR) therapy in medicine: Addressing the psychological and physical symptoms stemming from adverse life experiences. *The Permanente Journal*, 18(1), 71–77.

Shore, A. (2013). *The practitioner's guide to child art therapy: Fostering creativity and relational growth.* Routledge.

Spiegel, L. (2017). *Internal family systems therapy with children.* Routledge/Taylor & Francis Group.

Steele, M., Bate, J., Nikitiades, A., & Buhl-Nielsen, B. (2015). Attachment in adolescence and borderline personality disorder. *Journal of Infant, Child, and Adolescent Psychotherapy, 14,* 16–32.

Steinberg, L. (2014). *Age of opportunity.* Houghton Mifflin Harcourt.

Tinnin, L., & Gantt, L. (2013). *The instinctual trauma response dual-brain dynamics: A guide for trauma therapy.* Gargoyle Press.

van der Kolk, B. (2015). *The body keeps the score: Brain, mind, and body in the healing of trauma.* Penguin Books.

Vick, R. M. (2000). Creative dialogue: A shared will to create. *Art Therapy: Journal of the American Art Therapy Association, 17*(3), 216–219.

Willis, L. R., Joy, S. P., & Kaiser, D. H. (2010). Draw-a-person-in-the-rain as an assessment of stress and coping resources. *The Arts in Psychotherapy, 37*(3), 233–239.

Winner, E. (2000). The origins and ends of giftedness. *American Psychologist, 55*(1), 159–169.

Winnicott, D. W. (1971). *Playing and reality.* Basic Books.

Chapter 3

Late Adolescence and Young Adulthood

Individuals in this age group may develop a more critical awareness of societal issues, engaging in cultural discussions, advocacy, or activism contributing to cultural change and social progress.

Introduction

Developmental Markers

Chapter 3 focuses on the developmental period between 15 and 26. During these years, individuals undergo profound changes across various domains that shape identities, relationships, and perspectives. Adolescence is a transitional period between childhood and adulthood, marked by significant physical, psychological, and social changes.

Hall described adolescence as a period of "storm and stress", emphasizing the tumultuous nature of this stage. He highlighted biological changes as the primary driver for psychological upheaval during adolescence (Hall, 2004). Erikson's psychosocial theory proposes that individuals during these years face psychosocial crises of *identity versus role confusion*, and *intimacy versus isolation*. Erikson emphasized the importance of forming a coherent sense of self and personal identity during the earlier years and the ability for love and affection toward another as individuals move toward adulthood (Erikson, 1967). Anna Freud explored adolescent development through the lens of psychoanalytic theory, focusing on ego development and the navigation of conflicts between autonomy and attachment to parents (Freud, 1958). From Piaget's work, the shift from concrete operational thinking to formal operational thinking is prominent during these years. Piaget emphasized the development of abstract thinking and the ability to reason hypothetically (Piaget & Inhelder, 1969). Kohlberg's theory of moral development suggests these years show progress through stages of moral reasoning, transitioning from obedience and punishment to principles and abstract ethical values (Kohlberg, 1969).

Physical maturation and peak physical fitness occur during these years as well as the apex of brain development (Baressi & Gilbert, 2023). Siegel (2012) emphasizes brain maturation during these years, particularly in the prefrontal cortex responsible for higher-order functions like decision-making, impulse control, and social cognition, with expanded areas related to decision making and impulse control. Transitioning into adulthood and building personal identities are particularly influenced by social interactions that shape abilities to form

DOI: 10.4324/9781003324805-4

meaningful relationships, demonstrate empathy, and regulate emotions within relationships (Siegel, 2012).

These years highlight significant cultural development as well (Arnett, 2016). Familial heritage, traditions, and values help shape an individual's sense of belonging and identity. Exposure to diverse cultures through travel, media, and education plays a substantial role in development as young adults become more culturally aware, fostering cultural competence and adaptivity (Arnett, 2016). Individuals in this age group may develop a more critical awareness of societal issues, engaging in cultural discussions, advocacy, or activism contributing to cultural change and social progress.

Artistic expression is instrumental for personal growth and self-discovery (Lowenfeld & Brittain, 1987). Although many emerging adults stop engaging in artistic endeavors, individuals may continue to explore artistic mediums to express their evolving thoughts, emotions, and experiences. Life experiences, including social interactions, relationships, and personal growth, can fuel creative expression.

Setbacks

Individuals in late adolescence and early adulthood can encounter various setbacks that may impede their developmental trajectory. Vulnerability to mental health disorders such as depression, anxiety, and substance use and abuse is opened up through academic pressures, peer relationships, and overall life transitions (APA, 2022). The intensity of exploration of personal and professional identities might lead to confusion or difficulties in career paths and life goals (Erikson, 1967). Ambiguity and stress related to this identity development may also cause emotional distress and uncertainty.

Academic stress and financial stability are key functions of human development in Western cultures. Academic pressures in high school and potential higher education or vocational training can lead to performance anxiety or academic underachievement (Luthar & Barkin, 2012). Financial stressors including negotiating salaries, student loan debt, unemployment, challenges transitioning to financial independence, and down payments for major purchases including homes often fall during these years (Siegfried & Wuttke, 2021).

In establishing autonomy from parents, relationships may result in conflict that leads to emotional distress, and challenges in forming and maintaining intimate relationships and coping with breakups can impact emotional well-being and self-esteem (Arnett, 2016). These years also mark an increase in risk-taking behaviors, including substance use and unsafe sexual practices that can have negative impacts on physical and mental health.

Case Studies

The case studies in this chapter include clients ranging from 15 to 26 years of age. The art therapy settings included a university counseling center, hospital out-patient programs, a job center, and private practices. One client was seen in a juvenile detention center. Sessions included individual, group, open-studio, and family therapy. The duration of services ranged between three weeks to ten months.

The presenting problems for these clients were varied. Major issues included traumatic events including early life abandonment, past and recent physical and sexual abuse, a recent death of a parent, and struggles with sexual identity. Anxiety and depression, problems relating to others, hospitalizations, incarceration, and the inability to live independently or maintain employment brought other clients to therapy.

Primary approaches used with art therapy expanded with this age group and included developmental theories in the areas of psychosocial stages (Erikson, 1967); morality (Kohlberg, 1969), cognition (Piaget & Inhelder, 1969), and hierarchy of needs (Maslow, 1970), as well as Objects Relations Theory (Robbins, 1987), Psychoanalytic Theory (Johnson, 1989), and Attachment Theory (Bowlby, 1969). Approaches to therapy included: art therapy in a forensic setting (Gussak & Cohen-Libman, 2001), Acceptance and Commitment Therapy (Harris, 2019), Dialectical Behavioral Therapy (Linehan, 2015), Racial and Cultural Identity Developmental Therapy (Sue et al., 2022), Relational Therapy (Borden, 2009), Cognitive Behavioral Therapy (Beck, 2020), Person-Centered Therapy (Rogers, 1979), Strength-based Therapy (Berberian & Davis, 2020), Psychoanalytic Therapy (Jordan, 2017), Narrative Therapy (Dunne, 2016), along with the Expressive Therapies Continuum (ETC, Hinz, 2019) and Motivational Interviewing (Miller & Rose, 2009).

The clients in this chapter had complex and diverse challenges. Some of the challenges included a toxic relationship with a parent, childhood religious practices conflicting with their current beliefs, grieving the loss of childhood innocence caused by physical and sexual abuse at the hands of trusted family and friends, and grieving the loss of a loving parent. Because of these experiences, many of the clients were traumatized and developed inadequate coping skills.

Clients in this chapter needed to understand what happened to them in childhood and early adolescence was in the past and cannot be erased, but at the same time, they needed to realize those experiences did not define them now. They needed to feel safe enough to assimilate their past experiences and stop those experiences from detouring their mastery of current developmental goals. Those goals included choosing their friends and social groups, career decisions, and religious and moral beliefs. Major goals for these clients were developing autonomy and experiencing what it was like to live on their own without parental guidance and accepting responsibility and accountability for their decisions.

This age range of clients can also be resistant to therapy and show negative transference toward their therapists. Strategies used to break this reluctance to engage in a therapeutic alliance included therapists acknowledging clients' past, focusing on their future, and accepting the clients where they were developmentally. Other therapists presented themselves as co-therapists with the client and as co-creators with artmaking or as fellow artists co-creating alongside their client (Teoli, 2021), versus presenting themselves as an authority figure or an expert on what the client needed from therapy.

Promoting autonomy was a major therapy goal for this age group. Using a non-directed approach and letting clients select the materials and subject matter for their artwork and topics for discussion related to the work allowed them to practice autonomy in sessions. Some clients were encouraged to use journals to write reflections about themselves as well as for artmaking outside of art therapy sessions. This activity gave clients another way to act independently by taking some responsibility for their therapy. One author described the journals as a transitional object from art therapy to the clients' real-life setting.

Another issue clients dealt with in this chapter included meeting their career goals or making career choices other than the ones someone else selected for them. One client learned her medical condition may not be a barrier to future career choices. Another found his career in music, not as his parents' preference for him to be a music teacher, but in organizing a band of his own. Another client completed her career goal and became a certified nursing assistant.

When clients can be free from false beliefs and poor self-images, engage in self-care, learn from past experiences and mistakes, and realize their past does not define their present, hope for their future is possible. Therapy can be education in the form of learning about oneself leading to the ability to change (Rogers, 1979). Clients in this chapter became open to new ideas for shaping their lives in the future.

ADOLESCENT IN OUTPATIENT DIALECTICAL BEHAVIORAL THERAPY PROGRAM

KARA-LEIGH HUSE

With the onset of the COVID-19 pandemic and the culture climate of social media, American adolescents and their families are continuing to reach out for mental health support. Linehan's (2015) Dialectical Behavioral Therapy (DBT) has become an established treatment for assisting these clients in managing emotions, modifying behaviors, and decreasing self-harm. The following composite case study illustrates a 15-year-old, non-binary client's journey in an art therapy group. While completing the DBT outpatient treatment program, this client specifically utilized the art therapy group to practice DBT skills, express emotions, form identity, and increase self-awareness.

Developmental Concerns

In Erikson's stages of development, he categorized adolescents as individuals working towards forming their identity in comparison to their peers and the world around them. This *Identity versus Confusion stage* (1967) is prevalent now more than ever in adolescents. The presence of social media has contributed to even greater confusion and paradoxical clarity of identity for teens. They have an even greater insight into other adolescents' lives and are constantly comparing themselves, attempting to find their identity in the world. Providing adolescents with time to be creative, without the distraction of the internet, can help them gain necessary reflection into their identity. Moon (2012) stated, "the arts are a natural language for adolescents who are grappling with the deep concerns of their existence" (p. 13).

Approaches

DBT is effective in modifying behavior and thoughts for people who self-harm or have suicidal ideation (Linehan, 2015). Skills in DBT like mindfulness, emotional regulation, distress tolerance, and interpersonal effectiveness can all be practiced in the group art therapy setting. The group art therapy setting allows for the clients to evaluate their relationships with peers, the process of art-making, and appreciation of artworks (Moon, 2012).

While integrating DBT-informed art therapy (Clark, 2017) into this group, I promoted a strengths-based, humanistic approach, often making processing comments and focusing on the clients' strengths. The goal of utilizing art therapy in congruence with DBT is to give the clients a creative space to practice DBT skills in a group setting, and express their emotions creatively. "For adolescents in need of psychotherapy, art is not a frill or a time filler, but rather, a dynamic, validating, integrating, expressive, and entirely natural and necessary activity" (Moon, 2012, p. 12). The dialectical part of DBT is understanding multiple things can be true at once. Art-making is innately dialectical (Clark, 2017). A client can deem their artwork "bad" because it doesn't look realistic. However, not all artwork is realism and perhaps they enjoyed the process of making the painting, even though they did not "like" the result. I maintained the DBT practices of non-judgmental validation and being genuine in responses.

This Intensive Outpatient Program (IOP) is a DBT-based therapeutic program aimed to support the adolescent client and family by learning skills and addressing the whole client through various therapeutic avenues. The client attended art therapy groups, yoga, drama therapy, music therapy, DBT groups, family therapy sessions, and individual therapy sessions. During the art therapy groups, the floor counselors are also in attendance to support me with any behavioral needs during the group sessions. The materials available to the clients in the art therapy groups included markers, paper, colored pencils, collage images, oil pastels, watercolor, paint, glue sticks, and scissors (sharps are counted and only given when needed).

Client

Ace is a 15-year-old, non-binary client in the IOP with diagnoses of Major Depressive Disorder, Social Anxiety Disorder, and Bipolar II Disorder, with a history of self-harm. Ace was hospitalized for a suicide attempt earlier in the year and had been in a residential program after the suicide attempt. Ace then transitioned to a Partial Hospitalization Program (PHP) before ultimately moving into IOP and participating in the art therapy group. Ace was in IOP for ten weeks and attended eight art therapy groups (twice Ace was pulled from groups for different therapy sessions or appointments). The goals of treatment included decreasing thoughts of suicide and self-harm, learning to cope with anxiety and depression, building self-esteem, and promoting identity formation.

Initial Assessment

By the time clients get to group art therapy in this IOP, they have participated in intake sessions and assessments with primary therapists, and typically attended other group formats through inpatient and PHP treatment. When new clients arrive at the art therapy group, I introduce myself, explain my pronouns, provide an introduction into the goal of art therapy, and set expectations for the members of the group.

Sessions

Ace came to the initial art therapy group with a blunt affect and did not often elaborate or respond to questions. Ace expressed enjoying drawing and typically brought a sketchbook to school and the IOP, but often looked down at the artwork and rarely made eye contact. During Ace's first art therapy group, the group was asked to draw themselves as an animal. Ace drew a "bunny" and explained that like a bunny, both of them are "neutral and quiet". Ace used colored pencils to draw a cartoon-like bunny and did not wish to elaborate on the drawing.

In the second week of the art therapy group, Ace reported feeling "unsafe, afraid, and lonely" at the beginning of the session. The clients were asked to fold a paper in half and express their "outer-self" on the outside and their "inner-self" on the inside. Wanting to make the artwork larger, Ace used another piece of paper. Ace wrote "I'm sorry" and "I'm fine" on the outside of the paper. Saying "sorry" or "I'm fine" to people was often used to avoid sharing true emotions with others. On the inside of the artwork Ace drew a hand reaching for a star and around it wrote "I want to die" and "alone forever". Ace could not identify its meaning in the drawing, and did not share these words and the image with the group.

Worried Ace would self-harm, I requested to touch base after group. When asked about the artwork, Ace commented "fine". I worried about the term hiding emotional states and with encouragement, Ace agreed to check in with the primary therapist before the day was over.

During the next art therapy group, Ace reported feeling "worried, panicky, and depressed" about an upcoming family session and the pressures of schoolwork. To promote self-awareness and mindfulness, Ace was asked to create artwork representing gratefulness and mindfulness. Ace expressed a feeling of self-pride for getting good grades in school and responded with "good" when asked to identify the feelings elicited.

Feeling outside the comfort zone during another art therapy group, Ace was able to be present and flexible and eventually enjoyed creating a collage. The group was instructed to use colored construction paper to create a collage without using scissors. Not having complete control of the shape of the torn paper while practicing a kinesthetic action of ripping the paper to release energy (Hinz, 2019) caused discomfort. However, Ace was able to utilize distress tolerance and reported feeling "peaceful" at the end of the group.

In the next few art therapy group sessions, clients were working on identity formation through directives that helped them express interests, emotions, strengths, and how they perceive themselves. Ace created an album cover that represented hobbies, and a love for drawing and video games on the computer. While engaging in conversations with peers about the best computer games or music preferences, Ace expressed confidence when discussing the group's interests. In another group, Ace also created a coat-of-arms that represented personal strengths, including empathy, compassion, determination, and creativity. During this group, Ace gave feedback to peers, often commenting on the strengths seen in others.

In Ace's last art therapy session, the group was asked to identify a tree as a self-symbol and paint it. The group was encouraged to think about strengths and what makes a tree strong. Ace started working immediately on this painting and was very focused during the session. Ace ended up painting a tree representing hope, possibility, and growth. Ace expressed a need to continue to care for this tree. An explanation of needing to "prune" away relationships that no longer serve, watering the tree with coping skills, and recognizing resilience during weather changes were among the metaphoric tools that Ace took away from these group sessions. Ace also included seeds that had fallen off the tree and were beginning to grow from the ground, representing a desire to help others grow too. Ace expressed feeling "excited, hopeful, and anxious" about discharging from the program.

Outcomes

Bruce Moon (2012) reported four phases of art therapy treatment for adolescents, "resistance phase, the imagining phase, the immersion phase, and the letting go phase" (p. 99). In the initial art therapy session, Ace was resistant to the therapeutic process despite already using art-making in daily practice by carrying around a sketchbook. Ace participated in the directives but did not make eye contact or give insight into the artwork.

During the second art therapy session the *Imaging Phase* emerged entailing the denial of disturbing feelings. Ace wrote "I want to die", displaying enough trust in the group to paint this uncomfortable feeling, but then expressed to me "I'm fine", and not wanting to confront that feeling.

In the *Immersion Phase* Ace began to practice distress tolerance in the art therapy group by connecting and owning personal emotions. In the later sessions, Ace demonstrated leadership by honestly sharing emotions and making insightful comments about artwork, relating to peers, and giving constructive feedback.

Finally, in the *Letting Go Phase*, Ace's last art therapy session was focused on the mixed emotions around discharging from a program where experience, support, and meaningful relationships were established. During discharge from IOP, Ace expressed extreme gratitude for the art therapy group, sharing that it helped process personal emotions. Tending to the tree metaphor helped Ace to reflect on personal progress and hope for the future.

TAKEN BY A STORM

MARIA RICCARDI AND GABRIELLE GINGRAS

Setting

This is the story of an adolescent boy, Storm, who enjoyed his friends and had great capacity for empathy. He longed for intimacy and connection, but stormed out of situations when overwhelmed by painful emotion. It was difficult for him to set boundaries. Storm was referred to his school art therapy program for support in emotional regulation, developing acceptance, and leaning into goal-oriented action (Shukla et al., 2022). This case study will uncover his journey through individual art therapy, where he met weekly with a school art therapist over the course of 12 months. The sessions became a place of existential conversations, where the exploration of self, emotions, and identity empowered the client to change his relationship with his own story (Nadeau-Cossette, 2012).

Approaches

Narrative therapy stems from the sociopolitical contexts related to feminism, racism, culture, and the effects of colonization (Mori & Goldbeter-Merinfeld, 2019). The connection between time and history is fundamental within this framework, and its emphasis on context and culture can help patients better understand the complexities of their identity. As White (2007) expressed, clients often begin therapy with the assumption that some aspect of their identity, or the identity of others around them, is the source of their problems. "Identities can become colonized and saturated by problem stories, and narrative therapy assists clients in exploring new ways to look at old problems, reinforcing that their problems are separate from their personal identity" (p. 27). This framework allowed Storm to rewrite and re-appropriate significant events that took place in his life.

Using the Expressive Therapies Continuum (ETC) in conjunction with this narrative approach, Storm was invited to engage in free art-making. His choice of materials and subject matter revealed his preferred level of ETC and means of approaching new situations (Hinz, 2019). Storm's interactions with the materials, the stylistic and expressive elements of his final products, and his verbal and non-verbal communication were assessed. The completed artwork offered a visible representation of Storm's therapeutic journey, reflecting progress towards his goals and changes in his perspectives over time.

The Expressive Therapies Self-Inquiry (ETSI) scale for the art therapist was used to encourage self-reflection (Riccardi, 2023). This tool helped us evaluate our own preferences and aversions which could have impacted the art-based interventions with Storm. This self-knowledge, grounded in cultural humility, was a pivotal tool for strengthening bonds with this unpredictable teenager who often stormed out of the studio.

Intake Session

Storm is a 15-year-old Caucasian teenager, the youngest of two boys living with first-generation Italian parents. His parents stressed bicultural identity and retained some cultural norms of their homeland, while creating a heavy focus on their children's academic success. Valdivia et al. (2016) underlined that second-generation immigrants can demonstrate higher levels of acculturation and parental expectations than other groups. Due to his emotional outbursts and intense pressure to succeed, Storm developed a pattern of unhealthy relationship boundaries. He had difficulty creating safe attachment, and the main coping tactic for distress that he displayed was truancy. Storm also displayed low self-esteem and negative self-talk, focusing mainly on his shortcomings and challenges.

Storm reached developmental milestones within age-appropriate limits. He enjoyed sports, computers, art-making, and movies, and attended a sports-study program at the beginning of high school. He described himself as a creative boy with interpersonal skills. At the time of his initial treatment intake at ten years old, Storm was diagnosed with Attention-Deficit/Hyperactivity Disorder (ADHD; APA, 2022), along with some oppositional behaviors. He received art therapy services in conjunction with psychoeducation, which helped him and his family create adaptive coping strategies. Storm also experienced symptoms of anxiety and depression, and demonstrated frustration over academic failures and feelings of disconnect with his community, both of which led to a vicious cycle of problematic behavior.

Halfway through the current school year, Storm became completely disinterested, disengaged, and unmotivated. He did not attempt to justify his lack of academic motivation, and did not report the causes of these shifts. Along with this scholastic impairment, he experienced distressing and intrusive thoughts in the form of reprimands from teachers and family members. Storm developed aggressive behaviors and depressive symptoms. He lacked the ability to control his overwhelming emotions. Storm often drew in class when struggling to stay attentive, and knowing he'd have an excuse to get out of class regularly, was willing to start art therapy sessions at school.

Assessment

During the initial three-session assessment, Storm was asked to choose from collage materials, lead pencils, colored pencils, crayons, markers, oil pastels, natural materials, chalk pastels, watercolors, and clay. The materials were placed before him and arranged from most resistive to most fluid. Storm chose to start out using colored pencils. The first three images that Storm created featured symbols of protection, as if he was shielding a secret (Figure 3.1). Metaphors, humor, and form distortions conveyed a strong sense of emotions and mood. He demonstrated focus as he filled the interior of outlined forms. His free drawings revealed a predominance of outlines, indicating that Storm started working from the *Perceptual* component of the ETC, which focuses on line, pattern, and form. He also reproduced images from magazines. Then, he moved to the *Symbolic* component as the image took on personal and universal meanings. Storm was externalizing his worldviews, making the stories that he had inherited from his family, friends, school, and other sources visible. He was a storyteller, which revealed a slant towards the *Cognitive* component of the ETC, and seemed to be exploring new perspectives and problem-solving abilities through his characters' voices. Finally, the bright, high-intensity of colors in the first images alluded to contained emotions and a need for expression.

The first phase of intervention focused on the perceptual component, and the cognitive and symbolic levels. Leaning into these levels where Storm had strengths allowed him to bolster his inner resources. After the assessment, the art process included direction towards the *Affective* component, exploring the emotional aspects of his experiences and tendency towards repression (Hinz, 2019). A narrative approach underscored this developmental progression, allowing Storm the reflective distance needed to explore his old stories and to experiment safely with new ones.

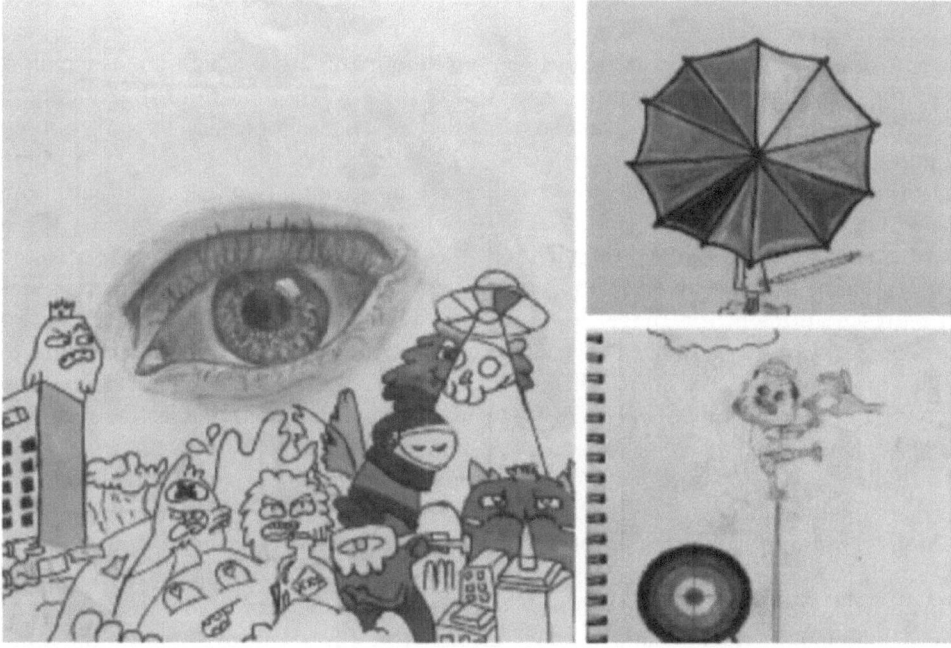

Figure 3.1 The Eye, The Umbrella, and The Dart Game

Collaborative Treatment Plan

Storm needed the space to unpack concerns around society and his identity. During the fourth and first treatment sessions, we reviewed his assessment images and discussed possible therapeutic goals with Storm. We explained that he had a unique ability for storytelling, and cultivating this skill could help him access new perspectives and better solutions. He understood that with better emotional access, he could learn to cope with challenging situations instead of running away. In his family of origin, emotions were not expressed, so Storm had learned to repress and shield them. Adolescent emotional development is marked by a gradually increasing ability to perceive, evaluate, and manage a multifaceted environment (Sharma et al., 2013). It was clear that Storm's emotional development was still maturing.

Intermediate Sessions: Movement Towards the Affective Component

As Storm became familiar with the structure of the ETC and basic material properties, he was encouraged to continue drawing to reflect on school perseverance. Storm's narratives no longer focused solely on his perceived shortcomings; they started to include a more balanced view of himself and his strengths. Throughout these sessions, Storm increased his investment in his well-being, increased his physical activity, and came regularly for art therapy.

Storm expressed discomfort when first encountering fluid mediums, but agreed to try them, even though he would not have the control that pencils allowed. This collaboration demonstrated a strengthening of the therapeutic alliance, greater vulnerability, and an important step towards emotional maturity. When he started to use more fluid media like watercolor pencils, watercolor markers, and oil pastels, he gradually added more colors to his artwork, expressing emotional cues.

The first time Storm finalized an image, he used fluid materials and high-intensity colors to cover the white space. He wrote a story to accompany his depiction of becoming a supervillain (Figure 3.2). He shared that he felt stifled by strict school rules, likening himself to the Joker from the popular *Batman* franchise. The addition of the cognitive intervention using writing allowed Storm to integrate conflicting elements, unify intellect and intuition, and generalize in new situations.

The images in Figure 3.3 were created with watercolor pastels. At times, Storm expressed frustration that he was not able to control the quality of these images. He formed a series of self-representations in the shape of waves. The addition of water into Storm's creative process identified a new need for self-compassion and self-discovery. According to Foucault (1966), individuals create themselves in a determinate manner in society, and consequently orient their lives to represent themselves in support of subjective forms of identity. Through these visual depictions of his story, Storm developed externalization skills that helped him separate his problems from his sense of self and cultivate a more positive personal identity.

Moving forward, Storm began to recognize more symbols in his art-making, using playing card suits to explore his experience of being kicked out of his first high school because of an incident. Using these suits he was able to express what he was unable to verbalize at that time (Figure 3.2). On one hand's knuckles, he wrote the word love, and on the other hand's knuckles he depicted the four suits of playing cards as symbols to name: happiness

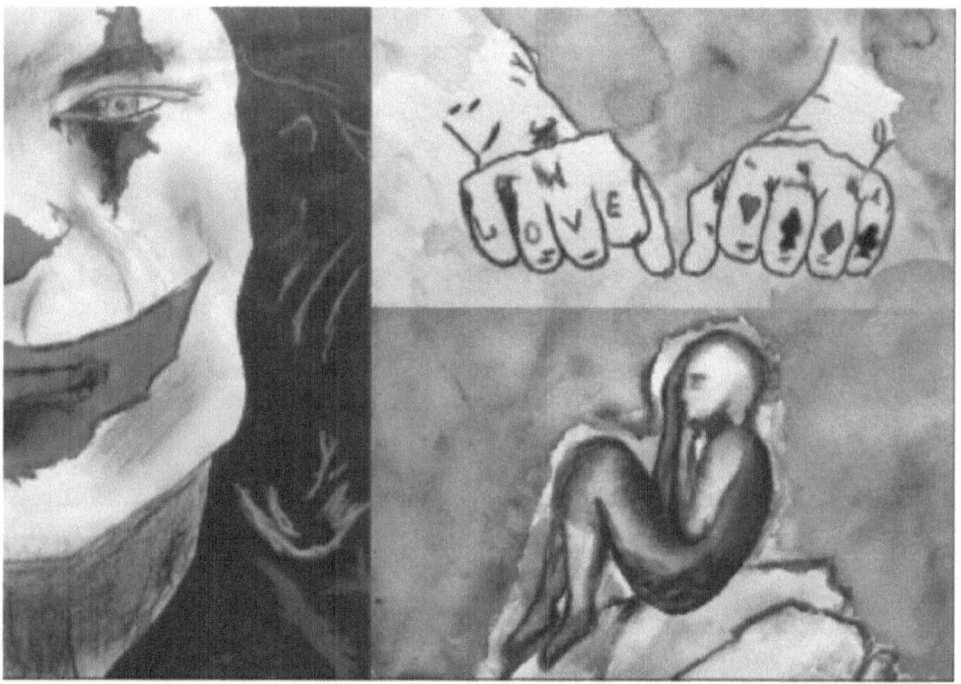

Figure 3.2 The Joker, the Deck of Cards, and Shielded

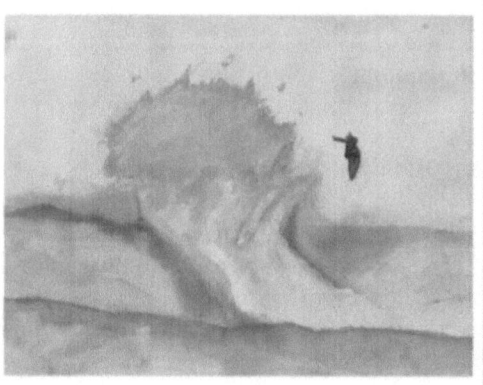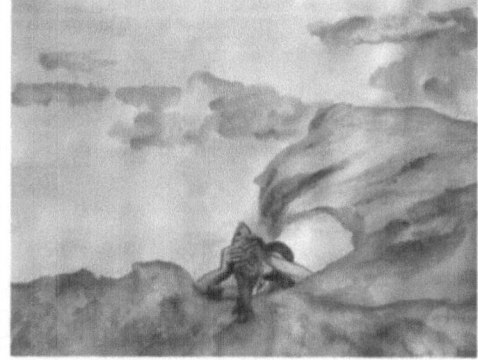

Figure 3.3 Surfer (by Storm) and Holding On (by the Art Therapist)

of being in a safe place, sadness of missing his friends, fear of not graduating, and anger of not being understood.

This was a complicated range of emotions for an adolescent to experience. He felt ashamed. He demonstrated increasing self-awareness and willingness to get help. He contemplated his habits such as daydreaming, escaping from classes, and was even considering using substances to cope with intense feelings. Research has shown evidence of a correlation between ADHD, mood, and anxiety, substance use, and personality disorders, and has demonstrated a decrease in co-occurrence with prevention and treatment (Katzman et al., 2017).

Storm was beginning to understand the growth possible through building emotional capacity, and experiencing therapeutic change. He was then encouraged to use a more sensory media, oil pastels. After completing a series of oil pastel images, Storm explained that he was scarred inside, and held onto a difficult memory (Figure 3.2). After completing the image, he indicated that he was feeling wounded. At this point in the process, Storm could describe his emotions, but not feel them. As he became familiar and comfortable with fluid materials, we encouraged him to reduce the use of forms and lines, believing this would help him evoke an emotional response. Staying close to the perceptual, cognitive, and symbolic levels of the ETC, where he was most comfortable, provided Storm with a feeling of safety while experimenting. Once he had more trust in the therapeutic process, he felt comfortable exploring new art materials and moving further towards the affective component. Storm experimented with a free flow of colored ink on a larger sheet, making no forms or outlines, and after several experiments with the media, Storm stood in silence, and held his breath. As his eyes moistened, he expressed grief by adding water as a finishing touch on the artwork. The art material was a gateway for Storm to share and externalize a story that he had been telling himself about loss and grief.

Later Sessions

Storm said that his ink-flow image represented his feelings during the experience of bereavement at the beginning of high school. He explained that after losing his grandfather, he became intensely lonely and depressed because he had not been able to talk about his grief. His silence resulted in another personal loss, when his best friend was expelled from school for something that Storm did. Storm described feelings of shame, guilt, and depression, and explained that he escaped these emotions using vapes and cannabis. Through discourse, he was able to deconstruct this narrative of self-blame, externalize these events, and explore new opportunities for growth.

In analyzing the images of the waves (Figure 3.3), Storm reflected on his use of surfer imagery, which showed both his interest in sports and his connection to strength through action. He created images of personal strength and energy through strong surfers symbolizing his yearning to finish high school. Toward the end of our sessions, Storm verbalized the importance of staying active, eating healthy, and cultivating the strength needed to come out of his personal storm. According to Ricœur (1991), stories appeal to the temporality that links together human experiences in the ways in which stories are told, and the affective dimension related to these lived experiences. Approaching termination, Storm elaborated on the story of losing his best friend, sharing his feelings surrounding loss, grief, and frustration. He shifted towards a positive affect, perhaps to help alleviate the heaviness of his disclosure and enthusiastically explored the strength and tools he had developed through art therapy. Storm came into his final sessions with a bright affect, being productive in art-making, and creating personal stories that he shared. He was understanding himself and his place in the world differently.

Storm was encouraged to experiment with different mediums, to write, and to play. He deepened his capacity for tough emotions like grief, and explored the perceived abandonment of his loved ones. He was able to experience the creative dimension, and, like the surfer, he became skilled at riding emotional waves. According to Sharma et al. (2013), he was able to develop a constructive personal identity by building on his strengths, setting new goals, and choosing his dreams. When sharing the image created during his last session (Figure 3.3), Storm revealed that he wanted to study in a creative field. He re-authored the story his family had told him about academic and career success. These yearnings eventually became reality when years after our work together, Storm finished high school and embarked on a career in web design.

Outcomes

Within the first weeks of treatment, Storm was encouraged to continue drawing in order to externalize his challenges and integrate principles related to school motivation. This allowed him to access a more balanced perspective and increase his investment in the art therapy process. He learned to discern struggles and strengths, find opportunities for growth in his dominant narrative, and create healthy boundaries in therapy. Within a month, Storm demonstrated the ability to structure past experiences, analyze and solve a problem, and learn self-control. This led him to think through past events, make sense of his experiences, and implement adapted boundaries.

During the second treatment phase, Storm used organizational patterns to create schematic representations of his feelings. Through exploring his personal narrative, he uncovered existing strategies for emotional regulation, identified anger triggers, and developed new tools for regulation and self-control. Within the last phase of treatment, Storm used stories, line, color, and forms to depict his feelings. Using the language of the arts, Storm cultivated a deeper capacity for feeling and speaking about difficult emotions. With greater emotional access and the ability to see other perspectives, his relationships improved too.

Conclusions

As art therapists, we have images for insight into patients' self-growth journeys. In viewing Storm's images, he was shielding his emotions and sorrow, leading him to feel like he had been caught up in a storm. Art-making and storytelling allowed him gentle discernment and the metamorphosis of veiled perceptions.

Storm's participation allowed him to step into self-compassion that led him closer to community and further away from isolated pain. The goal of school art therapy is to enhance emotional well-being, facilitate interactions, and increase capacity for expression through both verbal and non-verbal communication (Bosgraaf et al., 2020). Bat Or and Zilcha-Mano (2018), emphasized the importance of the therapeutic alliance in the context of art therapy as a gateway for the client to experience positive outcomes. Storm developed positive coping strategies and a renewed and secure relationship to self. This increased self-trust allowed him to tell stories that were not saturated with problems, created new possibilities for emotional regulation, and experiences of artistic success for him to enjoy.

EARLY ADOLESCENCE: TEEN WITH DOWN SYNDROME

SUSAN RIDLEY

Setting

The art therapy setting was an outpatient program providing a wide range of counseling services to a diverse population. Services ranged from individual and group therapy for clients of various ages, abilities, and disabilities. A selection of art materials was available in the counseling room for client use. Because of the limitations of space and storage in the individual counseling room, materials included markers, pencils, crayons, hard pastels, modeling clay, brush pens, collage materials including magazine photos and glue sticks. Tool adaptations were also available, for example, wide-handle scissors and sponge handles for pencils, markers, and brush paints for clients with physical challenges and fine motor limitations. These materials provide more control for clients because of their resistant and semi-fluid qualities (Hinz, 2019). They are also easy to use, familiar to most clients, and require just hand wipes for clean-up. A small table was provided in the counseling room for individual sessions, while the room used for group work had larger tables and chairs to accommodate more clients and a sink and access to water. While most materials were stored on site either in the individual counseling room or a storage space in the group room, special projects required bringing in materials such as wet clay, paints, printing supplies, or other projects when needed.

Session Planning

Kayla attended three one-hour individual art therapy sessions over the course of three weeks. The original intent was to engage in weekly art therapy sessions, however, after the third week, Kayla's mother chose not to continue. Her mother said that Kayla's behavior had improved, and her daughter wanted to attend an after-school program with her friends instead of coming to art therapy. Kayla's mother was not interested in making another appointment but said that if her daughter was experiencing any other issues then she would return.

Approaches

The theoretical orientation incorporated a combination of existential and person-centered approaches (Rogers, 2006). A strengths-based approach and utilization of narrative therapy also helped clients re-author their stories. Developmental considerations included Erikson's (1967) Psychosocial Theory and Maslow's (1970) Hierarchy of Needs. The Expressive Therapies Continuum (Kagin & Lusebrink, 1978; Hinz, 2019) was used to categorize media and materials to elicit specific psychological and emotional responses.

Case Study

Kayla was a 16-year-old American-born Caucasian female with special needs who was integrated into the mainstream of the local high school. She was born with Down Syndrome, which is categorized as an unspecified neurodevelopmental disorder in the DSM-V TR (APA, 2022). Down Syndrome is caused by a full or partial duplication of chromosome

21, which changes the development of physical characteristics and mental abilities including learning difficulties and developmental delays in motor skills, spoken language, and academics. There are often significant impairments in identifying basic emotional states, a lack of appropriate eye contact, and difficulties interacting socially (Martin, 2008). Due to social ineptness, individuals with developmental disabilities may appear disengaged, which may lead to difficulty in making or maintaining friends as they have difficulty in recognizing beliefs and predicting behavior in others. Additionally, individuals with developmental disabilities may be unable to describe or identify personal feelings, or have difficulty communicating strong emotions. Restricted, repetitive, and stereotyped patterns may present as a need for order and as rigid routine (Wallace et al., 2008). As children move through adolescence and into young adulthood, there may be a progressive deterioration of cognitive function which may impact their independence and autonomy (Mircher Clotilde et al., 2017).

Intake Session

Kayla was brought to art therapy by her mother because of recent outbursts of anger. Kayla's relationship with her older sister was described as very close even though there was a large age gap between them, and the sister lived in another state. Kayla also said that she had a close relationship with her parents, especially with her mother, "because she's the best". Her mother was present during all sessions and often answered for Kayla when she struggled to express herself. Kayla was asked to create a drawing of anything she wanted to do as an introduction. Kayla chose to draw a butterfly and said that it was "pretty, just like me". She used colored pencils on 8 × 11-inch white paper. Her mother said that Kayla often drew butterflies everywhere as they were her favorite. Kayla then proudly showed her notebook covered with different sizes of butterflies and flowers surrounded by hearts drawn in colored pencils. She added her drawing to her collection of butterflies when the session ended.

While Kayla was 16-years-old at the time of the session, her developmental drawing level was of a younger child around seven to nine years of age. According to Lowenfeld and Brittain (1987), standardized artistic developmental stages can provide information on whether the individual may be impaired or delayed, and if they need further diagnostic screenings or assessments. The artistic developmental stage of Kayla's drawing was schematic because of the set of symbols of definite objects and the relationship and space in her drawings. Kayla was very open when talking about her artwork. Although she was hesitant at first, she was fully engaged in the creative process. When she stumbled over her words, the images were very clear and helped her to communicate her thoughts and feelings. She followed the directives as requested and asked to continue art-making after completing her drawing.

Assessments

The Diagnostic Drawing Series (Cohen et al., 1994) was administered as prescribed over the second and third sessions. Kayla was given a 12-pastel-colored chalk box set and three sheets of 18" × 24" paper. Chalk lies between resistant and fluid materials on the Media Dimension Variables (MDV) and enables clients to express their thoughts without losing emotional control (Kagin & Lusebrink, 1978). According to Hinz (2019), three drawings

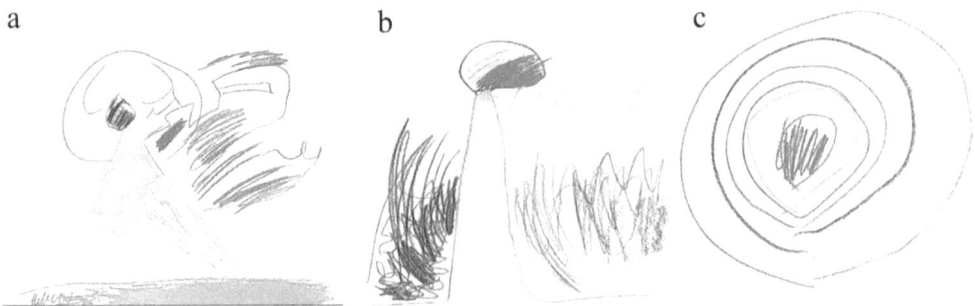

Figure 3.4 Diagnostic Drawing Series

are usually needed to assess client functioning and to identify themes in the artwork. The first directive was to "make a picture using these materials", which is considered a free drawing. The second drawing, "draw a picture of a tree", is considered a structured task. The third picture, "make a picture of how you're feeling, using lines, shapes, and colors", is a semi-structured task. After completing the three drawings, a short questionnaire was administered.

Figure 3.4a was described as a volcano with lava coming out. This made the client feel nervous about the volcano erupting. The colors represented nature "at the foot of the ocean" with people hiding in the volcano. The images represent "me, mom, sister, friends, and really scared". It was titled "A Volcano About to Erupt". Figure 3.4b was described as a colorful tree, a real tree that she had seen near her sister's house. Kayla liked all of the tree and didn't have anything more to say. Figure 3.4c was an image that she had seen somewhere. She was happy with the colors because they were similar to a target and represented "people playing games". Visual images in two of the drawings included the recurring shape, one was the volcano and the second, a phallic shaped tree. The images and colors chosen in the client's artwork suggested concerns around menstruation and potential interest in or engaging in sexual activity. Although Kayla said that she enjoyed creating artwork, she kept glancing at her mother seeking approval. Kayla was reluctant to discuss her artwork further or elaborate on the meaning behind the images. The presence of her mother in the session may have prevented her from talking about more sensitive issues.

Treatment Goals

While Kayla only attended three sessions, the treatment goals were based on the information gathered during intake and the art therapy directives.

Increase Communication Skills

One of the characteristics of Down Syndrome is physical difficulties with speech (i.e., swollen tongue). Helping the client to improve their communication skills may reduce feelings of frustration (Wetherby, 2006). Osborne (2003) and Evans and Dubowski (2007) believed that art was an excellent tool to bridge the communication gap between children with developmental disabilities because it did not rely on verbal communication or purely cognitive skills. For Kayla, art-making helped to enhance her communication skills and she would point to the images she created when she was unable to speak clearly. Art therapy can also help to sublimate anger and frustration to decrease the need for acting out behaviors which occurred during her second art therapy session. At the beginning of the third session, Kayla's mother reported that her daughter was no longer expressing anger towards her and seemed happier overall. Her mother also said that Kayla was drawing every day and seemed to use her art as a way to manage her emotions and to express herself. Hope (2008) described drawing as a way to help clients to develop, generate, expand, and communicate their ideas. Hopperstad (2010) suggested that children's drawings convey meaning and help them to articulate ideas and understandings in different ways other than verbal language. Using drawing as a means of communication can help clients process ideas, thoughts, and feelings (Adams, 2006).

Developing a Sense of Self

There is a complexity of developmental stages within the client between a child and an emerging adult. These bring with them a mixture of emotions and concerns about the future as the client moves from the dependence of childhood to the independence of adulthood. With a chronological age of 16 years, Kayla was in the *identity vs confusion* stage of Erikson's (1967) Psychosocial Theory, while her artistic stage of development was seven to nine years which focuses on *industry vs inferiority* and developing competence. According to the Hierarchy of Needs (Maslow, 1970), the desire for love and belonging through friendships, family, intimacy, and a sense of connection is the next stage after fulfilling physiological, and safety and security needs. Preoccupation with sexual identity can be seen in Kayla's artwork through phallic symbols and a focus on an erupting volcano which may represent concerns about her menstrual cycle or her increasing interest in a romantic or intimate relationship. Kayla often looked to her mother for reassurance and during the third session she smiled and whispered that she had a secret while her mother was preoccupied with something else. However, Kayla did not want to elaborate on what this secret was in her mother's presence and unfortunately, they did not return to therapy after this session. Emotions can be explored through art, helping the client to understand, process, and respond appropriately (Martin, 2009).

Improving Social Skills

It can be difficult for those with developmental disabilities to engage in joint attention with another person, and to focus on an object or action that is pointed out to them (Sholt & Gavron, 2006). Art activities can help to promote socialization and art tasks can help the client explore their self-image and form new patterns of relating to others (Gabriels, 2003; Waller, 2006). Art therapy directives can be used to discover the root of various conflicts in their lives, and can offer a relaxing and enjoyable atmosphere to practice social skills and taking turns. It can also help an individual with developmental deficits understand another person's point of view (Epp, 2008). Group art therapy can help the client socialize with others outside her family and art tasks can help the clients explore their self-images and personal ideations (Rogers, 2001). Asking the client to identify at least one positive attribute about themselves during each session can also help to reduce negative self-talk and frustration levels. Discussing the client's artwork can help them practice personal expression and refine their communication skills (Libemann, 2004). Art therapy can increase social awareness because it can help clients to think more abstractly by solving problems visually. While Kayla only attended three art therapy sessions, her choice to engage in an after-school program with her friends indicates a desire for social interactions. A referral to group art therapy was made, but Kayla's mother did not follow through with the suggestion. Unfortunately, therapy sessions are at the mercy of parents or legal guardians, and their willingness to engage in the therapeutic process.

Outcomes

Narrative therapy can help clients to examine the stories they tell about themselves and others and reedit the ending (Cashin et al., 2013). The use of art therapy can help clients explore their imaginations and turn their limitations into opportunities for growth. For Kayla, drawing butterflies and engaging in art-making was an opportunity to express her creativity, and gave her a voice when her words failed her. Giving clients a free choice of materials and activities can give them a sense of control while using more structured directives, such as painting your emotions, can help clients connect their emotions to colors and work on emotional regulation. Simple directives, such as painting your dreams, developing personal symbols or schemas, and using the drawings to tell stories, may help to improve communication between client and art therapist, and between client and family members. Drawing portraits of self or others can be an effective way of processing faces and understanding emotions as well as improving social skills and interactions (Betts, 2003). Although Kayla ended her participation in art therapy at this time, it is hoped that she will return to either individual or group art therapy sessions.

SPREADING MY WINGS: ANGEL

TAMI HARRIS

Setting

This case study was covered within my role as an art therapy consultant at a partnering organization. I have a contracted position as a mental health consultant with the Job Center where I provide short-term mental health support for students and staff. I also do crisis interventions, art therapy, and provide motivational interviewing in support of students graduating from the program with a high school diploma or a specified trade. Mental health services are voluntary, individual, and face-to-face. The average residency program is six to 18 months on campus. In my office, I keep a variety of artistic mediums (paper, various collage materials, canvas, pencils, charcoal, oil and chalk pastels, markers, and acrylic and watercolor paints). This is where I met Angel.

Approaches

Various therapeutic approaches were used during Angel's treatment including Rogers' (1979) Person-Centered Approach, Interpersonal Psychotherapy (Weissman et al., 2008), Motivational Interviewing (Miller & Rose, 2009), Expressive Therapies Continuum (ETC; Hinz, 2019), and Psychodynamic-Relational Therapy (Borden, 2009).

Intake Sessions

Angel was of Hispanic descent. She was a 17-year-old female who expressed a history of being bullied during middle and high school due to race. My first encounter with Angel was an initial introduction to art therapy and other services available. Our second session occurred following a crisis event that had taken place on campus two days after the introductory session. Angel was advised that services on campus were voluntary. I explained the scope of services, and limits to confidentiality. The reason for Angel's self-referral was to maintain mental health balance, establish positive coping skills, and obtain support. Angel's home was with guardians and a younger biological brother. Angel's mother died two years before and Angel had overall good social support, with no history of legal issues. She did not participate in any religious practices. Her highest level of school completed at the time of intake was the 11th grade. No special education resources were utilized, and Angel had no history of special resources for school.

Angel did have a history of mental health treatment, residential treatment, and was currently prescribed a battery of medication for mood, anxiety, and depression. She presented with a depressed mood, low energy, appetite and sleep disturbances, crying spells, feelings of sadness, hopelessness, and withdrawal. Additionally, Angel's behaviors included anger, irritability, punching walls or things, and an inability to walk away when someone disrespected her. At the time of intake, Angel denied homicidal ideation, but had recurring thoughts of suicide and had made previous attempts. She had multiple hospitalizations with six weeks being the longest stay.

At the time of her self-referral, she was struggling with nightmares, trying to avoid triggers, and experiencing hypervigilance. Angel had a history of sexual abuse, exhibited restrictive symptoms of an eating disorder, and was grieving the loss of her mother. Angel felt stressed out and experienced panic attacks. She also reported visual hallucinations and self-injury behaviors (i.e., cutting), nightmares, and having trouble falling and staying asleep. She also reported uncomfortable feelings regarding sexual thoughts and behaviors. Her typical coping mechanisms included listening to music, going outside, learning new things, and going to museums. Angel identified her strengths to include being a good communicator, a person who listens well, someone who has a sense of humor, acts as a motivator, and considers herself intelligent. Her goals at the Job Center included wanting to complete a Certified Nursing Assistant (CNA) certificate and obtaining a driver's license.

Assessments

Angel's assessment regimen included completion of several psychological measures and a formal interview. Angel's rapport and affect were appropriate, her speech and behavior were normal, but her mood was depressed and her judgment was only fair. At the time of assessment, she was experiencing mood swings, feeling depressed, and reported past self-harm and sexual assault by a family friend from the ages of six to nine. The perpetrator is currently in jail. Significant findings from the psychological assessments and interview led to diagnoses of Provisional Major Depressive Disorder, and Post Traumatic Stress Disorder (PTSD) according to the DSM-5 TR (APA, 2022). An outside referral was made specifically to address her PTSD. Angel only attended two virtual sessions with the outside therapist. She continued to see the offsite psychiatrist for medication reviews and continued to see me for art therapy sessions.

Sessions

Goals for Angel in Art Therapy Treatment

1. Crisis stabilization, create safety plan.
2. Stress management, identify and utilize positive coping strategies.
3. Emotional support, provide art therapy to express, process, and communicate emotional responses.

Angel met with me once a week or as needed. Early sessions focused on crisis interventions, stress management, and Dialectical Behavioral Therapy (DBT; Linehan, 2015) or mindfulness through art and talk therapy approaches. Angel continued to report incidences of self-harm and suicidal ideation. A safety plan was put into place and Angel's frequency of art therapy sessions was increased to two times per week until she was stabilized. After stabilization, she returned to weekly art therapy sessions. During the crisis stage, I used empathic exploration, stress management, and motivational interviewing by using painting to process emotions (Figure 3.5).

Figure 3.5 was the first painting that Angel made during art therapy sessions. Angel did not have skills to control her emotions at that time. I taught her the painting techniques of layering and she was able to express her sadness and anxiety onto the canvas. Angel titled

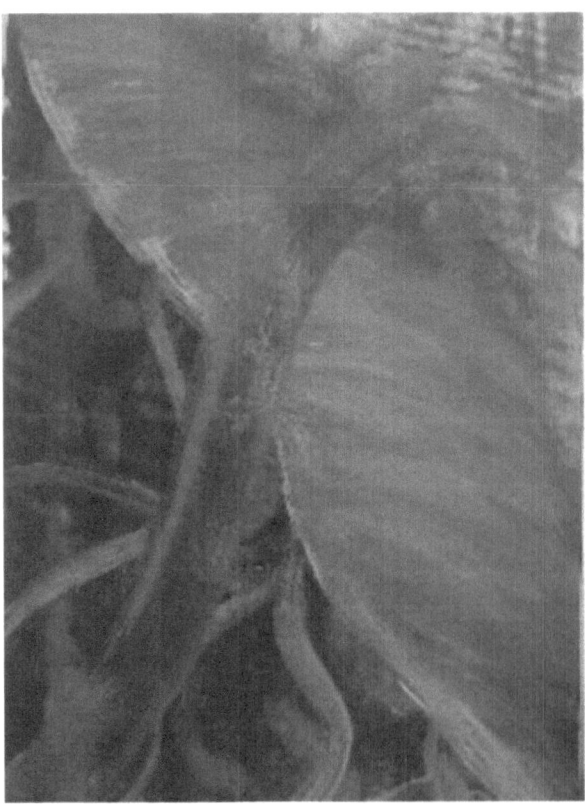

Figure 3.5 Pink Feather

the work "Pink Feather". She started off with red and blue paint, but the process grew from there. As rapport built between Angel and myself, she began to discuss her history of sexual abuse and plans to commit suicide on her upcoming birthday. Despite her depressed state, Angel remained focused on completing the program and improving her life. Looking back at the painting during her termination session, Angel would identify meaning and patterns that occurred during its creation. Angel would indicate the image demonstrated how she "wanted to be seen and heard". She noted that she "did not want this light" (the pink color) at that time. She thought she could take care of herself without help. In retrospect she recognized that she "was very sad" when the painting was first created.

As she continued to stabilize, Angel began going home on weekend passes and began creating artwork with markers, charcoal, and pencils. Sessions gravitated to motivational interviewing techniques with experimentations in the use of art. Figure 3.6 was created after Angel had developed some experience using charcoal. In her closing sessions, the emotional process and meaning of this image were further illuminated. She noted when she drew the wings she wanted something that would make her happy and okay. Angel noted she "was always focusing on other people and other things". The two wings are different, one represented her desire to be okay and have closure, the other "represented that freedom where I could just, like, go away". During the session when Angel created this image, she "was going to draw a person", but then "decided not to". There remain residual smudges that reminded Angel and me of the person who was once there.

At times Angel would express feelings of sadness and thoughts of self-harm but without a plan or attempts. I continued to use empathic exploration by creating art expressions alongside Angel and at other times Angel and I would create collaborative art expressions. These sessions allowed Angel the opportunity to embrace and process emotions with my support. Angel began expressing concerns about career goals and passions, so I provided assessments and art responses to begin focusing on strengths and career options.

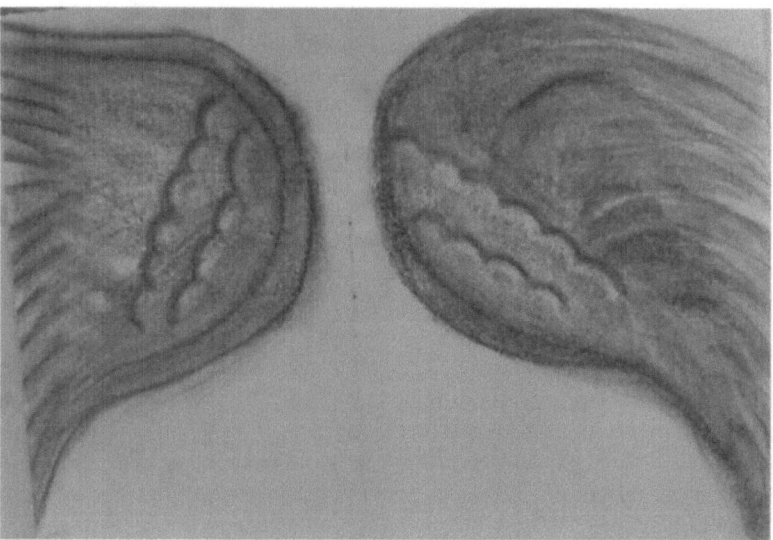

Figure 3.6 Wings in Charcoal on Paper

Angel had another crisis event where she expressed feelings of being out of control and was making slow progress in completing her clinicals. A second safety plan was put in place as a precaution. Within weeks, Angel regained mental stability and began to show art expressions containing writings and drawings with words of affirmation. Angel had established positive coping skills by identifying her triggers and establishing additional support from friends and family members. Typical teenage concerns arose including, role-identity, self-esteem, and relationships in general. These concerns were addressed in the weekly art therapy sessions that provided Angel an outlet to express current emotional states through the use of art materials ranging from fluid to restrictive per the ETC (Hinz, 2019). Sessions varied from directive to non-directive approaches depending on Angel's presented emotion. By the 21st session Angel was open to using new mediums and learning new techniques.

Art expressions became clearer and brighter colors were used primarily with markers (Figure 3.7). Angel had moved into a more healthy psychological space; it was as if her shadow had cleared. Angel maintained a sense of disbelief in her accomplishments as she had not yet received her diploma. Angel called her new level of status "All Star". Figure 3.7 began with the drawing of the girl and the faint shadow then appeared behind her. Angel and I did not talk much during the art-making process. I reflected on the work that we had done over the course of Angel's art therapy. Next, Angel added the text, "Inhale the Futuer [sic], Exhale the Past", which may have been an indication of her perseverance and readiness to move on. At the end of the session, Angel recognized how far she had come and began to cry tears of happiness. She elaborated by saying "I didn't know I could get better".

Outcomes

There were a total of 28 face-to-face hours of service that were provided over a six-month period. Angel displayed a significant amount of self-confidence and had excelled in completing her CNA, graduating with their high school diploma, applying for college, starting work study, and taking on a leadership role on campus. Angel also had a sense of sadness in having such accomplishments without her mother being present to witness. I suggested that Angel write a letter to her mother about her journey and where she is today. To process developing concerns, I had met with Angel seven more times prior to termination. Empathic exploration, stress management, and decision-making were processed through drawing materials.

Final and Post-Termination Sessions

During the termination session, Angel and I reviewed all the saved art expressions to reflect on her art therapy journey. She also added an additional response of closure to the dialogue that captured the essence of art therapy by reading a letter that she had since written to her deceased mother. Post-termination, Angel returned and reported she was finally able to accept everything good and bad. She embraced happiness and acceptance. She hoped to continue to save money, and to move into her own apartment. Her new goal was to continue advanced training in pharmacy.

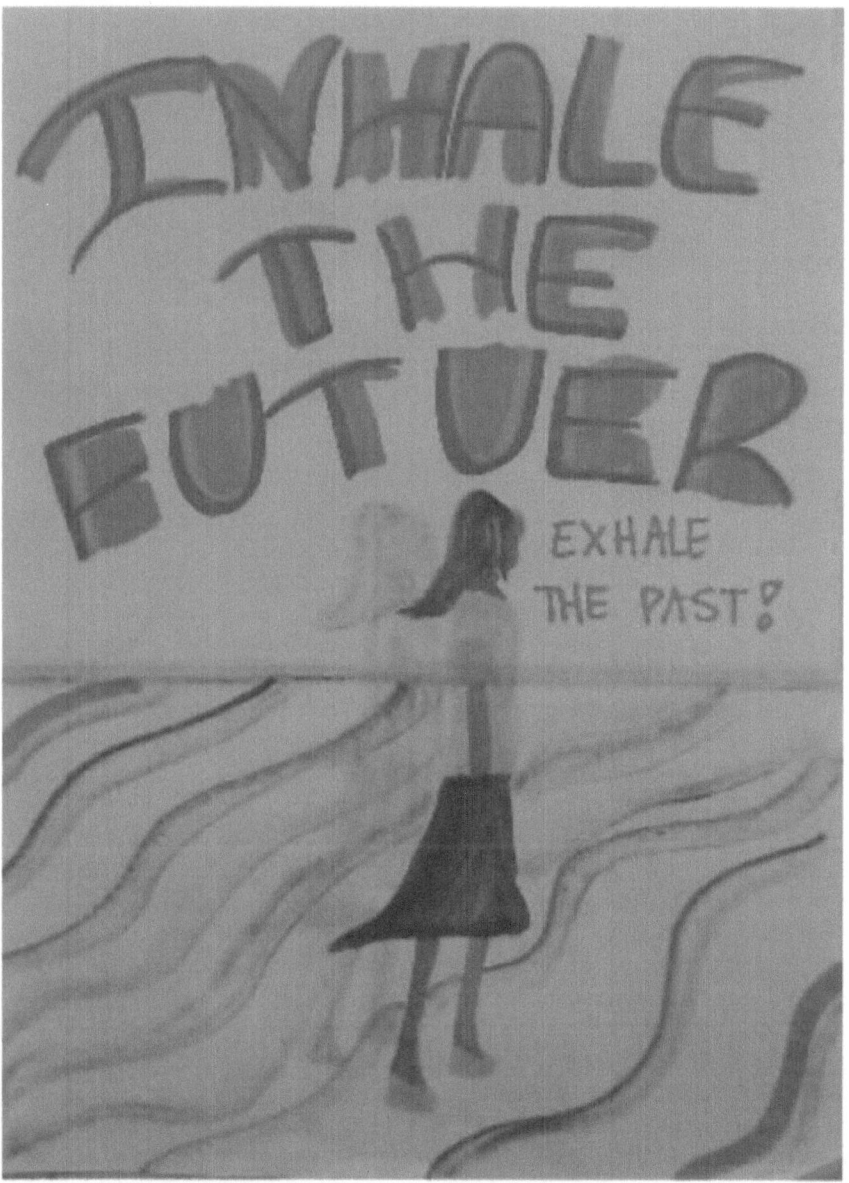

Figure 3.7 Inhale the Futuer [sic]

Conclusion

Ultimately, Angel moved to the top of her class with test scores and was well on her way to completing her CNA certification even though she expressed some anxiety in completing her board exam. Angel was eventually able to find closure regarding her mother's death by accepting the loss and having no sense of pain but comfort. She reasoned that they were both in a better place. Despite the significant improvements of Angel's mental capacity, she still had a sense of disbelief in her accomplishments and refurbished abilities. I assisted Angel in finding a sense of self-confidence in review of her art expressions. This provided Angel another opportunity to witness her ability to master new skills by learning alternative techniques to express emotions.

RODNEY: A CASE OF MID-ADOLESCENT FORENSIC ART THERAPY

NATASHIA P. COLLINS AND SAMANTHA CASTELLANO

Adolescence marks a developmental period defined by rapid physical, psychological, and social changes that produce challenging symptom presentations and unique considerations for the therapeutic relationship (Christie & Viner, 2005). Adolescents' moods may be labile, their emotions volatile, their defenses both fragile and rigid, and their relationships exploitative and self-serving (Henley, 2012). In fact, Henley (2012) believes that "many therapists avoid working with adolescents, given their propensity to be defiant, hurtful, ungrateful, and impossible to reason with" (p. v).

Despite the inherent challenges of working with this population, art therapists have guided adolescents through the art therapy healing process for many years (Bennink et al., 2003; Berberian & Davis, 2020; Kramer, 1993; Linesch, 1988; Moon, 2012; Riley, 1999). The benefits of art therapy during mid-adolescence are exemplified in the composite case of Rodney, a 17-year-old Black male residing at a Juvenile Detention Center (JDC). After a brief description of the setting, the art therapy approaches applied to Rodney's case will be explored in alignment with theoretical, developmental, and forensic considerations.

Setting

The JDC houses up to 29 juveniles, typically ranging from 13 to 18 years of age. Most residents are males from minority populations and lower socioeconomic neighborhoods; many are from single-parent households and are gang-affiliated. Adolescents within the JDC present with various criminal behaviors, with the most frequent charges related to armed robbery, grand theft auto, gun violence, murder, and possession and distribution of substances.

The art therapy setting ensures that services are safe, secure, and humanistic through environmental, relational, and procedural therapeutic security (Kennedy, 2022). Access to the JDC includes medical and security clearance, consisting of a wellness check, belongings search, and entrance through a metal detector and a series of locked doors. Art therapy services take place in a large multipurpose room with one secure door for entry and exit, and an open floor plan. The room consists of white cinderblock walls, high ceilings, and natural light streaming through large windows framing the roof. The space is free of obvious penal qualities (Kennedy, 2022) and is often decorated to reflect current or upcoming holiday celebrations. The environment is clear of moveable objects, no paper towels, soap dispensers, or garbage cans. Several small but sturdy weighted plastic tables are pushed together to form one large table where approximately eight people can sit. The chairs are also plastic and weighted, so they cannot be flipped, thrown, destroyed, or weaponized.

Relational therapeutic security is supported by the presence of at least one correction officer at all times. Correction officers are involved in the group process in various ways, ranging from observers to participants. As for safety within the treatment relationship, the art therapist negotiates interpersonal trust and a strong working alliance with clear limits and boundaries to manage risk.

Procedural therapeutic security involves following policies and procedures, especially orders regarding safety and the elimination of contraband art materials. Materials that are tacky, malleable, and unable to keep track of, like clay, Model Magic, or kneaded erasers, are prohibited, as pieces can be hoarded and used to jam locks. Sharps such as X-Acto knives and box cutters are also not permitted due to their weaponized nature. Procedural security also involves having a methodical system for the division and collection of materials, which is achieved through a numbering system and limiting available options.

Approaches

Theoretical, developmental, and forensic considerations influence art therapy with adolescents facing incarceration. Theoretical considerations are influenced by Cathy Moon's (2016) open studio approach. The developmental approach integrates Christie and Viner's (2005) biopsychosocial development model with Riley's (1999) perspectives on normal development in adolescent art. Forensic considerations evolve from Bennink et al.'s (2003), Gussak's (2016), and Gussak and Cohen-Liebman's (2001) seminal works on art therapy in a forensic setting. These integrated considerations informed a limited open-studio approach to art therapy with Rodney.

Limited Open Studio

Theoretical Considerations

An open studio approach to art therapy is identified by several factors, including an open-group format (rolling admission), non-directive interventions, and a free choice of materials (C. Moon, 2016). In the JDC, the open studio approach encompasses all of these group therapy considerations; however, it is also limited by therapeutic security. Admission to the art therapy group is not based on a formal intake (C. Moon, 2016). Correction officers determine attendance based on behavioral observations, including demonstrations of trustworthiness and the ability to maintain safety within a group setting. Regular attendance in art therapy is not guaranteed, as behaviors may change rapidly and discharges can occur during court appearances between group sessions.

Within the JDC, adolescents are faced with the juxtaposition of being stripped of choice, control, and autonomy while being developmentally driven to achieve such goals (Christie & Viner, 2005). By structuring the art therapy group without a directive, adolescents are encouraged to use creative autonomy and are provided with an opportunity to practice choice and control in the context of their art-making. The art therapist's goal is to produce an environment of democracy and equality where each group member can feel seen, acknowledged, and understood (C. Moon, 2016). Art therapists can support this goal by situating themselves as collaborators in the art therapy process rather than experts or authority figures (C. Moon, 2016). This approach to working with adolescents in the JDC reduces oppositional behaviors and empowers positive decision-making (Bennink et al., 2003).

Despite contraband restrictions, many art materials are approved during group art therapy in this JDC. Blank weighted paper and 2D drawing materials, including packets of markers, colored pencils, Sharpies, and graphite pencils; body outlines for tattoo design; sneaker and clothing templates for fashion design; coloring pages of mandalas, famous music artists, and other pop icons; lightweight table-top easels; canvas boards; and tempera and watercolor paints are permitted. Of utmost importance, the art therapist must ensure that the materials provided are of quality and in good working condition.

Developmental Considerations

Christie and Viner's (2005) brief biopsychosocial approach to development provides context to the physical, psychological, and social developmental needs of mid-adolescents. Development is positioned within a system of interrelated internal and external demands. While puberty and cognitive development are primarily internal demands and biologically determined, psychological and social development depend on external demands of environmental and sociocultural influences (Christie & Viner, 2005).

Biologically, mid-adolescent males are confronted with puberty, including growth spurts, voice deepening, maturing of reproductive organs, and the development of secondary sex characteristics (Christie & Viner, 2005). Mid-adolescent males may demonstrate psychological growth through increasing verbal abilities, abstract thinking, identification of law with morality, and development of strong ideologies. They may also view themselves as "bullet proof" (p. 301). The belief that one's vulnerability is bulletproof can lead adolescents to take substantial risks regarding substance use, personal safety, and treatment compliance. This belief can also result in denial that consequences apply to them. In reaching developmental goals, adolescents may feel challenged by authority, social morals and structure, human rights, responsibility, employment, spirituality, and the renegotiation of rules (Christie & Viner, 2005).

According to Riley (1999), the art therapy process and product serve as a mirror, a personalized depiction of the self (internally and externally), providing adolescents a space to develop their personality and identity. Art therapists can enhance adolescents' creative process through suggestions demonstrating respect for their worldviews, interests, and ways of reinventing meaning. It is developmentally normal for adolescents to assert a preference for drawing. The use of markers and stereotypic imagery, such as gang symbols or adolescent-culture logos, is expected when provided with opportunities for spontaneous image-making (Riley, 1999). This type of imagery aligns with adolescent need to conform to peer standards, keep adults at a distance, and assist with developing their mark of identity.

Considerations for Art Therapy in a Forensic Setting

Exacerbating characteristics of normal development, adolescents facing incarceration may display tendencies towards masking their vulnerabilities as a defense and for survival (Bennink et al., 2003; Gussak & Cohen-Liebman, 2001). Gussak (2016) asserts that disclosure of personal issues during therapeutic programming may lead to unhealthy and dangerous consequences, such as weakened ego strength, a rapid shift in mood or behavior, ridicule, retaliation, or domination by others. Art therapists who understand the "unspoken rules of the setting" (i.e., the need for privacy and identity; Gussak & Cohen-Liebman, 2001, p. 130) are more effective in supporting defenses, reducing suspicion, and decreasing vulnerability (Gussak, 2016). This may foster socially acceptable expressions of aggressive and libidinal impulses (Gussak & Cohen-Liebman, 2001).

Case Study

Rodney, a 17-year-old Black male, was raised by his mother in a single-parent household with three siblings, including two older brothers, Jamal and Mikail, and one younger half-sister, Shania. Rodney lived on the third floor of a multifamily home in an urban, lower-income neighborhood. Throughout his childhood, Rodney's mother worked two jobs to afford their two-bedroom house. Due to her work schedule, Rodney's mother was rarely home, leaving Rodney and his siblings unsupervised.

Rodney's father was incarcerated more than once during Rodney's childhood. Similarly, Jamal spent three years in a JDC when Rodney was nine, and he was incarcerated a second time, two years after returning home. During Jamal's second incarceration, Mikail enlisted in the Army and left home for basic training.

With his two older brothers out of the house, Rodney began spending most of his time at a local park with friends, or writing and recording music in a makeshift studio. Rodney began engaging in risk-taking behaviors and experienced several encounters with law enforcement. Rodney was discovered smoking marijuana in the park, skipping school, and shoplifting from a local convenience store. He completed several diversion programs to avoid incarceration but maintained a dismissive approach to attendance and participation. Upon completing his last diversion program, Rodney quickly resumed illegal and risk-taking behaviors. These behaviors came to a head on Rodney's 14th birthday when Rodney and two friends robbed a local convenience store. Rodney was arrested, charged with second-degree robbery, convicted, and sentenced to five years at the JDC.

Art Therapy for Rodney

While in his third year at the JDC, Rodney joined the art therapy group, which met once weekly for one hour. During the art therapy sessions, Rodney was reserved, quiet, and kept to himself. Rodney shared simple, respectful pleasantries with the art therapist, and he displayed a steadfast commitment to his work exhibited through focused concentration and consistent engagement. During art-making, Rodney seldom spoke with peers and shared little about himself. However, when provided with an opportunity to discuss his creations, Rodney shared aspects of life pre-incarceration and the connection between the art product and his family, relationships, identity, and hopes for the future.

During his first art therapy group, Rodney rifled through stacks of coloring sheets and selected a page with a large outline of Tweety, a cartoon canary in the Warner Bros. *Looney Toons* series. He requested to use colored pencils to complete the design, and he carefully filled in each section of the page, using varying pressure on the pencils to create dimension and shading. Upon completion of his artwork, Rodney titled the piece, "Tweetie".

Although a debated art therapy intervention (Carolan & Betts, 2015), this simple and structured coloring sheet provided control, familiarity, comfort, and a safe way for Rodney to begin art therapy at the JDC. The Tweety Bird coloring sheet created a foothold for therapeutic trust by enabling Rodney to begin with something he knew while venturing into a vulnerable process with which he was unfamiliar (Cozolino, 2017; Hinz, 2019).

As previously discussed, it is developmentally normal for adolescents to claim a preference for drawing materials and stereotypic imagery (Riley, 1999). It is also common for adolescents to select images reflecting familiarities (Bennink et al., 2003), such as their daily life, traumas, and dreams of a better world (Riley, 1999). While coloring, Rodney spontaneously explained that "Tweetie" is a nickname his grandmother gave his mother. Rodney spoke about the many Warner Bros. collectible items around his family home and shared aspects of his home life with the group, such as the challenges he faced growing up in his neighborhood. The stereotypic imagery in the coloring page inspired Rodney to explore and share facets of the sociocultural and environmental systems that inform his identity and worldview. Rodney's peers responded to his artwork by sharing their experiences with family and community, which facilitated a brief moment of connection and acceptance within the group.

Fire and Air

Nike's release of Air Jordans in 1985 is believed to be the catalyst of *sneaker culture* (Matthews et al., 2021). With many *sneakerheads* in the JDC, the art therapist directed the group to create a high top sneaker design using a template created with artificial intelligence (AI). This occurred during Rodney's sixth art therapy group. Rodney used pink, brown, and black markers to complete his design and repeatedly stated, "this is fire!" – a slang phrase for admiration. After completing (Figure 3.8), Rodney shared his sneaker design with the group, professing that he would buy a pair of his sneakers if they existed.

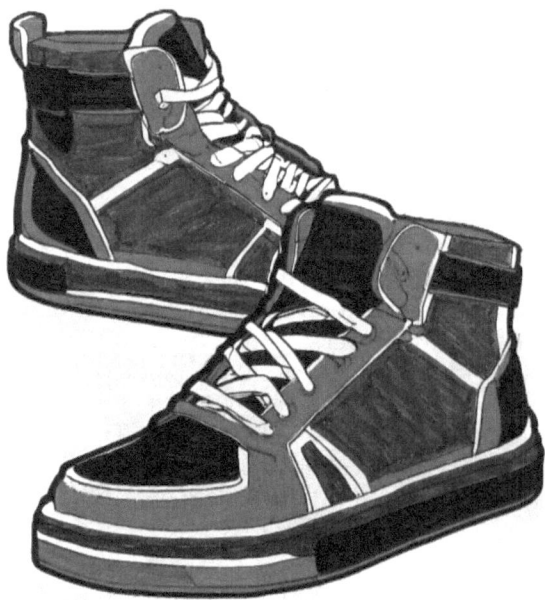

Figure 3.8 Fire and Air

Designing the sneakers led Rodney to reveal his goal of opening a clothing store, where he plans to balance his time screen printing with writing and recording music.

For generations, clothing has played a significant role in constructing and expressing identity (Crane, 2000). Clothing is a visible and symbolic representation of one's culture, degree of compliance with socially appropriate appearance norms, and social belonging (Crane, 2000). How adolescents dress and speak about fashionable brands, clothing, and accessories help shed light on who they are internally, how they want to be seen by others externally, and the popular cultural groups to which they want to belong. When considering the sneaker as a metaphor for a mirror, Riley (1999) explains, "To the outsider the [expensive athletic shoes] do not appear to be any different than a less expensive pair, but the label *is* the child" (p. 43). Conforming to peer group dress codes, musical choices, vocabulary, and hairstyles, are all attempts for adolescents to find social reassurance and identity (Riley, 1999).

Release Me

Rodney arrived at his 10th art therapy group following a court hearing and holding a marbled composition notebook for drawing and writing songs. Rodney's court appearance did not go as hoped – he reported frustration, anger, confusion, and uncertainty about his future. After settling into the art therapy group, Rodney shared a rap verse he composed about his court experience and requested to continue writing lyrics for the remaining 40 minutes of the group. Rodney worked quietly, looking down at his notebook with a furrowed brow. Every so often he could be seen mouthing words, tapping, rocking, and shaking his head as if he heard a melody to the lyrics he wrote.

Toward the end of the session, Rodney took a break from writing lyrics and in large letters across the top of his page he titled his song, "Release Me". Rodney accompanied the text with a small doodle of a chained heart (Figure 3.9). When provided with an opportunity to process with the group, Rodney shared the meaning of the song's title, lyrics, and doodle. In his own words, he explored themes of confusion, distrust, and lack of control.

Riley (1999) asserts that art-based journals, or a songbook in Rodney's case, are a developmentally appropriate intervention for adolescents. Journals can hold ideas, images, reflections, secrets, and patterns of "personal...codes" that allow therapeutic work to span beyond the session in the form of a transitional object (Riley, 1999, p. 61). Lyrics as *personal codes* contain metaphors that can consciously or unconsciously hide the true meaning of a song's emotional content, decreasing the vulnerability that comes from self-expression. Lyrical writing: (a) demonstrates respect for youths' worldviews, interests, and ways of reinventing meaning (Riley, 1999); (b) provides youth in a JDC with an opportunity for emotional escape (Gussak, 2016); (c) offers a discharge of feelings while maintaining behavioral self-control (Gussak & Cohen-Liebman, 2001); (d) conforms to peer standards while keeping adults at a safe distance (Riley, 1999); and (e) encourages youth to make their mark of identity (Riley, 1999).

Conclusion

Adolescents are notoriously challenging to work with due to rapid biological, psychological, and social changes contributing to mood swings; irrational thinking; defiant, defensive, or risk-taking behavior; and distrust for authority. Despite these challenges, art therapists have

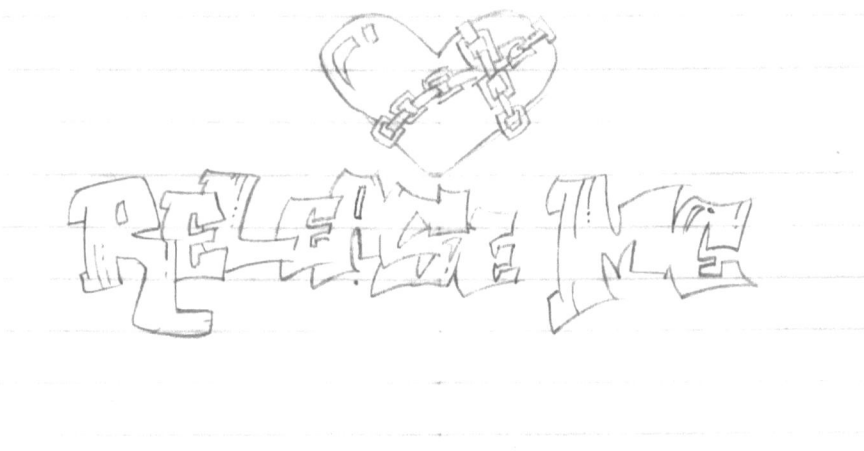

Figure 3.9 Release Me

supported adolescents' development and healing for many years. In the case of Rodney, a 17-year-old male residing within a JDC, art therapy provided, comfort through familiarity and a sense of belonging; opportunities for safe and appropriate control, expression, self-exploration, and socialization; and identity and goal development. Trust in the therapeutic relationship was built through collaboration, mutual respect, support for defenses, and clear boundaries within a limited open studio approach.

ADJUSTING TO COLLEGE LIFE

LISA THOMPSON-GIBSON

Setting

This case occurred in a Counseling and Psychological Services (CAPS) center at a midwestern, regional university that enrolls approximately 12,000 students at undergraduate, graduate, and professional school levels. CAPS delivers short-term, goal-focused services where students can be seen by a clinician every other week for 50-minute, individual therapy sessions. Services are rendered at no financial charge, since students contribute to a student fee structure to cover expenses. Students are stepped up for off-campus referral if presenting concerns are at a higher level requiring specialized or more frequent care.

Approaches

Therapy was delivered from a person-centered, strengths-based approach. Effective theoretical approaches with this client population include using developmental theories

(Chickering, 1981; Erikson, 1967; Kohlberg, 1969; Piaget & Inhelder, 1969) along with considerations toward Attachment Theory (Bowlby, 1969) and identity development using Racial and Cultural Identity Developmental Theory (Sue & Sue, 2013). Cognitive Behavior Therapy (Beck, 2020) and Acceptance and Commitment Therapy (Harris, 2019) are used to mitigate signs and symptoms of declining mental health and well-being. When rendering art therapy there are considerations toward the client's comfort with art materials and framing a treatment plan using the Expressive Therapies Continuum (ETC) to foster developmental growth and achievement of defined goals (Hinz, 2019).

Case Study

Rikah identified as an 18-year-old African American cisgender female who used she/her/hers pronouns. She was questioning her sexual orientation and did not identify herself in the binary. Rikah was a first-year student at a southern state university and had not yet declared her major. She lived on campus with one roommate whom she met upon arrival at school. Rikah's family lived in a middle-class, urban environment approximately five hours away from campus. She was the oldest of three children and was the first in her family to attend a four-year college. Her father attended a technical trade school and her mother attended a community college. Rikah was close with her family and they were invested in her success at the university. They financially and emotionally supported her and encouraged her. Rikah sometimes found that her parents did not understand what she was experiencing since they did not have a four-year college reference point to draw from in their own educational experiences. Rikah and her family identified as Christian and were members of an African Methodist Episcopal Church (AME). This was a key component to her identity and sometimes created tension since she was questioning her sexual orientation. She had no congenital or acquired disabilities. She did not have indigenous heritage and her nationality was American, from the United States.

Intake and Assessment

Rikah presented to CAPS for an initial assessment with the Assessment and Triage Counselor (ATC). She completed the required intake questionnaire before her appointment. During this appointment Rikah described feeling stress and uneasiness since arriving at campus one month prior. She had experienced changes in her sleep routine, especially having trouble falling asleep and staying asleep. She did not feel rested when she woke up. Rikah also said she had not had much of an appetite and had noticed a loss of three to five pounds without intention of losing weight. Rikah described feeling as if she was not herself and said that it had been difficult for her to meet and connect with people. She said it was the first time she had been in a community with more white people than black and brown people. This led her to feel irritable and frustrated. She said things with her roommate were going fine and they had an agreeable relationship, even though they did not have much in common. Rikah said her roommate was white and was from a small town about an hour away from campus. Her roommate went home regularly, leaving Rikah on her own. She had not yet declared her major and was hoping to eventually go into speech pathology. She regularly attended class and did not report academic concerns or stressors. Rikah said that she and her girlfriend broke up in the summertime before they both left for college. Rikah did not frequently hear from her ex-girlfriend, who attended a college elsewhere, but would see regular updates on Instagram about how her ex-girlfriend had "moved on". This added to Rikah's upset because she did not feel like she had "moved on" yet. She felt a bit hopeless and talked with her parents about what was going on since coming to college, and they tried to reassure her. They said that she should tough it out and it would get better. Rikah was close to her family and had not seen them for a visit since they dropped her off in August. She denied concerns regarding suicidal ideation (SI), non-suicidal self-injury (NSSI), or homicidal ideation (HI). She had no past or current experiences with SI, NSSI, or HI. When asked by the ATC what her goals were for counseling, Rikah said she would like to feel more like herself again, meet people with similar interests, and learn how to feel less upset.

The ATC offered Rikah the option of engaging in art therapy with the art therapist in CAPS. Rikah was intrigued and said that being creative had been helpful for her in the past. She said she liked making things and also used journaling off and on to get things off of her chest. Rikah agreed to try it. She had never experienced art therapy. Her only experience with therapy was in high school when she would talk with the school social worker when she had moments of upset.

Diagnostic considerations by the ATC based on the DSM-5 TR (APA, 2022) included: Adjustment Disorder with Depressive and Anxiety features, Persistent Depressive Disorder, Unspecified Anxiety, and Other Specified Trauma- and Stressor-Related Disorder. The ATC recommended symptoms be further assessed in therapy for diagnostic clarity and potential rule-out.

Early Sessions

When Rikah and I met for her first session, we reviewed administrative related topics to therapy like limits in confidentiality, scheduling and rescheduling guidelines, establishing goals for therapy, using assessments to measure progress, the therapeutic relationship, and guidelines if a referral would be needed in the future. Rikah had no questions about these procedures. She asked questions about art therapy and how it was different from talk therapy. After clarifying what Rikah could expect, I asked her if she would be willing to make art using an open directive. Rikah consented and I introduced her to the use of oil pastel cray-pas and a large 18 × 24 piece of white paper. Brief guidance was provided on how to use the oil pastels and then I explained that there were no specific expectations for the art piece except to enable us to get to know each other better. I asked Rikah to use lines, shapes, and forms to represent "What is the problem?" I explained that she could make something realistic or abstract, or something in between to visually represent what she had been experiencing. Rikah agreed and took a few moments to reflect on the prompt. She then began work using the oil pastels on the piece of paper. Rikah entitled the piece "*On My Own*" and interpreted the meaning of the drawing for me, explaining that she had drawn herself on one side of the paper while she had drawn everyone else in a group on the other side of the paper. Rikah's drawing was primarily monochromatic with blue color choices.

During the second art therapy session, assessment instruments were administered to gather additional quantitative data about Rikah's concerns. This included administering the Outcomes Questionnaire (OQ®-45.2) with a score of 83, which indicated moderately high symptoms above the clinical cut-off of 64; Generalized Anxiety Disorder (GAD-7) with a score of 12, indicating moderate anxiety symptoms; Patient Health Questionnaire (PHQ-9) with a score of 10, indicating moderate depression; Post-Traumatic Stress Disorder (PTSD) Checklist for DSM-5 (PCL-5) with a score of 13, indicating a non-clinically significant score for PTSD; and on the Adverse Childhood Experience Questionnaire (ACES), she scored 2 out of 9, indicating low risk.

I explained to Rikah that the OQ®-45.2 helped get a baseline understanding of her levels of overall well-being including sub-scores about symptom distress; her score of 42 was higher than the clinical cut-off of 37; in interpersonal relationships, her score of 21 was higher than the clinical cut-off of 16; and social role, where her score of 20 was higher than the clinical cut-off of 13. I reflected that the overall score suggested moderately high distress. I also shared results from the other assessments, highlighting that there were reported elevations in symptoms suggestive of depression and anxiety. This led to Rikah being asked to use art materials to describe how long she had experienced feeling this way. Rikah chose a large piece of paper and Mr. Sketch scented markers to illustrate her timeline showing when she started to experience these changes and what events had occurred. Rikah and I spent time deconstructing the art piece to better understand the chain of events that had led to her current concerns.

As a result of assessment findings from the two art directives, the assessment instruments, and her intake paperwork and clinical interviews, it was determined that Rikah's signs and symptoms met criteria for (F43.25) Adjustment Disorder with mixed anxiety and depressed mood (DSM-5 TR, 2022). Trauma was ruled out as a diagnosis since Rikah reported no concerns and the assessments revealed no elevations. The assessment results framed our work together. Rikah's goals and objectives were developed and are listed below.

Long-Term Goal

Improve skills in adjusting to attending college and living away from family. This goal would be accomplished with self-reports by Rikah using the OQ®-45.2 as a periodic assessment, regular art therapy directives, demonstrations of behavior change supporting reduction in OQ®-45.2 scores, self-report of improved well-being, and declines in reported distress.

Short-Term Objectives

1. Identify three activating or triggering events that result in declined coping.
2. Identify three new strategies for self-regulation and distress tolerance.
3. Develop three strategies for connecting with people with similar identities and interests.

Later Sessions

Rikah engaged in creating an art journal to track her progress toward adjusting to college and living away from her family. Her journal was an ongoing depository for work created in session as well as between sessions. Rikah brought her journal to each therapy session to either add to or process work that she had created on her own. This modality enabled her to experiment with alternative materials beyond those with which she was most familiar. She expressed interest in multimedia art and expanded her comfort on the ETC from gravitating primarily toward cognitive materials to other materials that enabled access to sensory, affective, kinesthetic, and creative outcomes (Hinz, 2019).

Art therapy supported Rikah in realizing how to actualize her long-term goal. She gained additional insight about how she became emotionally activated or triggered and experienced symptoms of anxiety and depression. This was accomplished by observing and documenting her day-to-day experiences in her journal. Additional knowledge about Cognitive Behavioral Therapy (CBT) and Acceptance and Commitment Therapy (ACT) principles helped Rikah achieve strategies for coping (Beck, 2020; Harris, 2019). Rikah learned that she was privileging distraction as her primary form of coping with distress. Through therapy, she diversified and showed an understanding of a multi-modal approach to distress tolerance. Rikah mapped out a physical fitness plan that she could use when feeling distress or disconnection. She also used a bullet journal format to accompany the fitness plan with nutrition and sleep hygiene guidelines. Rikah expressed an interest in learning yoga and found that this could be a platform for meeting people. She also did research about surrounding places of worship to find a location that would enable her to connect with a church community.

Later in therapy when Rikah's distress was reduced and her coping skills were improved, she expressed an interest in further processing the breakup from her ex-girlfriend. She also expressed an interest in gaining support around understanding her sexual orientation. She said she had gained an understanding that she was experiencing a sense of self-isolation since the breakup and wanted to improve her connection with others who were also questioning their sexual orientation. Rikah and I leaned into concepts of grief, and she was able to consider the reaction to the breakup as a grief response. This supported an expansion in coping skills and strategies for reaching out to others who had gone through similar experiences. I brought in concepts related to identity development to help Rikah explore aspects of herself. There was a focus on inner and outer work in art-making to illuminate how Rikah felt she was keeping important components of self to herself. This exploration process lent itself to discussing concepts of stigma, racism, sexism, and homophobia. Rikah resonated with the ability to create a collage mask using imagery to represent how she saw her inner identity and what she presented outwardly. This exploration strengthened insight that encouraged Rikah's ability to identify strategies for practicing authenticity and connecting with others who had similar interests and identities.

Outcomes

After attending 17 individual therapy sessions, Rikah and I agreed that it was time for termination. Rikah was confident in her help-seeking skills and her ability to seek out support through her family and newly developed social circle. At discharge, I provided Rikah with local referral resources and discussed options for re-activating services in CAPS if a future need occurred. We reviewed Rikah's trajectory through beginning, middle, and ending therapy as a means of reflecting on her progress. Rikah identified what she would like to continue to work on and said that making art had become a key component of her self-care repertoire. At the conclusion of therapy, Rikah completed a final OQ®-45.2 Therapeutic Alliance (TA) questionnaire where she provided feedback about our rapport; her score was 55/55. Throughout treatment, the scores on the TA averaged between 53–55, suggesting consistent strength in the alliance between client and art therapist.

During art therapy treatment, there was a reduction in quantitative assessment scores, suggesting improved well-being and decreased distress. Rikah's OQ®-45.2 score was reduced by 20 points, from 83 to 63, from beginning therapy to ending therapy. A 16-point reduction is considered clinically significant. Accompanying scores for the GAD-7 and PHQ-9 also reduced. I did not re-administer the PCL-5 since trauma was ruled out during the diagnostic process.

Rikah self-reported a higher level of well-being and satisfaction with her social role and interpersonal relationships. She indicated that she wanted to continue to focus on aspects of her identity, especially as an African American student attending a Predominantly White Institution (PWI) for her university experience. She indicated a level of improved satisfaction in her ability to cope with emotional distress and less intense episodes of anxiety or depression. She felt the origin of the increases in anxiety and depression were from adjusting to college. Rikah continued to perform well academically. She noted improvements in her daily functioning, including improved nutrition, sleep hygiene, and physical activity. I agreed with Rikah's self-assessment of overall improvement and encouraged her to self-monitor for a resurgence in symptoms so she could re-initiate therapy if necessary.

Conclusion

Young adulthood is a fertile ground for developmental transitions from adolescence to middle adulthood (Kuther, 2019). College counseling centers can serve as a pathway to support individuation, identity development, reconciliation, and integration of past experiences. The use of art materials with Rikah provided additional expressive pathways for her to build skills, expand her emotional regulation, and to develop insight into strengths and abilities. Art therapists interested in working with young adults in college counseling need to be skilled in developmental theory, college student development theory, culturally sensitive counseling, and assessment. There are a variety of mental health concerns that can emerge for the first time in young adulthood (Kuther, 2019). Art therapists who have a generalist approach to diagnosing will find that they will be well served in understanding the unique experiences that emerging adults have when enrolled in an institution of higher education.

SHARING A COMMON GROUND: ART THERAPY WITH A YOUNG ADULT

AMANDA LIGHTNER

Setting

The following case study was conducted in a private practice setting. The private practice is in the Midwest, in a capital city, near the downtown area. The practice is in a Victorian era house. Approximately a dozen therapists make up this co-op-style practice in which each therapist practices out of a room in the house. The room this case study was conducted in is a medium-sized room with wood floors and large windows.

The space of the room contains an art table which can seat up to four people, a comfortable chair, a locked file cabinet to secure documents and an additional large, locked cabinet for clients' artwork. A wheeled cart with a range of art materials is available for participants. Materials include: oil pastels, watercolor pencils, markers, and crayons; colored markers, pens, and pencils; graphite pencils (2H-6B); glue sticks; gum, pink, and artist kneaded erasers; a range of papers including, mixed media, watercolor, drawing, tracing, colored construction and colored tissue paper; small to medium size canvases; watercolor and tempera paints; collage materials, and polymer clay and tools. A sink was accessible in a nearby bathroom for water.

This case study, like other clients I work with in private practice, was self-referral. I receive an email or a telephone call directly from the potential client requesting to meet for therapy. I provide assessment, individual therapy, and treatment and discharge plans for my clients. During the therapeutic engagement, I coordinate care with other providers. A termination or closing session is included, so referrals and recommendations can be provided.

Approaches

Psychodynamic psychotherapy with a lens on early relational trauma and working with individuals who experience dissociation are explored in the case study. Psychodynamic psychotherapy focuses on a client's affect and expression of emotion. A therapist encourages exploration of a client's emotions and supports a client to describe and put words to their feelings. An exploration of the client's attempts to avoid distressing thoughts and feelings is encouraged by the therapist. A therapist supports the identification of recurring themes and patterns in the client's life. A discussion of the client's past experiences, especially early attachment relationships and how these relationships affect a client's current relationships is encouraged. A therapist supports the examination of the therapeutic relationship, specifically the transference and countertransference. The therapist supports a client to explore what is meaningful to them. A client is encouraged to speak freely with no prior agenda prescribed by the therapist (Shedlar, 2010).

Dissociation is a response to trauma. Dissociation provides an escape when there was no other source of escape available (Bromberg, 1998). In cases of early relational trauma, dissociation may be used by children as a means to respond to a dysregulated caregiver. I have found an openness in the therapeutic relationship to be a meaningful aspect of working with clients who have early relational trauma. As my client's art therapist, I provide symbolic framing and reflection of their experience and refrain from imposing my bias and general sentiments. These symbolic frames act as doorways to create a relational space for clients to escape through if needed. It is a means of interpersonal safety, as we move through the space of relational work together.

Case Study

Henry was a young adult who recently graduated from university. Art and music had a strong pull on this young man. He studied visual art at university and was employed as a musician. He was the middle child in his family. His father was a retired veteran and a fundamentalist preacher. He attempted to follow in the footsteps of his mother and sister who were both teachers. His work as an art teacher was not successful due to the interpersonal demands. During our work together, he would later disclose early relational trauma with his family of origin which appeared to affect his present ability to feel safe within his relationships.

Throughout the course of our work together, Henry remained in the care of his psychiatrist whom he met virtually. Henry had prior outpatient and inpatient mental health care. His prior hospitalizations were for manic episodes with psychosis. During our early time together, the psychiatrist who was on the treatment team diagnosed Henry with an anxiety disorder. His art therapy treatment was focused on this diagnosis. In later sessions, Henry was diagnosed and treated for a mood disorder. During the course of his art therapy treatment, I observed Henry show severe anxiety, dissociative states, manic episodes, and to report significant sleep disturbance.

Intake Sessions

Henry arrived at his first session carrying a number of objects. An item from his collection began to tumble from his grip, which he quickly scooped up before it hit the floor. I told him that I was impressed by his quick response and noticed he carried so much with him today. He agreed with an affirmative chuckle, as he appeared to appreciate my symbolic framing of his experience.

He was a stylish young man, with a slender frame and a tall looming presence. He collapsed into my office chair and forcibly began his session with a loud, disorganized account of the many difficult people in his life including family members, bandmates, roommates, peers, teachers, and colleagues. I attended to his irritable account with a calm and steady presence. During our first meeting, and throughout our work together, I was careful to use his words to reflect how difficult these people were in his life.

During our first meeting, he presented a disorganized and dysregulated self-state. I provided attunement to his affective states by offering reflection of his affect and his narratives in the moment. Clients with early relational trauma like Henry are not able to talk about what happened, they must show you. They must process their trauma or reenact their past experiences in front of you, which is called enactment, a form of dissociation used by individuals who have experienced and have unresolved early relational dynamics (Bromberg, 2011).

Being with Henry as he was meant that he was allowed to bring what he wanted to his art therapy sessions, both in what he wanted to talk about and what he wanted to show me. He brought art journals with sketches which he described to have been further developed and shown in a public setting during university. I wanted to know more about his sketches, which seemed an important and developed part of him.

Henry seemed to feel safe and well-regulated relating to me as a fellow artist. I stood ready to engage with his transference, as seeing me as an artist like himself, allowed for the establishment of rapport. While we explored the visual language of his art journals, I provided attunement, validation, and maintained a stance of consistent curiosity. Over time, he disclosed painful childhood memories with his family of origin.

Henry described a father who was threatening and forced his ideas upon him. A father who did not acknowledge Henry's feelings throughout his development. The psychodynamics of parental nonrecognition of emotions plays a role in the formation of dissociative structures in adults (Bromberg, 2011). It became apparent that Henry was affected by early deficits in his early relationship with his father. The objective with Henry would be one of constructing lost dialogues of his emotional states that were neglected in his early relationships (Robbins, 1987).

Early Sessions

In the continuum of early art therapy sessions, Henry stopped bringing his art journals. There appeared to be a shift in our work together as he articulated his thoughts and emotions in the moment. As this shift occurred, he chose to work with graphite pencils which

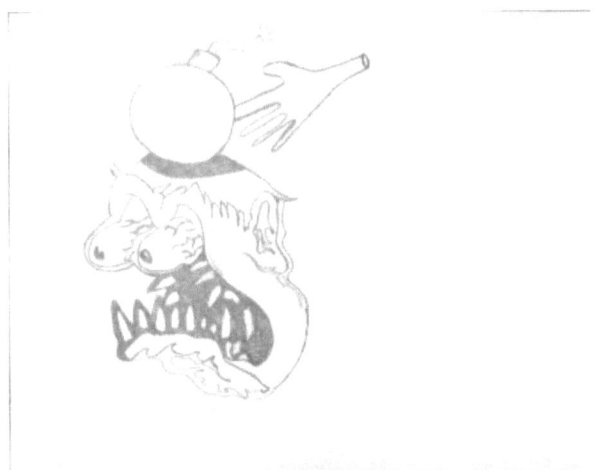

Figure 3.10 Henry's First Drawing in Session

provided a high level of control for him. He started the work shown below (Figure 3.10) with a graphite pencil on drawing paper. He applied much pressure to show me a threatening interpersonal experience with his father. He showed me what it was like to be with his father as he talked in a loud and booming voice. He described a father who was intimidating, threatening, and highly reactive.

In his drawing, a head dissociated from its body floats on an invisible plane. The affect on the face of the disconnected figure appears surprised and terrified as the bomb is deposited into it. The dissociated figure shows the internalized pressure from the reactive material, as evidenced by the eyes bulging out from his head. The drawing reflected the young man who drew it and his early childhood experiences with a father who symbolically dropped reactive material that later would release its energy to inflict damage internally.

His drawing quality showed implied energy as his pencil would impulsively and forcibly make contact with the paper. His pencil broke as he created the image and I felt frightened by Henry. I asked him if he would like another pencil and moved on quickly from the experience. I was not able to reflect this frightening moment back to him and instead worked towards managing the relational experience as a substitute for participating in it.

The art was used as a way to mask countertransference reactions and to keep Henry at a comfortable distance (Robbins, 1987). I felt frightened by Henry, and found myself distancing myself and restricting my affect. It was an impossible attempt to hide my strong feelings in the face of Henry's emotional dysregulation. I chose to focus on his use of art form to protect us both from his potentially explosive emotions.

Later Sessions

During his therapy sessions Henry was frequently agitated, irritated, and explosive, which resulted in highly charged interpersonal expression. I wanted to work towards a less threatening way for Henry to explore his strong emotions within the therapeutic relationship. I asked if he would like to create a landscape. A landscape would offer a healing dimension

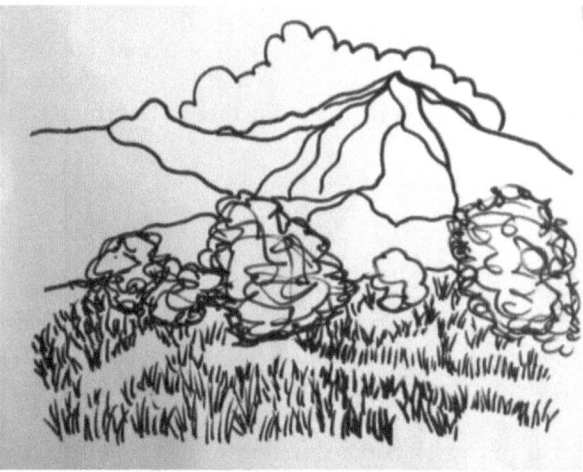

Figure 3.11 Henry's Landscape

of the integration of self-states within the page of the drawing. As Robbins (1987) cogently describes, the art becomes a container for the dysregulated client to organize dysregulated self-states within the therapeutic process (Bromberg, 2011).

Henry engaged with his drawing and used black markers to construct his landscape (Figure 3.11). The foreground of the landscape is covered with dark and low thick foliage. I wanted to know more about that part of his image. He shared that a person could get stuck in this part of the image and I stated I imagined it might be difficult for the viewer to see the person who was stuck.

Henry shared that it was toxic and dark, as he became tearful and frightened. I sat with him, acknowledged his tearfulness, and how difficult it was to look at this part. He started to sob. I sat with him while he experienced his emotions. He described that part of the image as having low energy. He related what it might feel like to move around in the image, describing further low energy aspects of himself, such as depressed movement and speech behaviors. I reflected how meaningful it was for him to share these difficult parts that felt stuck, the part that is toxic, dark, and alone.

We moved our focus to the horizon, far from the viewer were high peaks, which appeared disconnected from the lower landscape of the image. He shared, this part of the image could be dangerous and formed a feeling of being distant, almost like a god amongst the clouds. He said it would be difficult to come down from this part of the drawing and that he liked the feeling of being up there.

Outcomes

Henry reported a decrease in relational difficulties near the end of our time together. He verbalized feeling more understood and had a closer relationship with his partner. He showed progress from pre-constructed art works and isolated communications to communications within a shared context. He showed an observable increase in the ability to relate with me in-the-moment.

Henry engaged in art therapy for nearly ten months. He let me know he planned to be on the road again soon with his band. A closing session was set up so that Henry and I could say goodbye and review all his good work. We closed our work together as he remained in the care of his psychiatrist.

Conclusion

Art was a way to initiate contact and establish rapport with Henry. Art forms served as containers to work through charged interpersonal dynamics, as well as to organize and integrate self-states. Artworks become meaningful extensions of the therapeutic relationship that held difficult transference and countertransference reactions rooted in a client's early experiences.

During our last session, Henry said that our work had a different feeling than previous therapeutic work. I asked if he might say more, and he shared that "it was like they [previous therapists] were sending greeting cards all sharing a similar sentiment". I was touched by the insight and eloquence of this summary of our work together.

In my experience, the sentiments Henry referred to were those of his previous therapist's attempts to define his reality in their own words. It was not the objective to construct, nor define reality for Henry. It became clear to me the importance of using an art form to actively engage with Henry's internal self and object world. Henry's landscape provided a safe relational space to witness and acknowledge what is meaningful within the shared context of a common ground.

References

Adams, E. (2006). *Drawing insights*. The Campaign for Drawing.

American Psychiatric Association Publishing. (2022). *Diagnostic and statistical manual of mental disorders: Dsm-5-Tr*. American Psychiatric Association.

Arnett, J. J. (2016). *Human development: A cultural approach*. Pearson.

Barresi, M., & Gilbert, S. (2023). *Developmental biology* (13th ed.). Oxford University Press.

Bat Or, M., & Zilcha-Mano, S. (2018). The art therapy working alliance inventory: The development of a measure. *International Journal of Art Therapy, 24*(2), 76–87.

Beck, J. S. (2020). *Cognitive behavior therapy* (3rd ed.). Guilford Press.

Bennink, J., Gussak, D., & Skrowran, M. (2003). The role of the art therapist in a juvenile justice setting. *The Arts in Psychotherapy, 30*(3), 163–173.

Berberian, M., & Davis, B. (2020). *Art therapy practices for resilient youth: A strengths-based approach to at-promise children and adolescents*. Routledge.

Betts, D. J. (2003). Developing a projective drawing test: Experiences with the face stimulus assessment (FSA). *Art Therapy: Journal of the American Art Therapy Association, 20*, 77–82.

Borden, W. (2009). *Contemporary psychodynamic theory and practice*. Lyceum Books.

Bosgraaf, L., Spreen, M., Pattiselanno, K., & van Hooren, S. (2020). Art therapy for psychosocial problems in children and adolescents: A systematic narrative review on art therapeutic means and forms of expression, therapist behavior, and supposed mechanisms of change. *Frontiers in Psychology, 11*.

Bowlby, J. (1969). *Attachment and loss* (volume 1). Basic Books.

Bromberg, P. M. (1998). *Standing in the spaces: Essays on clinical process, trauma and dissociation*. Psychology Press.

Bromberg, P. (2011). *Awakening the dreamer*. Routledge.

Carolan, R., & Betts, D. (2015). *The adult coloring book phenomenon: The American Art Therapy Association weighs in*. https://www.3blmedia.com/news/adult-coloring-book-phenomenon

Cashin, A., Browne, G., Bradbury, J., & Mulder, A. (2013). The effectiveness of narrative therapy with young people with autism. *Journal of Child and Adolescent Psychiatric Nursing*, 26(1), 32–41.

Chickering, A. (1981). *The modern American college: Responding to the new realities of diverse students and a changing society*. Jossey-Bass.

Christie, D., & Viner, R. (2005). ABC of adolescence: Adolescent development. *BMJ* (Clinical research ed.), 330(7486), 301–304.

Clark, S. M. (2017). *DBT-informed art therapy: Mindfulness, cognitive behavior therapy, and the creative process*. Jessica Kingsley Publishers.

Cohen, B. M., Mills, A., & Kijak, A. K. (1994). An introduction to the Diagnostic Drawing Series: A standardized tool for diagnostic and clinical use. *Art Therapy: Journal of the American Art Therapy Association*, 11(2), 105–110.

Cozolino, L. (2017). *The neuroscience of psychotherapy: Healing the social brain* (3rd ed.). W.W. Norton & Co.

Crane, D. (2000). *Fashion and its social agendas: Class, gender, and identity in clothing*. The University of Chicago Press.

Dunne, P. (2016). *The narrative therapist and the arts* (2nd ed.). Possibilities Press.

Epp, K. M. (2008, January). Outcome-based evaluation of a social skills program using art therapy and group therapy for children on the autism spectrum. *Children & Schools*, 30(1), 27–36.

Erikson, E. (1967). *Identity and the life cycle*. W.W. Norton & Company.

Evans, K., & Dubowski, J. (2007). *Art therapy with children on the autistic spectrum: Beyond words*. Jessica Kinsley Publishers.

Foucault, M. (1966). *Les Mots et les choses: Une archéologie des sciences humaines*. Gallimard.

Freud, A. (1958). Adolescence. *The Psychoanalytic Study of the Child*, 13(1), 255–278.

Gabriels, R. L. (2003). Art therapy with children who have autism and their families. In C. A. Malchiodi (Ed.). *Handbook of art therapy* (pp. 193–206). Guilford Publications.

Gussak, D. (2016). Art therapy in the prison milieu. In D. E. Gussak & M. Rosal (Eds). *The Wiley handbook of art therapy* (pp. 478–486). John Wiley & Sons, Ltd.

Gussak, D., & Cohen-Liebman, M. S. (2001). Investigation vs. intervention: Forensic art therapy and art therapy in forensic settings. *American Journal of Art Therapy*, 40(2).

Hall, S. (2004). *Adolescence: Its psychology and its relations to physiology, anthropology, sociology, sex, crime, religion and education*. Elibron Classics.

Harris, R. (2019). *ACT made simple*. New Harbinger.

Henley, D. (2012). *Foreword to the first edition*. In B. L. Moon (Ed.). *The dynamics of art as therapy with adolescents* (2nd ed., pp. v–vii). Charles C. Thomas.

Hinz, L. D. (2019). *Expressive therapies continuum: A framework for using art in therapy* (2nd ed.). Routledge.

Hope, G. (2008). *Thinking and learning through drawing*. Sage.

Hopperstad, M. H. (2010). Studying meaning in children's drawings. *Journal of Early Childhood Literacy*, 10(4), 430–452.

Johnson, D. R. (1989). On the therapeutic action of the creative arts therapies: A psychodynamic model. *The Arts in Psychotherapy*, 25(2), 85–99.

Jordan, J. (2017). *Relational-cultural therapist (Theories of psychotherapy series)* (2nd ed.). American Psychological Association.

Kagin, S. L., & Lusebrink, V. B. (1978). The expressive therapies continuum. *Art Psychotherapy*, 5(4), 171–180.

Katzman, M. A., Bilkey, T. S., Chokka, P. R., Fallu, A., & Klassen, L. J. (2017). Adult ADHD and comorbid disorders: Clinical implications of a dimensional approach. *BMC Psychiatry, 17*(1).

Kennedy, H. G. (2022). Models of care in forensic psychiatry. *BJPsych Advances, 28*(1), 46–59.

Kohlberg, L. (1969). Stage and sequence: The cognitive-developmental approach to socialization. In D. A. Goslin (Ed.). *Handbook of socialization* (pp. 347–480). Ran McNally.

Kramer, E. (1993). *Art as therapy with children* (2nd ed.). Magnolia Street Publishers.

Kuther, T. L. (2019). *Lifespan development lives in context* (2nd ed.). Sage Publications.

Liebmann, M. (2004). *Art therapy for groups: A handbook of themes and exercises.* Brunner Routledge.

Linehan, M. M. (2015). *DBT skills training manual* (2nd ed.). Guilford Press.

Linesch, D. G. (1988). *Adolescent art therapy* (1st ed.). Routledge.

Lowenfeld, V., & Brittain, W. L. (1987). *Creative and mental growth* (8th ed.). Macmillan.

Luthar, S. S., & Barkin, S. H. (2012). Are affluent youth truly "at risk"? Vulnerability and resilience across three diverse samples. *Development and Psychopathology, 24*(2), 429–449.

Martin, N. (2008). Assessing portrait drawings created by children and adolescents with autism spectrum disorder. *Art Therapy: Journal of the American Art Therapy Association, 25*(1), 15–23.

Martin, N. (2009). *Art as an early intervention tool for children with autism.* Jessica Kingsley.

Maslow, A. H. (1970). *Motivation and personality.* Harper & Row.

Matthews, D., Cryer-Coupet, Q., & Degirmencioglu, N. (2021). I wear, therefore I am: Investigating sneakerhead culture, social identity, and brand preference among men. *Fashion and Textiles, 8*(1).

Miller, W. R., & Rose, G. S. (2009). Toward a theory of motivational interviewing. *American Psychologist, 64*(6), 527.

Mircher Clotilde, C. C., Marey, I., Rebillat, A.-S., Cretu, L., Milenko, E., Conte, M., Sturtz, F., Rethore, M.-O., & Ravel, A. (2017). Acute regression in young people with Down Syndrome. *Brain Sciences, 7,* 57.

Moon, B. L. (2012). *The dynamics of art as therapy with adolescents* (2nd ed.). Charles C. Thomas.

Moon, C. H. (2016). Open studio approach to art therapy. In D. E. Gussak & M. L. Rosal (Eds). *The Wiley handbook of art therapy* (pp. 112–121). John Wiley & Sons, Ltd.

Mori, S., & Goldbeter-Merinfeld, E. (2019). *Pratique de la thérapie narrative: comprendre et appliquer.* De Boeck Supérieur.

Nadeau-Cossette, A. (2012). *L'intégration socio-scolaire des adolescents immigrants* [mémoire de maîtrise, Université de Laval]. Dépôt institutionnel de l'Université Laval.

Osborne, J. (2003). Art and the child with autism: Therapy or education? *Early Child Development and Care, 173*(4), 411–423.

Piaget, J., & Inhelder, B. (1969). *The psychology of a child.* Routledge.

Riccardi, M. (2023, February). *The Art Therapist Self-Inquiry (ATSI).* World Art Therapy Virtual Conference. https://www.artstherapies.org/course/world-art-therapy-conference

Ricoeur, P. (1991). *Temps et récit.* Ed. du Seuil.

Riley, S. (1999). *Contemporary art therapy with adolescents.* Jessica Kingsley.

Robbins, A. (1987). *The artist as therapist.* Human Sciences Press, Inc.

Rogers, C. R. (1979). The foundations of the person-centered approach. *Education, 100*(2), 98–107.

Rogers, N. (2001). Person-centered expressive arts therapy: A path to wholeness. In J. A. Rubin (Ed.). *Approaches to art therapy: Theory & technique* (2nd ed., pp. 163–177). Brunner-Routledge.

Rogers, S. (2006). Evidence-based interventions for language development in young children with autism. In T. Charman & W. Stone (Eds.). *Social & communication development in autism spectrum disorders: Early identification, diagnosis, & intervention* (pp. 143–179). Guilford.

Sharma, S., Arain, M., Mathur, P., Rais, A., Nel, W., Sandhu, R., Haque, M., & Johal, L. (2013). Maturation of the adolescent brain. *Neuropsychiatric Disease and Treatment, 9,* 449.

Shedlar, J. (2010). The efficacy of psychodynamic psychotherapy. *American Psychologist, 65*(2), 98–109.

Sholt, M., & Gavron, T. (2006). Therapeutic qualities of clay-work in art therapy and psychotherapy: A review. *Art Therapy: American Journal of Art Therapy, 23*(2), 66–72.

Shukla, A., Choudhari, S. G., Gaidhane, A. M., & Quazi Syed, Z. (2022). Role of art therapy in the promotion of Mental Health: A critical review. *Cureus, 14*(8),e28026.

Siegel, D. J. (2012). *The developing mind: How relationships and the brain interact to shape who we are.* Guilford Press.

Siegfried, C., & Wuttke, E. (2021). What influences the financial literacy of young adults? A combined analysis of socio-demographic characteristics and delay of gratification. *Frontiers in Psychology,12,* 663254.

Sue, D., & Sue, D. (2013). *Counseling the culturally diverse: Theory and practice.* John Wiley.

Sue, D. W., Sue, D., Neville, H. A., & Smith, L. (2022). *Counseling the culturally diverse: Theory and practice.* John Wiley & Sons.

Teoli, L. (2021). Companioning artmaking: Creating art alongside clients in group art therapy. *The Arts in Psychotherapy, 75*(1), 101806.

Valdivia, I. M., Schneider, B. H., & Carrasco, C. V. (2016). School adjustment and friendship quality of first- and second-generation adolescent immigrants to Spain as a function of acculturation. *Journal of Adolescent Research, 31,* 750–777.

Wallace, S., Coleman, M., & Bailey, A. (2008). An investigation of basic facial expression recognition in autism spectrum disorders. *Cognition and Emotion, 22,* 1353–1380.

Waller, D. (2006). Art therapy for children: How it leads to change. *Clinical Child Psychology and Psychiatry, 11,* 271–282.

Weissman, M. M., Markowitz, J. C., & Klerman, G. (2008). *Comprehensive guide to interpersonal psychotherapy.* Basic Books.

Wetherby, A. (2006). Understanding and measuring social communication in children with autism spectrum disorders. In T. Charman & W. Stone (Eds). *Social & communication development in autism spectrum disorders: Early identification, diagnosis, & intervention* (pp. 3–34). Guilford.

White, M. (2007). *Maps of narrative practice.* W.W. Norton & Company.

Chapter 4

Mid Adulthood

Midlife is a period of psychological and emotional development during which individuals may experience desires for change.

Introduction

Developmental Markers

Between ages 27 and 60, individuals continue to experience substantial development across various domains shaping their identities, relationships, and perspectives. During these years, adults are seen as at peak performance. However, physical changes such as a gradual decline in muscle mass, bone density, and metabolic rate begin in the late 20s and continue through midlife (Barresi & Gilbert, 2023). Vision is often impacted in the 40s and 50s. Menopause for women and andropause for men occur, marking significant hormonal shifts (Barresi & Gilbert, 2023).

Socially, healthy adults have separated from their parents and have embarked on developing an independent life. During these years, adults tend to establish and refine long-term relationships. Marriage, parenthood, and career advancement characterize this period (Lachman, 2004), as well as expansion of social networks and an emphasis on generativity and contributing to the welfare of future generations (Erikson, 1967). Adults learn to balance career commitments, family responsibilities, and personal pursuits while navigating societal expectations and cultural norms (Lachman, 2004). They experience increased emotional stability and a better understanding of emotions along with enhanced emotional regulation and resilience gained from overcoming challenges and navigating life experiences. This leads to enhanced moral reasoning and ethical decision-making (Kohlberg, 1969). Increased awareness and engagement in social issues can also lead to community involvement and civic engagement during these years (Erikson, 1967).

Cognitive skills continue to develop throughout adulthood and expertise is common in one's profession or area of specialization (Jenkins et al., 2008). Adults have increased ability for reflective thinking, wisdom, and integration of knowledge from life experiences. Achieving a sense of flow in adulthood can be found in work, hobbies, and personal pursuits (Csikszentmihalyi, 1997). Engaging in activities that align with one's skills and interests can enhance the likelihood of experiencing flow. Contrary to the belief that creativity declines with age, research suggests that adults can continue to enhance and express their creative abilities (Cohen, 2006). Continued learning, exposure to new experiences, and a

DOI: 10.4324/9781003324805-5

willingness to take risks contribute to fostering creativity in adulthood guided by a wealth of life experiences (Kohlberg, 1969).

Setbacks

Between ages 27 and 60, individuals may face various setbacks that can impede their developmental trajectory. Career stagnation, job insecurity, or unexpected career changes can lead to stress and dissatisfaction (Jenkins et al., 2008). Financial setbacks, such as debt accumulation or economic downturns, can affect long-term planning and cause distress (Jenkins et al., 2008). Societal pressures regarding success, achievement, and societal norms might create feelings of inadequacy or failure (Berg et al., 2010). Balancing work, family responsibilities, and caregiving duties can lead to stress and burnout and can lead to relationship changes like marital conflicts, divorce, or breakups that might impact emotional well-being and stability (Jenkins et al., 2008).

Midlife is a period of psychological and emotional development during which individuals may experience desires for change (Cohen, 2006). These times are often characterized by a reassessment of life goals, values, and achievements. Onsets of health issues, chronic conditions, or disabilities can significantly impact daily functioning and quality of life (Barresi & Gilbert, 2023). Coping with physical changes, menopause, or andropause might affect self-image and emotional health. Reevaluation of life goals and meaning are associated with midlife transitions and can be challenging (Erikson, 1967).

Navigating cultural expectations and generational differences can be challenging (Berg et al., 2010). Social equality and understandings of social structures and disadvantages also have bearings on the psychological health of adults during these years (Umberson et al., 2014). These challenges can significantly impact individuals' well-being and require supportive interventions or coping strategies to navigate effectively through this stage of life.

Case Studies

The case studies in this chapter include clients in their late 20s through their 60s. The art therapy settings included working bedside in hospitals with in-patients and chairside at an infusion clinic with out-patients. Other settings included private practice for individual and family therapy and at an art therapy open studio for groups. One client was able to receive art therapy services throughout her medical treatments, starting in the hospital and later as an out-patient at all the other settings listed above. The duration of services for these clients ranged between five months to five years. There were major medical issues for some of them, including cancer or a mental health diagnosis. Other clients came to therapy after a failed suicide attempt, a serious accident that left them in a wheelchair, and issues surrounding childhood sexual and physical abuse in which one client reported a history of extreme dissociation.

Working with this population included using therapeutic approaches and models and focused on theories of practice. Approaches included Person-Centered Therapy (Rogers, 1979, 2001) with Internal Family Systems (IFS; Schwartz, 1995), the Expressive Therapies Continuum (ETC; Hinz, 2015), as well as mindfulness, trauma-sensitive (King, 2016), and integrative body-comparison (Hass-Cohen et al., 2022) based therapeutic models. Theories included Existential (Yalom, 1980), Constructivism (Piaget & Inhelder, 1969), Maslow's (1943, 1970) Developmental Hierarchy of Needs, stages of psychosocial development (Erikson, 1967), Chakras (Wauters, 1997), and Archetypal Psychology (Schmanke, 2018). Journals were also used with this adult age group. Clients reported they found value in journaling as a safe way to express their strong thoughts and feelings while coming to terms with their past and present experiences. Other clients viewed journals as a tool that recorded personal histories of healing and recovery.

In midlife many seek to redefine themselves by returning to school, pursuing new careers, finding new spouses, and in some cases pursuing dreams from their youth. It is an age of significant productivity, especially for those who work in creative fields (Wallas, 1926). It is a time of reevaluation and change as seen in the case studies in this chapter.

The changes for some of the clients were prompted by outside circumstances like an accident or a serious illness. Other changes came from within when clients' present circumstances were severely impaired by painful past experiences, or when clients came to the realization that a life is a finite measurement of time and, therefore, dreams and goals are to be met now rather than later.

As these clients worked with their therapists, many of them made progress in redefining themselves beyond their identities as a cancer survivor, an accident victim, or an abused child. By giving clients an understanding of constructivist concepts (Gergen, 2015), clients gained insight into how they could reinvent themselves and alter their purpose in life. Clients were able to come to terms and assimilate their past without allowing it to solely define who they are today.

Midlife is a time when self-care is important (Rura, 2020). In one case study, a community center serving impoverished, middle-aged women, established an online art therapy wellness group. The main purpose of the group was to prevent potential difficulties caused by being isolated during the pandemic. This goal was accomplished, and the group also helped these women establish a support network in the neighborhood. In the group, they discussed new purposes and goals for themselves as roles in families began to change. The program continues today as art therapy is now recognized as a valued resource at the center.

During midlife, thoughts of mortality prompted others to take on the role of a mentor for the next generation of leaders, and to think about the legacy they leave behind when they are gone (Erikson, 1967). Therapy with this age group was complex. It included encouraging self-care and altering the narratives of their lives, after they experienced significant and painful changes. Therapy also helped clients find a new purpose to pursue in the second half of their lives.

BURNING WITH SHAME: AN ADULT DEALING WITH SEXUAL ASSAULT TRAUMA FROM CHILDHOOD

KATHERINE JACKSON

Intake

Jenny was a 28-year-old heterosexual Caucasian woman of Irish descent who self-referred to my private practice. She had recently been married to her high school sweetheart and did not have children. Jenny was college educated and taught second grade at a local elementary school. She initially came to art therapy specifically to work on her overwhelming feelings of shame, guilt, and depression, which were beginning to complicate her ability to be fully present in her marriage. She frequently had bouts of crying and was no longer interested in physical intimacy with her husband. Jenny was the oldest of two girls and came from an intact family. Her parents were Irish Catholic and had immigrated in the 1980s due to political turmoil in Ireland. They had encouraged cultural and religious beliefs on Jenny and her sister by attending weekly Mass and providing a Catholic private school education. Jenny had mixed feelings about her faith and considered herself more spiritual in nature.

After the intake, Jenny revealed that she had been sexually assaulted by a classmate in high school when she was 15 years old. She believed that the sexual assault was most likely her fault, because she did not scream or fight the young man off. She was able to connect her shame, guilt, depression, and loss of sexual interest in her husband with this event without prompting, which was a strength of insight. Jenny reported that she had attempted to tell her mother when the event happened and her mother suggested she just move on and said, "boys will be boys". She told no one else and was now having memories and flashbacks. This "boys will be boys" statement was deeply offensive and hurtful for Jenny, but due to her naivete about sexual assault, she buried it inside her psyche, and shortly thereafter met her high school boyfriend whom she later married.

A wellness, strengths-based approach was chosen as the best approach to art therapy. The intent was to integrate trauma work and psychoeducation about childhood sexual abuse. Jenny was in the *New Couples* stage in the Family Life Cycle (McGoldrick et al., 2008), and the *Intimacy versus Isolation* stage in Erikson's (1967) developmental stages.

Early Sessions

At the first art therapy session, Jenny and I made a treatment plan to work on her suppressed trauma of sexual assault, and address feelings of shame, guilt, and depression. Psychoeducation would play a role in helping Jenny learn about trauma and her feelings. I gave Jenny large drawing paper and chalk pastels. I wanted to use the *Affective/Perceptual* level in the ETC (Hinz, 2019), with the intention of expressing feelings. I chose materials that were not too fluid, fearing that too much affective output might shut Jenny down emotionally. In her first image (Figure 4.1), she drew what she called "Pandora's Box" and said she was afraid of what might be revealed once she began expressing herself in therapy. The open box revealed round, billowing, organic shapes that were colored yellow and red. Jenny also drew lightning shapes to show her fear of a metaphorical "storm" about to be unleashed. She expressed that most of her life she had wanted to be a "good girl" by going to church, making good grades, getting a good job, getting married, and having children. She was deeply concerned about her lack of physical intimacy with her husband and was convinced it was related to unresolved sexual trauma. I attempted to normalize her feelings and suggested we take therapy slowly, letting the process unfold as we worked together. I suggested some breathing techniques, such as box-breathing, based on exhaling and inhaling four times (Weil, 1999) to help in the event she became anxious as difficult emotions and memories surfaced.

In the next session, Jenny explored masks as a defense. She used masks in order to maintain her façade of being a "good and kind person". Her mask was of a sad face, clownish in nature with shades of blue and gray. I wondered if Jenny was hiding behind her mask as much as she thought. Maybe her feelings were more transparent to others. She later spontaneously drew an image entitled, "Shame Fingers Pointing" (Figure 4.2). Jenny was having

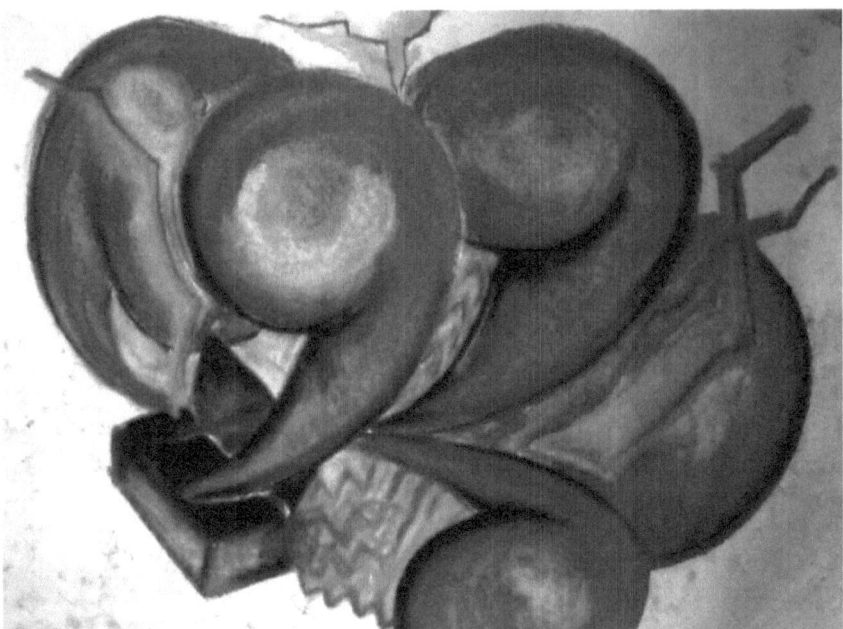

Figure 4.1 Pandora's Box

hyper-critical feelings of shame. She expressed that she felt like a "bad person" because of the sexual assault. In this powerful image, Jenny is surrounded by pointing fingers and she is curled up in a fetal position in the center of the mandala-like shape. I took the opportunity to validate her feelings but also shared psycho-educational information about the fight, flight, and freeze responses which are common in trauma (van der Kolk, 2014). She acknowledged that when the assault occurred, she felt paralyzed and could not move or speak. Jenny had mistakenly thought that because she was literally frozen in her responses that she was a bad person and had somehow let the assault happen. She visibly relaxed in our session once she learned that freezing is a protective response and is common in cases of sexual assault.

Mid-Point Sessions

Over the next several sessions, Jenny continued to use chalk pastels, she loved the fluid nature of the medium and felt she could express herself well. She was able to draw other pictures of her shame and began to see her deep rooted guilt through the eyes of her religious teaching. She drew a powerful image depicting a person on fire running away from a group of judging, black-robed, nondescript, human forms. She entitled this "Burning with Shame" (Figure 4.3). Jenny clearly identified her feelings about her sexual assault, shame, and fear that she was not being a good wife to her husband. From my clinical view, there were many layers of shame and self-judgment that Jenny had been experiencing. Once she began to open her metaphorical Pandora's box, many of the suppressed feelings and hyper self-criticism began to tumble out.

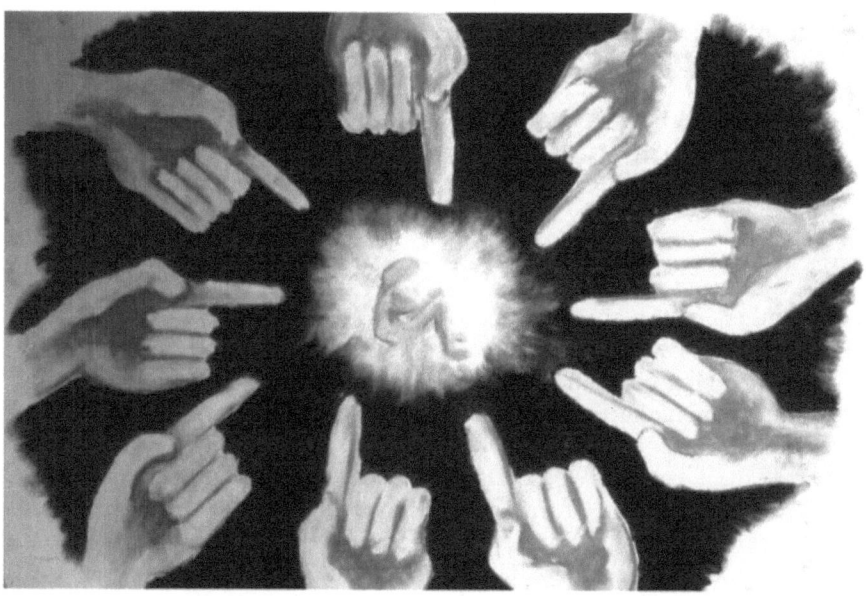

Figure 4.2 Shame Fingers Pointing

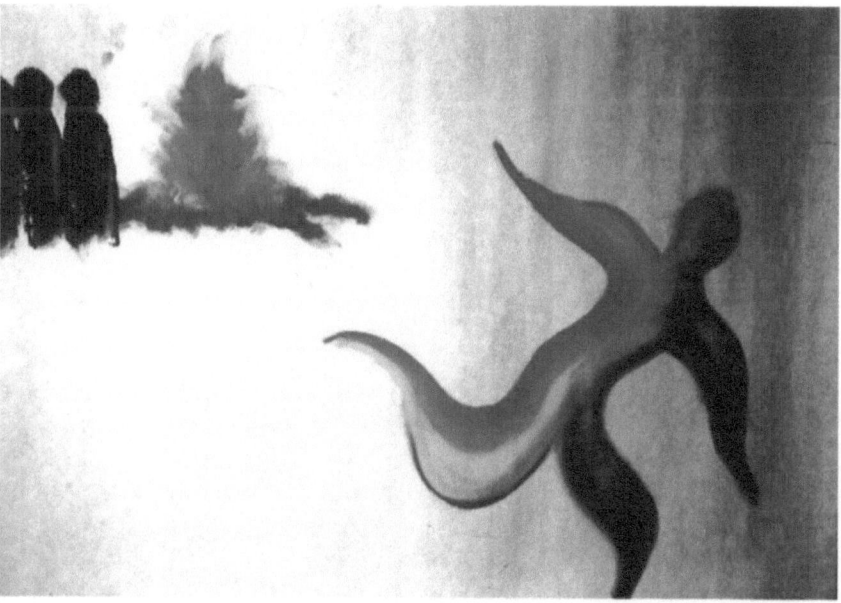

Figure 4.3 Burning with Shame

In subsequent sessions, Jenny began feeling less depressed and lighter as she continued to use art therapy as a safe space to vent and express her innermost feelings. In working with trauma, creative expression through art-making is seen as having the potential to safely bring into awareness, while containing and transforming aspects of personal experience that are hard to access verbally (van der Kolk, 2014). The spontaneous imagery about shame seemed to free up unconscious material, allowing Jenny to give voice to her symbolic imagery and the pain trapped inside.

Termination

Jenny made several other images about shame and judgment over the course of several months. Then impulsively one day she drew a seed pod that was cracking open. She said she had a dream of seeds breaking open and releasing some kind of healing energy. I encouraged Jenny to explore the image further. Dream images and symbols can be harbingers of deep changes occurring in the unconscious (Swan-Foster, 2018). In Figure 4.4, Jenny drew a dark, circular pod shape she named "Seed Opening". Yellow and orange colors escaped from the cracked opening at the top of the seed. The contents of the seed look fiery like molten lava, but for Jenny, it remained a positive image. I was reminded of the symbolism of the Phoenix rising out of the ashes of fire. On one side of the seed were blue swirls, which she said represented blue skies ahead. On the other side were steps, representing her new journey into healing.

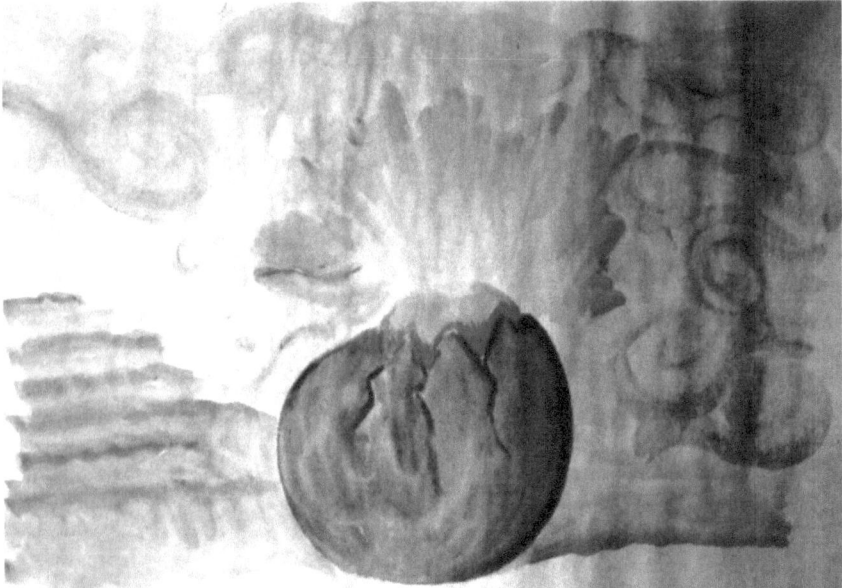

Figure 4.4 Seed Opening

Conclusion

I worked with Jenny for about nine months on a weekly basis. Her transformation was apparent as she reported increased insight, less depression, and no residual feelings of shame and guilt. My hope was that Jenny would come to find meaning in her painful experience and release herself from blame. Through loosely structured art-making, and psychoeducation about trauma and abuse, Jenny was able to find happiness in her relationship with her husband and general satisfaction in her everyday life. As Dollinger et al. (2011) stated, "traumatic experiences can profoundly affect the concept of self and the perceived relation of self to the world outside" (p. 203).

CHALLENGES OF ABILITY: A CLIENT'S STORY

REBECCA REINHOLZ

My Story

I am the third born of four children. My mother works in higher education, and my father is a software engineer. I was diagnosed with Cerebral Palsy at 18 months. We were a middle-class family and I was lucky to have the privileges that I did. I had a good medical team and received timely treatments when they were needed.

Medical treatment has been a part of my life since I can remember. My first surgery was at age four and a half, and then I had more surgeries during eighth grade and the 11th grade. I attended Physical Therapy (PT) until I started first grade and went back to it in seventh grade. I have been in PT consistently ever since. Some abilities wax and wane; for example, my left hand is still not as dexterous as my right. As I've gotten older, I have watched some of my abilities decline. While I walked without any braces or assistance when I was younger, I now wear an ankle brace when I have to walk outside my home and sometimes use a wheelchair to conserve energy and limit pain, giving me more freedom to be out in the community. As my abilities have changed, I have become more aware of the limited accessibility in our community, even over 30 years after the Americans with Disabilities Act was passed. Because of this, I now advocate for accessibility in my community.

As I grew older and came to realize that I was not as able as my siblings, I started to think of myself as broken. Throughout my growing up years, I compared myself to my siblings and became self-critical. I internalized my "brokenness". Throughout my journey, there was little in the way of mental health support. I thought of myself as a weight on my family. I even learned to drive to stop being a burden on my family.

As my medical care continued, I censored with whom I shared information. I didn't think people would understand. I did not share my diagnosis with friends until I was in the 10th grade. Not knowing whether I was protecting myself or others, I became psychologically frozen and couldn't talk about it. More recently, I noticed that the Adverse Childhood Experience Survey (ACES) does not include medical trauma as an indicator.

My first mental health diagnosis was major depressive disorder in my senior year of high school, and my first inpatient mental health treatment stay was at age 17. I really struggled during my last semester of high school. I was finally excused from my gym class. I had a real connection with my math teacher but had to drop AP math, among other classes, during my last semester. Looking back, my guidance counselor wasn't very helpful. I wish she and other adults in my life at that time would have advised me to reconsider attending a college far away from home.

Because of my connection to a physical therapist earlier in life, I decided to pursue a degree in it. I was accepted to a college in an urban setting close to 400 miles away from my family. Physical therapy required a graduate degree, so the program I entered was a bridge program where the last year of my undergraduate work would serve as graduate studies. When I started, I was successful in my coursework, but was not able to start my clinical work.

My first suicide attempt was during my first semester away in college. After that, I was no longer allowed to stay in the dorms overnight for the rest of the semester. My parents came to campus to support me and arranged for me to stay in hotels to finish the semester. I met with the Dean, who was helpful in making the arrangements.

I took the spring term off, returned home, and started seeing a regular psychiatrist. The psychiatrist had me complete a psychological evaluation. I participated in a partial hospitalization program (PHP) for my mental health and learned about Dialectical Behavioral Therapy (DBT). This was my first experience in DBT, since then I've probably worked through all the modules at least four times. DBT gave me a lot of insight into my own mental health conditions and really allowed me to see what were symptoms of my mental health instead of my own perceived character flaws. To this day I still wrestle with the concept of Radical Acceptance in regard to both my mental and physical health conditions.

I decided to return to school the following fall. I felt stronger and still wanted to pursue a career in PT. When I arrived, I was connected with the school counselors in the counseling center who proved to be helpful during my studies. I had two girlfriends in school who were also great support.

During the end of each semester, I struggled. I was tired, wiped out, and couldn't study. My disability services counselor taught me grounding skills and tried to help every time I got to this part of the semester. Often, I became suicidal and cried. I felt like I was making a mistake.

I was constantly seeing a therapist on campus since freshman year. During my last semester at school, I was doing telephone sessions with my therapist at home. All my decisions began to be degree driven. At one point, I emailed my primary professor and told her I needed to meet. I never told her I was planning another suicide attempt, but she saw through my façade and recognized I needed immediate help. I was thinking about how to hang a noose. She took me to the emergency room right away, and my dad drove down to bring me closer to home because the medical unit near my school was one that did not adequately suit my needs. It was an inner-city emergency room where they were not particularly responsive. When I was finally seen, the psychologist on duty knew me, and agreed to discharge me to my dad. Dad took me to an inpatient behavioral health hospital closer to my home. I stayed at the hospital for two weeks, then spent two weeks in residential treatment. This was my second stint in residential and insurance cut out after two weeks. After that, I spent over a month in PHP at the same hospital. My faculty mentor called to check on me while I was in residential treatment and told me she missed me. The faculty wanted to ask if I was going to make it back that semester. Intuition told me I was done.

My first exposure to art therapy was in the residential treatment program at the mental health hospital near my home. My first project was a self-concept mask, art therapy helped me to see what was going on in my life. My mask inside was black and white with a thin gray line representing me. The outside was intended to express myself to the world, it was yellow fading to blue with splatter paint to represent the humor I use to deflect my pain. I explored how I really felt. The mask seemed like an exercise to me at the time. Two years later, when I redid the mask (Figure 4.5), I found so much more meaning. The inside was dark representing pain and the poems were written during a particularly dark time in my life. The outside was shiny and showed me how much I keep to myself.

Building an effective treatment team took some time. I needed regular counseling and worked to find the right person. There were ups and downs through this time. In 2015, I was seeing a male therapist who I had been with for five years while I was at college. I followed orders and attended sessions with him weekly. One day I told him I was feeling asymmetrical. He responded by asking if my breasts were the same size. I told him that was a very personal question. In reality I was feeling asymmetrical due to my CP affecting only the left half of my body. During our next session, I told him that his comment made me feel uncomfortable and I never saw him again. In the upcoming years, I would be diagnosed with an eating disorder (ED). I have considered that this comment may have contributed to my negative body image. During these years, while working on getting stabilized, I also underwent Transcranial Magnetic Stimulation, and Electroconvulsive Therapy which gave me energy.

When I returned formally from college, I was enrolled in a Comprehensive Community Services (CCS) program with the help of the Aging and Disability Resources Center (ADRC). The ADRC did not have the right resources to help me unless I wanted to pay $500 a month for medications. Through them, I was connected with my current treatment team.

Early in 2019, I was admitted into residential eating disorder therapy. The art therapist there introduced me to the Japanese art form of Kintsugi where a broken vessel is reassembled.

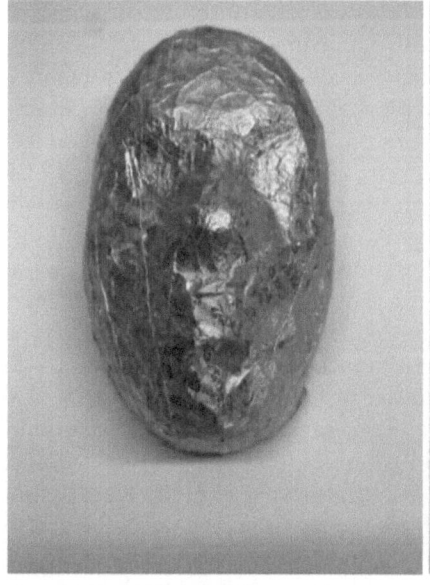 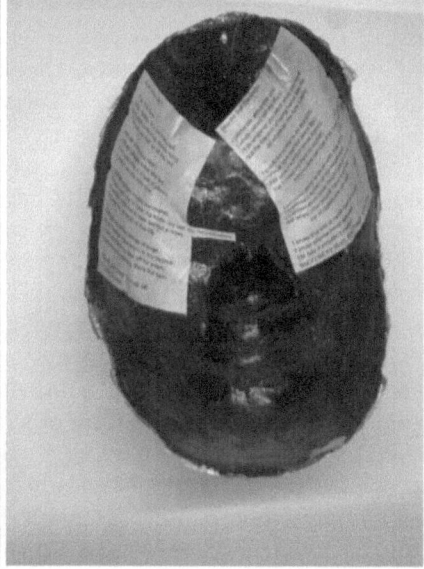

Figure 4.5 Inside/Outside Mask

I made a rebuilt broken mug that represented the complex emotions I was experiencing from my physical trauma. I also wrote a poem about my experience of being broken.

In an effort to find some value in life, I started volunteering at a nearby hospital. My first assignment was visiting patients. I dreaded this, and before long, I let the coordinator know how I felt. She then connected me with a crochet group that was run by an art therapist at the cancer center. The group was primarily made up of cancer survivors who crocheted lap blankets to be distributed to cancer patients undergoing treatment in the clinic. I met weekly with the group and started to get connected. I became a part of a team there.

Through the crochet group, I was given the opportunity to participate in an art show for employees, volunteers, and family members. I did not identify as an artist, but in talking with the art therapist, I realized I had the re-assembled mug and could enter that. I entered, and I won! This art show was my first contact with the rest of the art therapy team.

COVID-19 came during the time the art show was displayed at an associated large medical center. The crochet group had to transition to virtual meetings. When the crochet group went virtual, so did all the other art therapy groups offered by the medical art therapy team. I connected with two other art therapy groups during this time. Both were open studios; one was three hours, and the other was two. Participating in these groups gave me the opportunity to engage more fully in art therapy and learn about myself. This is also when I learned that art therapy was available for outpatient 1:1 treatment. The lead art therapist for the open studio groups became an integral part of my treatment team. She attended group meetings with my CCS team and arranged for me to work individually, virtually with an art therapy intern.

I found working individually with an art therapist supported me in grounding and seeing my experiences. I learned about the value of working on long-term projects and how using certain materials worked to help me learn about myself and become more mindful. I became able to talk things through using art to enable words; the pictures opened dialogue. Participating in art therapy also helps with talk therapy. I prefer long projects that keep me coming back, allowing me to focus and learn. Once, I was introduced to the wheel of emotions and created illustrations and found quotes for each emotion.

After my time with the art therapy intern, I looked for an art therapist with whom I could continue to work. I was introduced to a social worker who used art, but it became obvious that working with her was not the same as art therapy. I have been able to connect with an art therapy clinic where I am able to have weekly, individual art therapy sessions. The virtual studios have also continued, and this has allowed me to stay engaged. Through the virtual studios, I also met another art therapy intern who has a disability. I found this encouraging, and we do talk about physical happenings, and it makes me feel like I am not alone. It's like we were meant to meet. These art therapy groups have become maintenance. They are a place where I can share with others and get feedback from multiple people. The groups have also helped me to build a therapeutic art practice at home. For instance, I do paint by numbers and crochet regularly at home outside of the groups. The groups also helped me to explore triggers in myself and in others. Early on there were times I found I had to tiptoe, when I became uncomfortable. I would get quiet, then when things became too much for me, I would exit the group. Now I am more comfortable and have learned that there are others with sensitivities and needs. Insight into others within the group helped to build tolerance and empathy.

Throughout the process of understanding my abilities, I have learned to speak out more. I write testimony telling my story for *The Mighty,* a community of connection for people with chronic illness, disability, mental health concerns, and more. I know it's not my "job" to tell my story, but no one can listen unless someone is talking. I have also contacted leadership in local shopping centers advocating for benches, handicap buttons for lobbies and bathrooms, and bringing attention to areas where people who are able may not have recognized the needs of those of us with varying abilities.

Since COVID-19, aside from my ongoing participation in art therapy, other parts of my life have changed as well. I rented my first apartment and adopted a cat; his name is Kai. Kai attends my virtual groups with me and is likely my favorite life addition. I went back to in-person volunteer work at the hospital as part of the support team in the vaccine clinic. After that, I went back to the cancer clinic as soon as we were allowed. There I visited with patients and made sure they had the resources they needed to stay comfortable. I took a leadership role in distributing the lap blankets we made during the crochet group. I have joined athletic teams in sled hockey, wheelchair rugby, basketball, and lacrosse. I have also started treatment with Ketamine every four weeks. My therapy appointments have been reduced from twice to once a week, and I have gone three years without inpatient treatment.

STONE BY STONE: REBUILDING THE INNER HOME WITH AN ADULT SURVIVOR OF SEXUAL TRAUMA

VALERIA KOUTMINA

Setting

This case study delineates one group member's progress during participation in an art therapy group for survivors of sexual trauma. The group met weekly in-person at an urban North American art therapy studio for several years prior to the COVID-19 pandemic, and virtually from 2020 to the end of 2022. A full range of materials was available to participants in the art therapy studio, and material kits were sent out to virtual participants to mimic this range. Kits included drawing and watercolor pencils, oil pastels, paper, glue sticks, brushes, and air-dry clay. Sessions were conducted in an open-studio, process-driven format. Session structure included verbal and visual check-ins at the beginning, followed by sharing and discussion of pertinent themes, feelings, and events in clients' lives. Recognizing major resonance among clients, I would propose that group members take their thoughts and feelings into their artwork, adding some suggestions for doing so. This was "always an invitation, not an expectation", as one group member remarked. Long-term thematic directives and material-based metaphoric interventions were offered when the group members indicated openness to a deeper group process. When meeting in person, the group would often close with a few words of affirmation or reflection from each participant. A box of beads and trinkets was passed around at the very end and participants were invited to take a tactile representation of their insight. During virtual meetings, clients were offered a visual check-in opportunity using the whiteboard on Zoom and verbal or gestural check-outs at the conclusion of each session.

Developmental approaches, embodied interventions, and mindfulness techniques were applied throughout the course of treatment. Archetypal psychology, especially work with the Inner Child, Critic, and Shadow (Schmanke, 2018), Internal Family Systems (Schwartz, 1995), mindfulness, and trauma-sensitive therapeutic methods (King, 2016) informed the work. Integrative body- and compassion-based methods (Hass-Cohen et al., 2022) were gently introduced through art-making when clients indicated readiness to engage. I was transparent with clients about theories and their applications in order to encourage their trust and agency in the therapeutic process. Psychoeducation and visual exploration of the developmental hierarchies: the ETC (Hinz, 2015; Kagin & Lusebrink, 1978), Maslow's (1970) Hierarchy of Needs, and Chakras (Wauters, 1997) informed the sessions, leading to greater embodiment, self-awareness, and establishment of intra- and inter-personal safety in the therapeutic container. Art therapy assessments were utilized in an informal manner, and Emily made unique use of the House-Tree-Person assessment (Buck, 1948; Hammer, 1958) and its metaphors. Themes of fragmentation and integration arose early in Emily's treatment.

Client

Emily is a Caucasian woman in her 40s. She was the second of four siblings growing up in an Irish, Catholic family. Emily has multiple nieces and nephews, and often spends time with three of them. Both Emily's parents are deceased, with the mother's death being most recent in 2020. Emily currently lives in a metropolitan North American city where she works in healthcare. She joined the art therapy group in the summer of 2019.

Intake Session

Emily presented as excited, inquisitive, and actively engaged in the individual intake session. It took her about a year after first contact to feel ready to join the group. Emily indicated that she had experienced sexual and emotional trauma in early life and adulthood, and was hospitalized several times due to symptoms of depression and anxiety, including episodes of extreme dissociation. The most recent incident of sexual assault occurring in Emily's 30s precipitated recall of the earlier trauma. Because she was symptomatic, Emily's experience was that of the identified patient among her family members, who seldom voiced or acknowledged their feelings. Emily shared that her relationship to her body was complicated by trauma. Feelings of shame, discomfort with taking up space, and disordered eating led to fluctuations in weight and distortions of body image (Tripp, 2016). Emily sought an art therapy group after being introduced to it in the hospital. She shared she would often journal and draw her feelings, valuing this manner of expression as well as the record of recovery it provided.

Speaking about her internal and lived experiences was difficult for Emily, as was entertaining the notion of being seen and heard. She identified concerns about feeling flooded or dissociating when she began telling her story. She expressed fear of losing control. Art-making and writing became vehicles for the feelings Emily struggled to express and embody. Emily's demeanor was serious and somewhat self-conscious during our first meeting. I sensed she was acutely aware of her body in space and my perception of it, but her affect remained open and warm throughout the meeting. Emily indicated that she was keenly interested in the psychotherapeutic process and had considered the possibility of becoming an art therapist before choosing social work as her vocation.

Early Sessions: Looking at the Fragments

Emily arrived on-time for her first session with the group and took a seat to the left of me. From this position, she could see the entire studio, including the door and anyone who might enter the space, while also feeling security from the wall behind her. I felt this position also indicated her alignment with me and openness to guidance, as I was able to interact with her directly without addressing the whole group. After introducing herself to the group members and receiving their welcoming remarks, Emily worked in silence. The group was exploring the co-created therapeutic container while addressing challenges to presence and participation such as fear, anxiety, and post-traumatic symptoms. Participants were invited to return to previous works or generate new ones in order to process current feelings and responses to the group dynamic, and relationships between their own internal parts (Schwartz, 1995). Potential approaches to working with conflictual or split-off emotional content were explored verbally. I offered a concrete example: folding a piece of paper into sections representing the parts in conflict, and attempting to separate, tolerate, and eventually integrate the images into a new composition. The group session was conducted as an open studio to encourage exploration, choice making, and creative problem-solving. Emily was shown the tools available in the studio. Using caution not to overwhelm, I offered her drawing and colored pencils first, mindful of the need for materials to be familiar and accessible. Over the course of the session, Emily expressed her self-state through drawing. As the piece began to take shape, so did the pile of art supplies surrounding her. This prevented others from having a clear view of Emily and her work.

Her posture and demeanor had the quality of hiding in plain sight. Emily seldom spoke during the early sessions. She created delicately drawn symbolic representations of her feelings and was able to eventually articulate that she felt fragmented, dissociated, and anxious about her capacity for containment and wholeness in the aftermath of trauma. Figure 4.6 depicts a self-portrait featuring fissures across the face and neck, with a heart-shaped hole in the left cheek, where the stoic façade is cracked. One of the eyes and the mouth are tightly closed, indicating potentially limited ability to see and speak. Emily returned to the symbols of cracks and fissures again and again. They were used to denote dissociation, crumbling foundations created by the dysfunctional family of origin, and disconnects between aspects of identity. Figure 4.6 illustrates Emily's identification with feelings of brokenness at the start of treatment, a message she received frequently, first from her family and then from others in her life. Emily noted ambivalence about expressing herself with spoken words or actions, as she did not yet feel safe to do so. Feelings of rage and shame were especially difficult for Emily to access, and she often included writing in her early works to ensure the meaning was clear. These writings indicated self-doubt and distrust in her art expressions and a desire to exercise control over the narrative.

Emily produced several projects in the studio that featured self-portraiture and depictions of feminine figures like fairies and trees that resembled the female body. Women and fairies were always drawn nude, a feature quite incongruent to Emily's outward presentation, but indicative of her sense of vulnerability. Often figures were hunched or in fetal positions, alone and surrounded by darkness. Figure 4.7 is an image Emily produced after approximately one month in the group. She stated that the picture depicted her internal state at the start of treatment on the left, and how she wished to feel on the right. The womb-like purple cocoon around the figure on the left later became a frequent feature of Emily's works. She described it as a depiction of her boundaries, and would often create an image of it on the whiteboard during remote sessions. Still early in treatment, Figure 4.7 was painted with watercolor and featured stark contrasts, bright colors implying affective expression, and well-formed figures which communicated feeling through postures. Emily had shifted from the *Cognitive/Symbolic* level of the ETC into the *Affective/Perceptual*

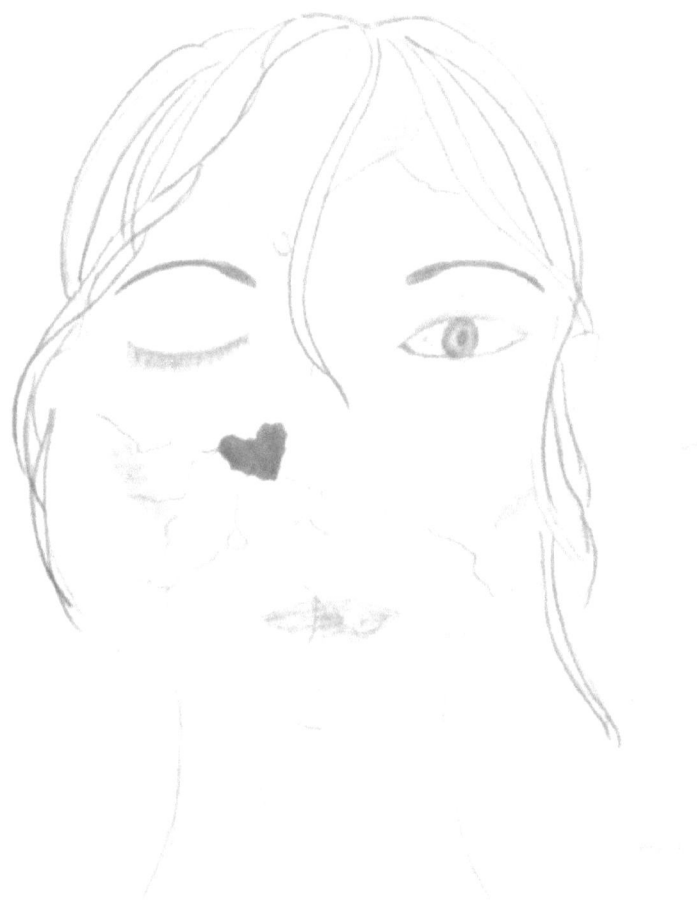

Figure 4.6 Self Portrait with Fissures

dimension, "fluid media and bright or intense colors evoke Affective functioning", while the inclusion of form and figure bespeak perception (Hinz, 2015, p. 45).

Gradually, I began introducing Emily to tactile materials like yarn, clay, paint-sticks, and physical processes, such as cut and torn paper collage, large-scale drawings, and sculpture, that would provide opportunities for self-soothing and sensory integration while engaging the whole person in the creative act. Hinz (2015) found "the healing functions of Sensory work include discovering, valuing, and expressing inner sensations, as well as increasing tolerance for internal and external sensation" (p. 44). This is congruent with Emily's goals as her long-term treatment trajectory included learning to acknowledge, tolerate, accept, integrate, and appreciate the various parts of self and experience. Short-term objectives included building rapport and establishing conditions of safety within herself and in the

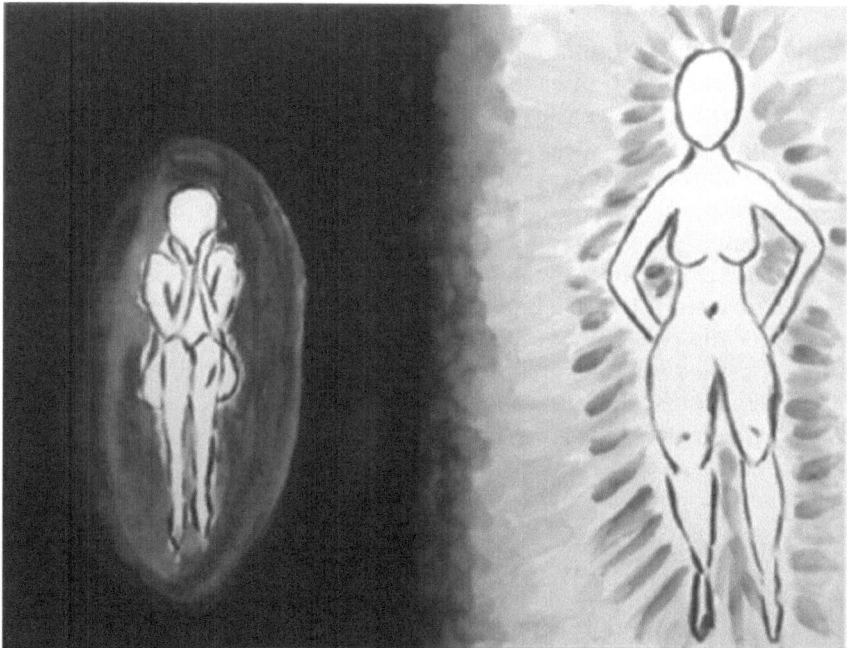

Figure 4.7 Emily's Past and Future

therapeutic environment, identifying and learning to tolerate strong affects, and gaining compassionate insight into trauma responses.

A shift became palpable in Emily's relationship to overwhelming negative thoughts and feelings when she chose to use a self-box as a container and asked me for a hole punch. Over the course of several sessions, Emily worked diligently on writing out a comprehensive list of negative thoughts and associated feelings. Then she tore up the paper. I anticipated she would want to put a protective seal between herself and these negative feelings. To my surprise, having cathartically expressed and processed these words, she chose to "re-home" their torn bits in a small cardboard box, putting some holes in the lid. Emily stated that the box served as a container for these feelings and ideas, and that "as all living things, they need room to move and air to breathe". Emily had tamed the negative cognitions and emotions and came to be their benevolent keeper, regaining control, a sense of containment, and compassion for formerly overwhelming, threatening psychic content.

Later Sessions: Rebuilding

As treatment progressed, Emily became curious about expanding her tight "purple circle" (Figure 4.7) to include more sources of socialization and support. She became verbally engaged in group sessions, often commenting on her progress in self-advocacy and expression. Emily's works became bigger, her gestures more expansive, and the materials more visceral, indicating an embrace of expression on the lower, embodied levels of the ETC (Hinz, 2015). She seemed more comfortable taking space and being seen in action. The barriers to visibility she had formerly erected were slowly removed.

When sessions were moved to an online platform during the COVID-19 pandemic, Emily welcomed the new format. Themes of optimal environments, inner space, and the concept of home frequently arose in the group's work during lockdown. Notions of identity, cultivation and affirmation of instinct, intuition or inner-knowing, discernment, integration, and letting-go rose powerfully up for exploration within the group. Group members developed symbolic and visual vocabularies based on the metaphors of gardening and home introduced through art-making directives. Many sessions were dedicated to working with the idea of the self as a home for experiences, cognitions, feelings, memories, and sensations. Emily's work continued to acknowledge the rifts and fissures she so poignantly identified earlier in treatment, but her relationship to them was now vastly changed. She began noticing self-limiting beliefs and sifting the external messages she had received from her authentic-core-identity. With both her parents now deceased, Emily experienced a sense of permission to express herself more freely, to take up space, and to trust herself. The materials she chose were more fluid (i.e., watercolor, inks, even acrylic pouring), indicating a burgeoning capacity for taking risks and regressing safely, knowing that she is capable of containing and managing any spills. Emily was also often seen working rhythmically, rocking and moving her torso and arms when engaged in large-scale drawings using paint sticks. "Vigorous art activity with the Kinesthetic component can give clients the opportunity to let go of inhibitions and control, or can allow clients to experience alternating inhibition and disinhibition" (Hinz, 2015, p. 44). Emily seemed better able to allow herself to move through the range of art materials and internal experiences (Figure 4.8).

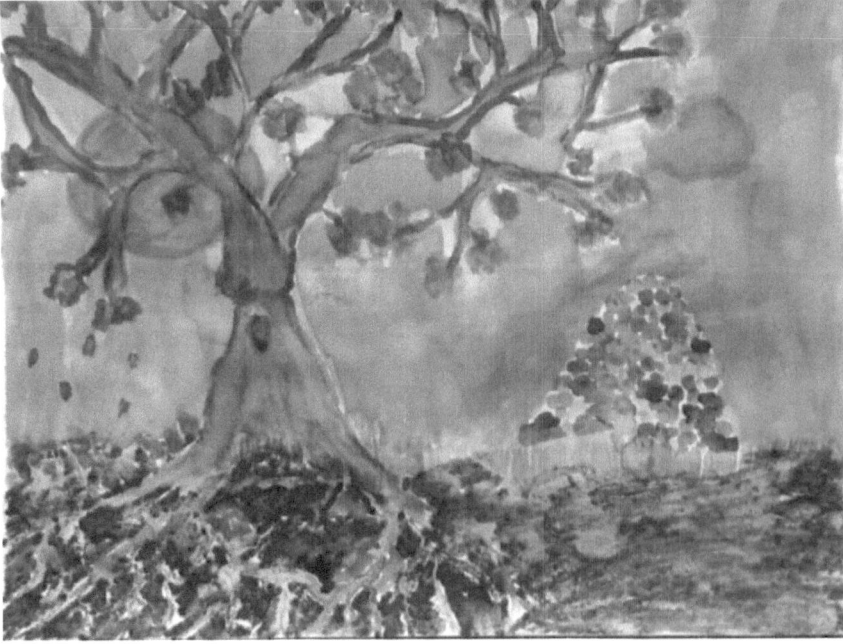

Figure 4.8 Removing Obstacles, Rebuilding Foundations

Emily created this painting based on a sketch she made in one of our group sessions, where I invited participants to become the "discerning gardener". Sessions began with a guided visualization. I asked participants to imagine planting seeds and growing the garden of their lives by engaging in the intentional processes of weeding, pruning, working the soil, and cultivating the things they wished to thrive. Emily once again created the image of a feminine tree with a knot-hole. The tree's roots ran deep underground, supporting and nourishing it. During the guided visualization, Emily discovered multiple stones blocking the roots' path, so she excavated them, bringing them into the conscious light of day and making a pile next to the tree. To Emily, the stones represented obstacles she has encountered in life, but she did not wish to discard them. Emily stated that they may be used to "fortify and shore up" her foundations and to continue building her inner-home. She expressed gratitude and relief at having discovered a sense of safety within herself, and communicated the understanding that her resourcefulness and ability to transform and re-purpose obstacles was key to her survival and continued growth. The painting includes the "purple circle" of the moon, as well as the sun shining above in the distance. Half of the tree is lush and verdant, while the other half is shedding its leaves, signifying cyclical loss and new growth in the process of recovery from trauma.

Outcomes

When contacted to collaborate on the creation of this case study, Emily was passionate about calling the later/current phase of her treatment "rebuilding". She defined her progress in art therapy thus far as a journey toward "greater knowing", which included intuitive and somatic sensing. She traced her trajectory from fragmentation and feelings of brokenness to greater awareness and acknowledgment of the exiled or split-off parts, their eventual acceptance, integration, and appreciation, resulting in a sense of authenticity, agency and wholeness. Speaking to me about the "broken foundation" she stated:

> It's not who I am but it's what I have been given to work with. I can sort through it, cultivate it, modify it, solidify it, and mold from it that which I need to stabilize my present and engineer my future.

Emily continued participating in the group under the guidance of another therapist after my departure from the organization. She reported that creative expression had become integral to her continued progress in managing feelings of inadequacy, shame, fear, confusion, and anger. During our time together, Emily gained traction in her recovery from trauma by integrating earlier experiences and working through all of the levels of the ETC to develop greater creative coping skills and internal supports. In conversation with me, she stated that she still thinks about the pile of stones in Figure 4.8 and feels there is further work to be done realigning them in ways that support her. She has benefitted from both group art therapy and individual Ketamine-assisted psychotherapy.

THREE ACCESSES OF ART THERAPY IN CANCER CARE

JILL MCNUTT

This case study explores the application of art therapy for a 45-year-old female undergoing treatment for stage 2 colorectal cancer. The study covers initial art therapy sessions during the patient's chemotherapy treatments in an outpatient infusion clinic, subsequent outpatient art therapy in a mental health context, and eventual transition to an open art therapy studio. The study aims to demonstrate the therapeutic benefits of art therapy in support of emotional expressions, (dis)stress reduction, self-care, and social engagement throughout the patient's cancer journey.

Colorectal cancer treatment involves a combination of treatment approaches. These approaches vary according to the stage and severity of the cancer diagnosis. Pamela's treatment regimen included surgery and chemotherapy. The cancer diagnosis came as a surprise to Pamela, who did not know of any cancer in her biological family. Upon diagnosis, Pamela was referred to an oncologist and a surgeon. She saw the oncologist at a large metropolitan medical center where she would undergo three months of chemotherapy. It was during her chemotherapy treatments when I met Pamela and introduced her to our art-on-a-cart art therapy program.

Setting

Patients have multiple points of access to art therapy within the large metropolitan medical center where these art therapy services were provided. Art therapy is provided bedside for hospitalized patients, chair-side in infusion clinics, outpatient in either 1:1 or family formats, or in groups in the form of open studios.

My art supplies are brief, but intentional. The cart includes: 1¼-inch clear glass gems, magazines (National Geographic are my favorite to carry), images cut from magazines, inspirational words cut from magazines, a small bottle of Elmer's glue, a purple glue stick, origami paper, a handful of pony beads, waxed string, an expired deck of playing cards, a small set of watercolor paints and a brush that holds water, small watercolor paper (up to 8 inches), a box of polymer clay cut into quarter-inch squares in a variety of colors, empty, cleaned, and sanitized medication bottles, direction sheets for baking polymer clay, scissors, inspirational mandala coloring pages from a book authored and drawn by a former cancer patient, 12 brush markers, 24 woodless color pencils, a package of model magic, body outlines in various poses on 8½ × 11-inch paper, a box of animal spirit cards by Steven Farmer, and a plastic clipboard. All supplies are cleaned and sanitized before loading the cart. A segment of the cart is dedicated as a "used materials" area indicating that materials there need to be cleaned and sanitized before being used again.

Approaches

Art therapy is a therapeutic approach that utilizes creative expression to support individuals in addressing emotional, psychological, and physical challenges. In the context of cancer care, art therapy provides a unique avenue for patients to explore feelings, enhance coping skills, and improve overall well-being. Art therapy offers a non-verbal and symbolic means of expression that allows patients to discover and address fears, anxieties, and hopes (Nainis et al., 2006). Art therapy provides a safe space for exploration, externalization of emotions, cathartic release, and increased self-awareness. Art therapy interventions using guided imagery and mindfulness-based art techniques have been shown to lower stress levels, enhance well-being, and improve quality of life in cancer patients (Thyme et al., 2009). Art therapy helps patients develop coping skills and build resilience in the face of cancer-related challenges. The goals of the art therapy program were developed through qualitative interviews with cancer patients (McNutt, 2018). The goals include building hope, strength, and resilience; mindfulness and interactive distraction; introspection and self-learning; and growth through experience. Glinzak (2016) studied art therapy participation patterns among patients who used art therapy inpatient, outpatient, during infusions, and in open studio sessions, and found that patients who are inpatient, or in infusion tend to use art therapy for the first two goals and patients seen as outpatient or in open studio tended toward the latter two goals.

Theoretical approaches in art therapy with adult cancer patients can focus on, but are not limited to existential, psychodynamic, and constructivist perspectives. Each theoretical frame provides different lenses through which clients are understood. The perspectives also provide frameworks for planning therapeutic processes. The existential perspective emphasizes concerns such as meaning-making, life purpose, and issues of mortality (Luzzatto & Gabriel, 2000). Through art therapy, patients can explore personal values, fears, aspirations, and purpose and meaning throughout the cancer journey. The psychodynamic perspective emphasizes exploration of unconscious processes, past experiences, and interpersonal dynamics to gain insight into present thoughts and behaviors. This perspective is useful in exploring psychological conflicts and emotions. Art-making within the psychodynamic perspective provides a symbolic language through which unconscious material can be explored and insights can be gleaned (Moon, 2016). The post-modern constructivist perspective emphasizes the subjective construction of reality and recognizes the influence of social and cultural contexts (Luzzatto & Gabriel, 2000). This perspective encourages patients to create and reinterpret their narratives and identities in response to the cancer experience. Patients using art therapy as part of their cancer treatment have the opportunity to recreate meaning through art-making, storytelling, and metaphor. Regardless of the approach, patients are encouraged to find new perspectives, create alternative narratives, and develop a sense of agency in navigating the cancer journey.

Client

Pamela was a 45-year-old divorced mother of three teenage girls. She worked in the service industry where she held positions from bartending to dishwashing. She lived in a small suburban community not far from the medical center. Pamela was the only child of two newly retired parents. Neither parent had a history of major medical conditions. Pamela was divorced for almost five years at the time of diagnosis, and her ex-husband and his wife agreed to spend time with the girls while Pamela underwent her treatments. Pamela had no history of mental health treatment, but her youngest daughter had difficulties with learning and had an individualized education plan. Pamela expressed guilt regarding reduced time with her children, holding her parents back from traveling, and not being able to help at the restaurant where she was employed.

Intake Sessions

Pamela's initial sessions were in the infusion clinic as she was receiving chemotherapy. Her appointments were scheduled on alternate weeks, and she was sure to schedule her sessions while art therapy was available. Pamela's official prognosis was positive, but she was often overwhelmed by what she would call the "big-C" of cancer. She saw cancer as a killer, and sometimes doubted what she was learning. During our first session, I offered her a flat glass gem and some magazine images to make a *hope stone*. Hope stones are a common process used in the clinic to help patients remember their strengths, acknowledge their hopes, and support ongoing resilience. The process includes cutting a magazine image, and an aspirational word out and gluing them to the back of the glass gem in such a way that the image becomes magnified when looking from the top. Pamela selected an image of three pink roses and the word "family". During our weeks together in the infusion clinics, Pamela's physical and emotional state ebbed and flowed. Some weeks she became fluent in art participation and created small watercolor paintings, usually of simple flowers; she learned to fold origami cranes; and created emotionally charged cards for each of her daughters. Other weeks, she simply selected an animal card from my deck, and we talked about how the selected card and associated reading reflected her current situation. Throughout the four months of her chemotherapy treatment, she laughed some, smiled often, and cried when necessary.

Outpatient Sessions

It was almost a month after Pamela had completed chemotherapy that she made her first appointment for outpatient art therapy. When she arrived for her appointment, Pamela wore her hair down, was dressed in jeans and a loose-fitting blouse. She wore make-up and had her nails done. This was a change from her casual chemotherapy wear. Her cancer screenings all showed clean results, she had returned to her role as primary parent of her three daughters, had returned to work, and her parents felt safe enough to travel out of the country. When Pamela returned to art therapy, she reported not having a desired direction, but felt she needed to continue making art. For the sake of finding direction, I had her draw a bridge. She used pencils first, then applied color using watercolor paints, and finally added strength to lines on the left side of the bridge with a fine-tip, permanent black marker. The bridge was well constructed, made of stone. It spanned the banks of a shallow but fast-moving stream. The sky was painted in a soft blue with scattered clouds of gray. The grass field on the left side of the bridge was detailed and included flowers. The space beneath the bridge, the right side of the bridge, and the landscape that existed on the other side of the bridge was undefined and blurry. Pamela may have been trying to create distance in relation to proximity of the viewer. When I asked her where she would place herself in the drawing, she indicated that she would be sitting in the grass and smelling the flowers.

Pamela was able to reflect on current life events including her parents' retirement moves, her daughters' middle and high school events, and celebrations that were taking place at her employment. However, she had difficulty discussing the positive prognosis her Oncologist and Surgeon were sharing with her. During our second session, I wanted to get a picture of how she experienced emotions. I introduced a variety of body shapes on regular printer paper. In our clinic, we have a collection of 21 different poses. Pamela chose to use the body outline of a balance beam walker (Figure 4.9). I invited her to imagine her emotions as colors as they existed within her body and then depict them onto the body form. Pamela

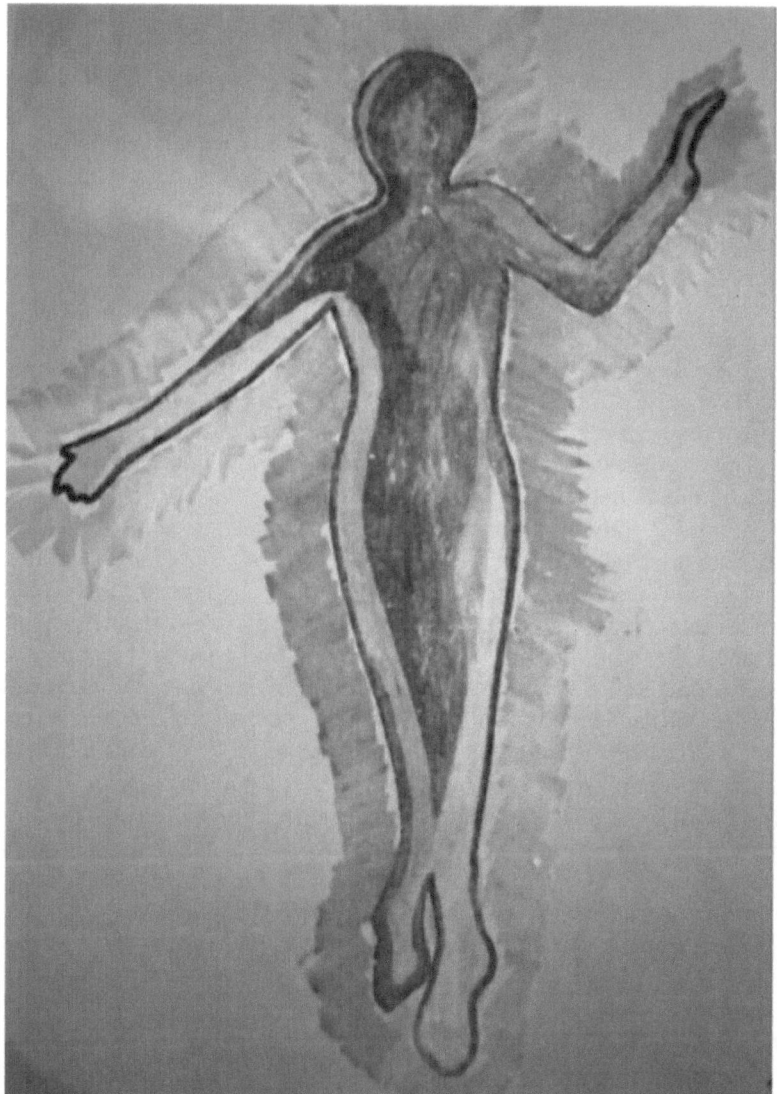

Figure 4.9 Balance Beam

used brush tip markers and filled the space within the body shape and included what she called an aura around the outside of the figure. She then indicated that the emotions were there, but they were not as bright or visible as the markers indicated. She then used a white oil pastel to soften the colors of the image. The colors in the hands of the figure were not dulled with the white. This may indicate her ability to be present for others, not so much for herself. In describing the emotional image, Pamela indicated feeling heart palpitations sometimes; bad dreams, but not nightmares, that would prevent her from falling back asleep; and feelings of confusion when more than one person in her life needed something along with subsequent irritability. At this point, it started to become clear that Pamela may be experiencing anxiety due to her cancer diagnosis and treatment.

During Pamela's third session, I asked her to try collage making. Specifically, I asked her to create a three-part collage that demonstrated past, present, and future. She complied, and began sifting through magazines. She found several images to represent her past, including a young girl image that reminded her of herself, images that showed loving couples to represent her parents, and a baseball player with a dirty uniform to represent her ex-husband. The present included images of young women engaged in dance, sewing, playing a guitar, and brushing hair. These images were said to belong to her and her three daughters. The future section included images of her daughters and desired families that would represent her grandchildren. It was notable that her depiction of the future did not include herself. Pamela and I set each of the three images up on the opposite side of the table, so we could reflect on them together. She described each of the images and noticed that she did not see a future for herself. Her fear of the "big-C" had frozen her development. She had difficulty finding personal purpose outside of caring for her daughters and her parents. Even her ex-husband had a higher priority over her own self-care. We discussed the possibility that she was suffering from anxiety, most likely due to her cancer diagnosis.

Pamela and I discussed options moving forward. We determined that the most productive long-term goal would be to rediscover herself and spend time enjoying her own life. One area that we decided to work on was her internal narrative of the "big-C". This process would take some evidence, and a concretized understanding of the current state of cancer treatment. I gave Pamela a small sketchbook that we stock regularly in the studio for patients. We requested help from her oncologist, her surgeon, the librarian of the medical library, and the rest of the treatment team. Pamela was to journal and sketch after learning each new piece of information regarding her specific diagnosis and prognosis. The second area we chose to work on was getting reacquainted with herself. I suggested painting a self-portrait, but Pamela thought that would be too challenging. Instead, she identified a flower that represented herself. The flower was a morning glory as she felt more alert during the mornings and faded out later in the evening. We prepared a canvas and found a few images of morning glories for her to paint from. Acrylic paint was the chosen medium for this process.

As the weeks progressed, Pamela continued to attend individual art therapy sessions for another six weeks. Each week, she would present the progress she was making in her journal and add another layer of acrylic paint to her morning glories. Pamela would point out strengths and weaknesses of the morning glories that were also true of her own life. During what would be Pamela's second to last individual session, she talked about her eldest daughter's impending graduation. Pamela expressed pride in her daughter's accomplishment and wanted to make special plans to celebrate. When she returned the next week, Pamela had planned a trip to Disney World for the family including herself, her daughters, and her parents. She was excited and shared memories of her own trip to Disneyland when she was younger. She shared plans of sharing those experiences with her daughters, particularly visiting the Pirates of the Caribbean. This was the first time Pamela had shared plans for the future that included herself. That day she put the finishing touches onto her morning glories (Figure 4.10), which she indicated would be taken for framing and hung on her living room wall. We also reviewed her journal. Pamela had begun to believe her prognosis. At the close of sessions, I invited Pamela to attend our Open Art Therapy Studios that occurred every second and fourth Friday from two until six pm.

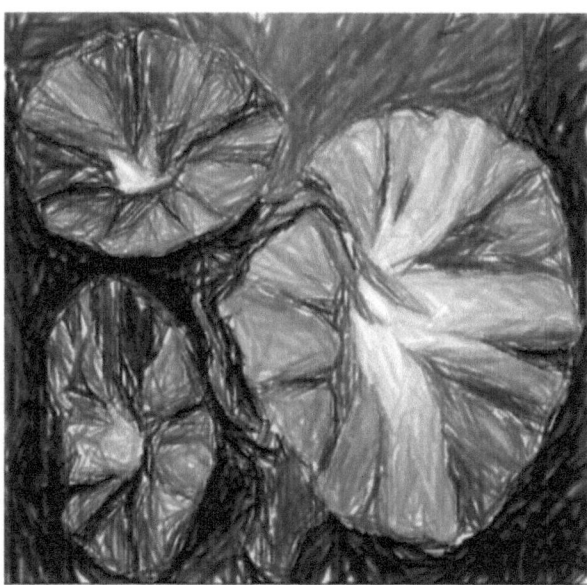

Figure 4.10 Morning Glories

Open Art Therapy Studio

The open art therapy studio provides patients with a supporting community and the opportunity for social connection. The sessions foster a sense of belonging, shared experiences, and mutual support among participants. The group dynamic encourages peer validation, empathy, and interpersonal relationships. Open studio sessions are open to patients, survivors, family, caregivers, staff, and the community. Each studio begins with an optional, featured process so that newcomers are at ease in joining. The studio supply options are wide and include almost any media except chalk pastels and raw clay.

Pamela's first open studio session was about two months following her outpatient sessions. She came alone and engaged in the featured process of still life painting. She joined a grieving mother accompanied by her granddaughter at a table and began sketching. The still life at the table was a bowl of apples with one apple outside the bowl. The grandmother sat with Pamela and explained that her daughter did not survive her cancer and that she was now the guardian of her granddaughter. Pamela's expression was swift, she moved her hand to her heart, jaw dropped, mouth edges pointed down, and told the grandmother how sorry she was for her loss. The grandmother shared that she and her granddaughter had been coming to the open studio for about six months. The grandmother explained how making art together helped them to create a new relationship that remembered her daughter and honored her place forever in their hearts. Pamela was encouraged by this interaction; she held compassion for the mother and daughter of her companions but also identified herself as a survivor.

Pamela attended the next three open studio sessions with her youngest daughter. They came to the open studio right after the eighth-grade daughter was out of school. They participated in the featured process each week and went home for dinner. On Pamela's fourth time at open studio, she and her daughter announced that they would not be returning. Pamela felt it was time to focus on family and make plans for the future. Pamela dropped in after her next oncologist meeting. She and her daughters were preparing for graduation, and her parents were on their way home from Germany. At this session Pamela reached into her pocket and pulled out the small glass stone with three flowers and the word 'Family' that she had made during our first session. She held the stone to her heart, and simply said thank you.

Results and Outcomes

Through her work in art therapy, Pamela recognized her anxiety and fear of the "big-C". She worked systematically in her journal, and reflectively in her self-portrait through morning glories (Figure 4.10). Pamela was able to express her needs, confront the narrative of the "big-C", and developed trust in her own future. Pamela experienced a reduction of both distress and anxiety symptoms. Her relationships with her daughters and her parents became more intentional and meaningful. Pamela may not continue in art-making, but she will continue to be a mother and a daughter.

For Pamela, art therapy in the infusion clinic served as an avenue for relaxation and interactive distraction. It supported her resilience, helped keep up her strength, and provided her company on a journey she chose to undergo without family. The transition into outpatient services allowed Pamela to explore her personal fears and patterns. The outpatient setting allowed time for us to reflect on her circumstances, create a treatment protocol, and renarrate non-helpful internal dialogue. The open studio served as a transitional connection to art therapy while she separated from art therapy services.

Conclusion

Pamela used art therapy to help normalize the cancer journey from diagnosis through the more rigorous and immediate stages of treatment. Art therapy and our relationship were easily available for her at any juncture of her care. The trust developed within the therapeutic relationship helped Pamela to engage holistically in the art-making processes. She was able to identify non-functional internal scripts and hear conflicting evidence. She learned the importance of self-care and balance in caring for others. This is a crucial aspect of her continued health and well-being.

ART THERAPY REMOTE GROUP: MIDLIFE ADULTS

HEATHER DENNING

During the COVID-19 pandemic, art therapists needed to reconsider what an art therapy setting entailed and expand to include remote sessions. Online art therapy became more common and expanded options for those experiencing stress (Biro-Hannah, 2021). Additionally, the need for art therapy services for those isolated during the pandemic prompted community agencies, not necessarily tied to clinical services, to consider how the arts could support the wellness of community members.

This group case study addresses midlife adults seeking wellness-based art experiences provided remotely by an art therapist and arranged and hosted by a community agency addressing poverty and empowerment. Programming at this agency included literacy, nutrition, preschool enrichment, and financial assistance with rent and utilities and did not typically offer art therapy. However, agency directors sought ways to combat isolation for community members enrolled in their programs and initiated contact with a local arts center that connected me as an art therapist to the agency on a contractual basis. A remote, group program, *Art for Wellness* was developed with the goals to decrease isolation and promote general wellness for community members. Thus, this group case study addressing midlife adults may be non-conventional, but has become more common and provides a narrative of ways art therapists are being called to serve the community and its needs.

Setting

The setting was each participant's home and a space within that home designated for artmaking during this group. Spaces ranged from a corner table in a bedroom to a full basement and home art studio with access to many art supplies. I facilitated the sessions in my home remotely in an isolated corner of a room with an art space situated in front of a bookshelf, a medium-sized table, a laptop computer, and the needed art supplies within reach. Care was taken to maintain a clinical boundary by removing any personal photographs, but at the same time a couple decorative items were within view to avoid presenting a dull environment. Both natural and overhead lighting illuminated the space for a clear view of the art supplies and me.

The format was an eight-week series of remote group sessions occurring once a week and lasting for an hour and a half. A two-week pause occurred between session four and five due to winter holidays. Once beginning, the sessions were closed groups offering consistent membership. All participants, except one, completed all sessions. It was unknown why the individual who stopped attending terminated. The groups occurred through the Google Meets platform. A program specialist employed within the community agency assisted by initiating and monitoring the remote platform for each session. She also co-led the initial check-in portions of the sessions. Each of the sessions was structured with an opening check-in question, introduction and directions for the art task, artmaking time, and then sharing and discussion of the art created.

I ordered the needed art supplies in advance of session one and packaged together items for participants to pick up at the community agency. The art supplies were financed by a grant and made available to the participants at no cost. The supplies included: watercolor paints with a medium-sized round brush, round diffusing paper, cardstock, blank note cards with envelopes, decorative papers, glue sticks, a pre-cut round loom, colored markers, repurposed magazines, and strands of colored yarn. Participants were asked to provide their own pencil, scissors, ruler or straight edge, and additional collage materials of their choice.

Approaches

The approaches integrated a variety of theories primarily suited to the participants' age range and my clinical training and competencies. I had extensive prior experience working with adults in group art therapy sessions within a community mental health setting. Concepts of Yalom and Leszcz's (2020) therapeutic factors of group were fostered to recognize universality and promote group cohesion. Bruce Moon's (2016) 13 essentials of art-based therapy groups were referenced and used to support the group's purpose. "Making art in the presence of others reduces isolation and creates a sense of community" (Moon, 2016, p. 8). Existential approaches in working with adults in midlife accentuate purpose, meaning, and mortality (Moon, 2016; Yalom & Leszcz, 2020).

Clients

The following client descriptions are composites of participants served through the *Art for Wellness* group. Six individuals participated in the group. All presented as cisgendered women mostly in their 50s, although the group was open to participants of all genders. Five of the participants appeared to be of European American descent and one African American descent. All resided in a midsized, Midwest city, and lived below or close to the federal poverty level. None were working full time. The women were receiving forms of financial assistance from the county, state, or federal programs aimed at supplementing incomes and combating poverty. They were involved in other programs provided at the agency.

Three of the six participants disclosed having a history of mental health symptoms which were anxiety and mood related. They also openly discussed being in therapy. Most of the women were actively involved in caretaking of family members, some across multiple generations. All expressed some interest in art or creative outlets with varying levels of experience and a variety of art mediums. All the participants were attending voluntarily and learned about the group through promotions from the community center or their case manager.

Intake Session

A program specialist at the agency completed the initial screening and registration for the group participants. Criteria included being age 18 and older, living within the county where the agency was located, and having an income below or close to the federal poverty level. Participants responded to flyers, social media posts, and email promotions distributed by the agency. Case managers within the county did refer several of the participants. A full clinical assessment was not obtained due to the setting and services provided. Several of the participants disclosed mental health histories and had clinical assessments completed at other agencies. Participation did not require records of prior diagnostics or treatment.

Early Sessions

Introductions occurred during the first session. I described the purpose and goals of the group which included coping with isolation during the COVID-19 pandemic and using art to promote general wellness. I also explained that participants did not need to be artistically trained to participate and that the main goals were to use art to connect to others during a period of social isolation.

A general release of information was signed prior to session one between the agency, participants, and myself since I was contracted to provide services. I reviewed the language in the release as it included information about photographing artwork. As an art therapy educator, I also asked permission to share participant images for educational purposes with a signed release.

The limits of the group services were described due to the remote platform and programming offered by the agency. It was explained that while mental health themes might surface in the art and discussions, a mental health crisis could not be fully evaluated, and participants would be referred to community mental health crisis services or their mental health providers. Contact information was shared for the county crisis services if needed.

Sessions one through four included the following art tasks: a vision board, a Zen doodle mandala drawing, construction of an art journal, and creation of artist trading cards (Stirnemann, 1997) with the theme "message of support" (Figure 4.11). Each task was structured with the materials and prompts. I provided some examples of each task and for the art journal construction, an additional template showing the design was provided. The rationale for a structured approach with media and prompts was related to the timing of the group and its remote nature. The directed approach allowed the participants comfort in building the group space and getting to know each other.

All participants were moderately to highly engaged with the art materials. One participant reported the lack of knowledge on technology prevented her from being on camera, so it was difficult to evaluate her engagement level with materials. During the first two sessions, participants quietly worked and then discussed their art when prompted. By the third and fourth sessions, participants were more familiar with each other, and discussion was more spontaneous. Common topics of discussion centered on limits placed during the pandemic, health issues, caregiving for a spouse or grandchildren, and coping with stress. All participants except one appeared visibly on camera and shared their art.

Figure 4.11 Art Therapist's Example Artist Trading Cards

Visual themes related to nature surfaced in both the vision board and artist trading card sessions. Most of the women reported some connection to nature as helping them cope with stress and isolation. Images of birds and themes of nurturing were noticed. Many commented on enjoying the group and the benefits of being creative and focusing on themselves in a time where caretaking of family members presented both social connection and mental strain or worry.

Later Sessions

During weeks five through eight, the following art tasks were facilitated: a relaxation landscape inspired by artist Heather Galler (2014), a nature weaving on a provided loom, watercolor painting on diffusing paper, and creation of handmade note cards incorporating "a letter of support to oneself"." Five of the women remained from the first four sessions. Because I was now more familiar with the group members and the themes that emerged, I continued the focus on self-care, connection to nature, and promoting wellness. It was also noted that more direct feedback and discussion between participants occurred versus earlier sessions when discussions were initiated by the program specialist and myself. Engagement appeared to increase in both the artmaking and discussion. It was noticed that more spontaneous communication occurred while participants were creating art. This communication did not always center on themes of the art or personal symbolism of imagery, but instead increased self-disclosure occurred regarding specific health concerns and family relationships. These discussions illustrated Yalom's concept of universality as participants learned they shared similar experiences (Yalom & Leszcz, 2020). Many of these concerns are related to midlife adult development where self-care can decrease, impacting overall well-being (Good, 2016).

Media that was less structured was used during the second portion of the group as we gained more familiarity with each other and shared prior art experiences. Considering group development, less structure is generally required during later stages of group therapy (Toseland & Rivas, 2017).

Outcomes

The outcomes described are my observations of themes within the group's artwork and discussion. No quantitative tool was used to measure the outcomes. Participants did verbally provide feedback at the end of session eight. All remaining five participants reported the group as being beneficial for several reasons: gaining support from other women facing common challenges with caretaking, feeling less stress and distraction from worry while creating art, and reconnecting to art as a creative practice. One participant, who identified as an artist, felt empowered by sharing her own knowledge on art techniques and resources with the group, including me. All participants expressed interest in attending future *Art for Wellness* programs whether in a remote setting or in-person.

Conclusions

The *Art for Wellness* group appeared to accomplish its purpose and goals to decrease isolation experienced by adults during the COVID-19 pandemic. The group offered midlife adult women the opportunity to connect while creating art and share their experiences during the pandemic. Many stressors were verbalized relating to the pandemic but expanded to their role as women and caretakers within their families. Participants were able to provide support to each other while engaging in the creative process. The theme of reconnecting to nature was reinforced in both group discussions and art. This imagery was visible with collage media and in a tactile manner during a nature weaving art task.

Biro-Hannah (2021) observed Yalom and Leszcz's (2020) therapeutic factor of universality while facilitating an online art therapy group during the pandemic. This included universality as participants were able to share their common pandemic-related experiences. Biro-Hannah continued by noting the facilitator was also experiencing the pandemic, which supported a communal relationship between the facilitator and the participants. These findings resonated with my experience as a midlife woman in her 50s facilitating the *Art for Wellness* group. Through interaction and co-creation within a remote platform, verbal and non-verbal communication offered a connection at a time when we all needed each other.

ART THERAPY AND PAIN MANAGEMENT

JILL MCNUTT

Setting

This case study explores the use of art therapy as an intervention for pain management in a 53-year-old woman diagnosed with fibromyalgia. She was referred to the health counseling center within a large medical system. The office was conveniently situated in the lower level of the medical center where she saw her primary care physician regularly for fibromyalgia. The health psychologist referred Anita to art therapy to help focus on mindfulness and address any underlying emotional aggravators of her pain. Fibromyalgia is a chronic condition characterized by widespread pain, fatigue, sleep disturbances, and tenderness in specific areas of the body with heightened sensitivity to stimuli. The cause of fibromyalgia is not fully understood; it is believed to involve abnormalities in the processing of pain signals, leading to an amplified response to stimuli in the neurological system (Wolfe et al., 2010).

The art studio was equipped with a wide range of art supplies stored in cabinets around the periphery of the room. A large table for working with eight chairs sits in the middle of the room. There is a sink for clean-up just outside the room. Anita scheduled bimonthly sessions with her physician and art therapy together to avoid additional travel.

Approaches

The theoretical perspective for this case is an integration of person-centered, psychodynamic, and mindfulness-based approaches. Psychodynamic elements allowed exploration of underlying emotional issues contributing to pain, mindfulness to aid in cultivating present-moment awareness and coping strategies, and person-centered to provide individualized attention, acknowledgment, and unconditional positive regard (Rogers, 1979).

Intake Session

When Anita first came into art therapy, she had no idea how art therapy could help. She indicated that she was unable to be creative due to the pain and could not see any benefits for participation in art therapy for the future. I explained that art therapy could help with interactive distraction, mindfulness, and exploring new narratives. Anita agreed to set up some appointments, while maintaining her doubts.

Anita was married and reported her husband had little compassion for her situation. She had two adult daughters, both married with two children each. Both lived within an hour and came to visit at least every other month. As per Anita's report, her husband saw these years of grandparenting as an exciting time of life and was resentful that her pain was negatively impacting his ability to spend time with their grandchildren.

Anita's art therapy assessment involved an intake process including a review of her medical history, pain experiences, and coping mechanisms. I used two art-based assessments: the draw-a-person in the rain drawing (DAPR; Willis et al., 2010) to address her coping skills, and an informal drawing to understand the subjective nature of her pain experience.

The DAPR

Anita's person in the rain was strapped to a chair and unprotected except for hands being raised to block the face from the rain (Figure 4.12). The rain was drawn in choppy consistent lines. The image itself was drawn in the center third of the paper on the upper half. The rest of the paper was left blank. Anita reported that she did not have control over the pain or the stress that rained down on her.

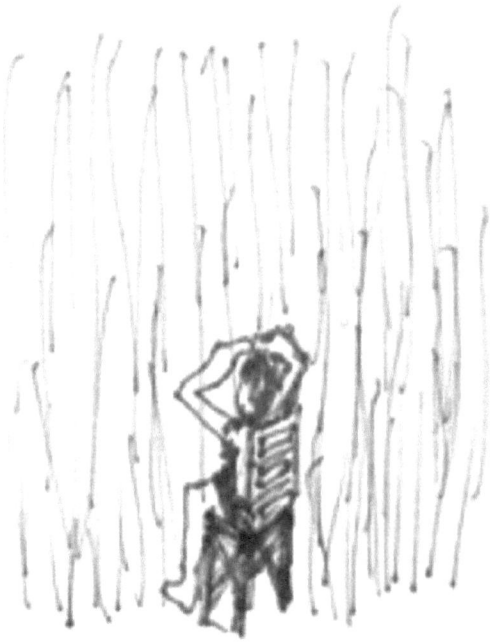

Figure 4.12 Person in the Rain

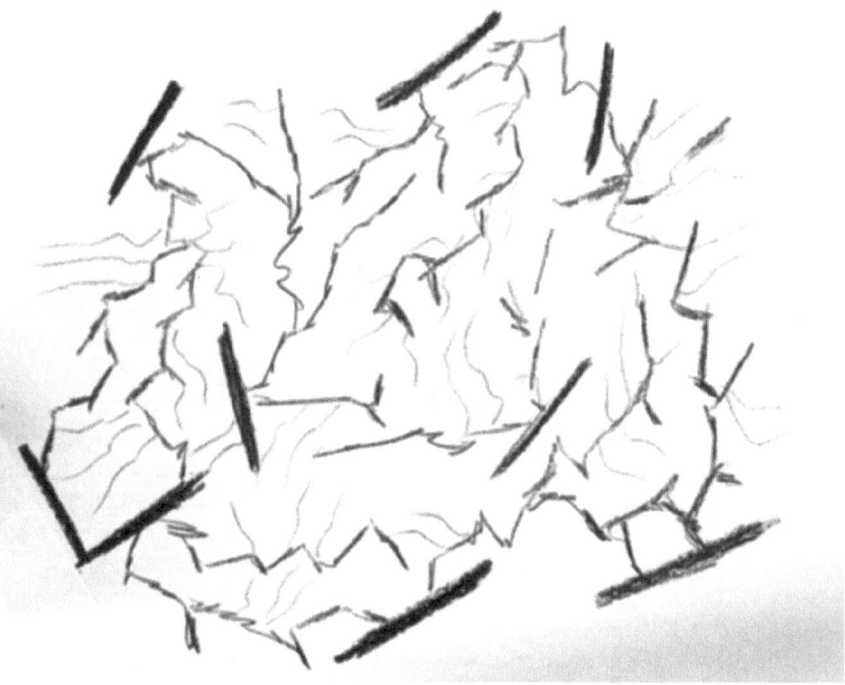

Figure 4.13 Anita's Pain

The pain drawing (Figure 4.13) and discussion led to the discovery of psychological and perceived blocks. The initial description focused on Anita's attempts to approach tasks like washing dishes, preparing meals, vacuuming, etc. Each time she undertook these tasks, the pain would block her ability to engage and complete the task comfortably. Continued discussion led to the husband's perceived dissatisfaction with the marital relationship and engagement with grandchildren. The discussion also reflected our client and art therapist relationship, as each suggested art process was turned away as likely inducing pain.

I noticed during the drawing assessments that Anita was experiencing pain. She gripped the pencils tightly, her shoulders and elbows were pulled in tightly to her side, and she seemed to have a grimace on her face. I considered the structure of the ETC (Hinz, 2019) and projected that Anita was almost singly experiencing the current situation through the sensory component. Using her tight grip, she applied pressure when drawing lines and made her strokes with jerky movements. Both drawings were done quickly and spontaneously without cognitive reflection. Although the DAPR showed a narrative, it was one that was imposed by the directions given within the instructions.

To help ease her discomfort, I invited Anita to sit back in her chair and get her body into as comfortable a position as possible. I invited her to close her eyes and focus on her breathing. I offered guided relaxation but she was resistant to listening and following verbal directions. She was able to come to a state of relaxation when I simply and slowly counted backwards from ten.

When her stress level subsided, we engaged in a conversation about goals. Together we decided to focus on addressing frustration, focusing on pain reduction, improved emotional well-being, and enhancing coping skills. I further recommended couples counseling or having the husband join us for some sessions. This recommendation was met with strong hesitation. Anita explained that her husband was the worker in the family and could not take time off work for these kinds of explorations.

Sessions

To provide a sensory experience and create a product Anita might enjoy, I introduced her to a marbling process using shaving cream and liquid watercolor. Anita had difficulty pressing the button on top of the shaving cream can, so I sprayed the shaving cream into the butcher pan. Anita then chose three colors and drizzled the liquid watercolor onto the shaving cream. I provided her with a wooden stick to drag across the colors, creating a marbled pattern. She then took six-inch square pieces of watercolor paper and gently pressed it into the shaving cream. Using a plastic spatula, Anita then gently scraped the dimensional shaving cream from the paper. She then wiped down the table and looked at the marbled paper. The colors were bright. I explained the colors would soften as they dried. Anita turned her head toward me and smiled. I simply nodded my head and opened my hand toward a stack of watercolor papers on the corner of the table. Anita continued and in that session she made two dozen squares of marbled watercolor paper.

When Anita returned two weeks later, she was excited to see how the papers looked when they were dry. She referred to the papers as backgrounds and started to imagine trees and flowers within the marbled surfaces. I brought out the liquid watercolors, paper, and a few large brushes to help Anita learn to create brushstroke paintings. I chose the larger brushes remembering Anita's difficulty with holding and manipulating the pencils. The larger brushes provided a wider handle so she would not have to grip it so tightly. I taught Anita about charging the brushes with color and demonstrated some basic stroke principles. I invited her to experiment with the different brushes and colors on blank paper before deciding what to do with the marbled squares. She spent that entire session playing with the brushes and did not mention her pain.

After spending the prior session practicing brushstrokes, Anita came to the next session ready to apply her new-found technique to the marbled squares. We took out the materials, and she was able to imagine into each separate, marbled square and determined what to place on each. Some squares had flowers, some trees, and one had a heart. Anita experienced some pain during this session as she struggled to get the brushstrokes exactly where she wanted them. With this watercolor as the process, it was easy to direct the conversation toward flow and letting the image and the process determine outcomes. Anita learned that when she hurried, or tried to make the image look perfect, she experienced stress and this made her pain symptoms worse. Each time her pain took over, we stopped and took time to step back. Each time she was able to re-start the process. At the end of that session, Anita had three completed flower images, two trees that she found acceptable, and the one image of the heart which she planned on giving to her husband. She had four unsuccessful attempts that she deemed unsalvageable and tossed them into the garbage on her way out, saying, "sometimes I have to just let things go". When Anita returned for her next session, she indicated that the heart art she gave her husband sparked a non-pain related discussion.

As time went on, Anita continued to trust her own experiences with art materials; she even built an affinity to play without direction or focusing on outcomes. Art-making became a functional distraction from the pain and allowed space for emotional exploration. Artmaking also became a tool for mindfulness practice focused on cultivating present-moment awareness, and helping to manage pain-related stress. Gentle art-making processes facilitated the verbalization of emotions associated with her condition and allowed for a deeper understanding of the mind-body connection. This empowered Anita to actively engage in her pain management.

Outcomes

Anita continued to come to art therapy for a period of about six months. Over the course of art therapy, Anita reported a reduction in perceived pain intensity, an increased ability to manage flare-ups, and an improved relationship with her husband. Anita's experience in mindful participation in artmaking underscores the effectiveness of art therapy in pain management for individuals, particularly with fibromyalgia. The integration of a person-centered focus, attention to the isomorphic nature of art participation, and mindfulness-based techniques in art therapy offered Anita a holistic method to address the complex interplay between her emotions, perceptions, and physical sensations in chronic pain.

TAMYRA

ERIN HEIN

Setting

I met Tamyra at an outpatient infusion clinic in an urban midwestern hospital. It is a smaller clinic, with the capability of serving a maximum of 11 patients at one time. Most of the patients who are seen in this clinic sit in one of nine recliners that are situated along the outermost wall of the clinic in sectioned off pods of two or three chairs. Each chair has its own personal television on a telescoping arm. A few patients will go into one of the two rooms located along the north wall of the clinic. Working with patients means bringing a small stool up next to wherever they are seated and working chairside or bedside individually while they are receiving treatment. This often means we do not have a private place to work as there may be another patient in the chair opposite or on the other side of a small half wall that separates the pods. Sessions are usually informal, with an intake and assessment built on conversation. The therapeutic time frame is often shorter as I may see a client as little as one time due to a shift in their chemotherapy schedule, or as many as four times a month for three to four months if their treatment goes as planned. There is always the chance that things may suddenly get worse and the patient is not feeling up to creating art that day, or the patient may pass away, terminating the therapeutic relationship abruptly.

When working with patients in the infusion clinic, there are four main areas of growth found to be beneficial. The first of which is interactive distraction (McNutt, 2018). A lot of the patients in the clinic are dealing with angst and distress caused by their related disease. Giving the patient an opportunity to actively distract from anxiety or pain can assist in reducing the focus on these feelings within the body. The second area is building hope.

When faced with a life-changing diagnosis, such as cancer, patients may feel ungrounded and unsure of what the future may bring. Creating reminders of hope for the future can help patients focus and, therefore, feel more grounded. The third area is introspection and self-learning. It is during this step that we encourage the patients to take a step back and focus on what kind of emotions they are really having, where the roots of those emotions may be growing from, and what patterns of behaviors those emotions cause. It is only when we understand those emotions and behaviors that we can work out how to prune unhealthy behaviors and allow healthy habits to flourish. The last area is transforming and re-identifying with the self. When patients have spent weeks to months going in and out of clinics and doctors' appointments, they can often assimilate their whole identity to being only a patient. It is through this step that the patients attempt to rediscover themselves and redefine their identity. An example of this would be John Doe is a cancer patient; however, after redefining himself, John Doe becomes John, an avid bicyclist who loves to barbecue and he has cancer.

Within this infusion clinic setting, I have a large plastic box in which I carry a small variety of supplies. I make sure that this box has the supplies necessary for a variety of projects that can assist in working towards the aforementioned areas of growth. There are also two cabinets that hold a larger quantity of supplies in case the box needs replenishing, or a patient requires a different directive to accomplish the goals they have set for themself. All available supplies would include six-inch square origami paper, glass stones about an inch in diameter in circle and oval shapes, old magazines that have been donated over the years, scissors, liquid and stick glue, air-dry clay, small glass bottles ranging from three inches to one inch tall, polymer clay in a rainbow array of colors and cut into quarter-inch blocks, plastic tools for modeling and shaping the clay, pre-printed coloring sheets with mandala or geometric designs, crayons, markers, colored pencils, shrink film, sandpaper, student-grade watercolor paper, watercolor paint pans, soft paint brushes, watercolor crayons, tempera paint sticks, elastic cord, jewelry clasps, and a variety of beads.

Approach

When working in the infusion clinic, I work from a person-centered approach. Natalie Rogers (2001) wrote that this approach emphasizes the worth of every individual and mandates that they are all treated with respect for who they are as a person. This theory also believes that each patient has the ability to guide their own journey through the therapeutic landscape and has an innate desire for personal development. In order to be a therapeutic presence working from this theoretical approach, one must "be empathic, open, honest, congruent, and caring, as [one] listens in depth" (N. Rogers, 2001, p. 164). This means that every patient we see has the capability and the internal drive to work towards their goals, and we as art therapists must listen closely with respect and an open mind. We must strive to communicate our acceptance of who the patient is as a person through our active listening. Feeling heard and accepted leads to feeling understood and empowered to find solutions (N. Rogers, 2001). We can also extrapolate that if the patient is the guide on a personal journey, and we want the patient to find individual solutions, this would lead to understanding that the patient knows best what is in the artwork. Natalie Rogers (2001) puts it as "if the client happens to like the therapist's interpretation of the art, then he or she will return again and again to find the meaning from the authority figure – the therapist – rather than develop the ability to find meaning for him- or herself" (p. 168). A therapist can ask leading questions, as if to shine a light on certain incongruities, but we must allow the patient to be the one to determine what their artwork is telling them.

As this work does take place within a hospital setting, there is an added layer within the work. The person-centered approach must take place within the medical model. Medical art therapy is when an art therapist uses the media and creative process as a way to provide therapy to patients who are going through a bodily illness and are undergoing medical treatments (Keselman & Awais, 2018). Healthcare often prioritizes the physiological illness and symptoms, which means that the psychological symptoms caused by the illness can often receive a lower priority. When a patient has to be in the hospital, either as an inpatient or outpatient, they are surrounded by sounds, language, and even an environment that is unfamiliar, which may cause more stress (Keselman & Awais, 2018). This is why it is important for a person-centered model of art therapy to be found within medical hospitals. The art therapist can combat the psychological stress and uncertainty by helping the patient feel heard and understood, this way the medical professionals can focus more on the physical issues with less interference from the psychological ones.

Client

Tamyra is an African American woman in her mid-60s. She was being seen in the infusion clinic for Intravenous (IV) infusion chemotherapy as a treatment for a breast cancer diagnosis. Tamyra was a friendly person who was open to talking with anyone around her, be it a staff member or a fellow patient. Like many of the patients I saw in the clinic, she was a little skeptical of me when I first appeared in front of her with my box of art supplies. This may be reflective of the fact that Tamyra is a Black woman and I am a Caucasian woman.

Research demonstrates that the African American population has a long history of conflicts and mistreatment within the mental health field, a predominantly Caucasian field, which has resulted in wariness and skepticism when it comes to mental health professionals. Most African American individuals would rather consult and discuss their mental health issues with family members, close friends, or even those in their religious community before working with a therapist (Curtis-Boles, 2017). Aburizik et al. (2023) commented as well that the *Strong Black Woman Schema* often pushed by society stereotypes, defines Black women as being "resilient, strong, and unemotional" (p. 934) to the point that they may be encouraged to never break down and never need help from anyone. This kind of thought process may be encouraging to some, but may also be oppressive to others by not allowing them to show their human feelings. These factors can often make many of the Black women patients I approach skeptical of what it is I am offering them and what it would mean for them to participate. I have found that open and honest communication gives patients the choice to participate or not. Using this approach, I have been able to break through most of the skepticism and gotten conversation and participation in art therapy in return. With Tamyra, my consistency, openness, and acceptance helped her feel more comfortable in forming a therapeutic relationship with me.

Intake Sessions

I introduced myself and offered the choice of art therapy two separate times before Tamyra finally accepted. My initial intake with her was very informal through conversation and visual clues. We sat and discussed her life and family. I learned that she had three adult children as well as one teenage granddaughter that she helped raise. Tamyra never mentioned a spouse but did mention that her parents were both deceased.

The nurses had informed me prior to meeting with Tamyra that she had a breast cancer diagnosis. While I sat and chatted with Tamyra, I noticed that she sat upright and on the edge of the recliner rather than settling down into it. She was also moving her hands around a lot and when she did put her hands down, they would grasp onto each other. A nurse came to get her vital signs and asked the typical questions that the nurses ask every patient. During those questions Tamyra mentioned experiencing some pain at the site of where she had been receiving radiation therapy. Tamyra also mentioned throughout our discussion that she was nervous about what might happen during treatment and the potential outcome.

Observations, comments from the patient, and information from the nursing staff helped formulate my preliminary assessment of her presenting issues. Tamyra had breast cancer and was experiencing anxiety about the diagnosis. She was feeling ungrounded about the outcome of treatment. She was also experiencing some pain and discomfort in the affected area of her body. As Tamyra became comfortable in the therapeutic space, her ability to strike up meaningful conversations displayed a desire for companionship, and to not feel alone while going through these anxiety-provoking treatments.

Because therapeutic encounters in the infusion clinic may only last one session, I use a very informal assessment method that takes place during initial conversations. In meeting with Tamyra, I learned that her anxiety and feelings of being ungrounded seemed to be the top issues of concern. I verified this by asking if she felt worry and stress were top priorities we should try and work through. She agreed. Our short-term objective was to create art that would help actively distract her from anxiety.

We determined that creating art while she was waiting to receive her IV medications would be more effective than waiting for when her infusion would begin. Often when patients arrive in the clinic, they first get their blood drawn, then wait for results to return. After that, nurses are able to start the pre-medications which must be given before chemotherapy. The nurses wait until after these lab results are back because if certain numbers are too low, they may have to add other medications to the treatment. For example, the patient may need extra magnesium. If other numbers are too low, such as the patient's white blood cell count, they may not be able to get the chemotherapy at all for fear of wiping out too much of the immune system. Waiting for lab work can often take anywhere from 30 minutes to an hour and a half and is dependent on how busy the staff is in the lab. This period of waiting was often when Tamyra noticed the most anxiety as it held the uncertainty of whether her numbers would be good enough to still get her medications that day.

Tamyra voiced concern about the feeling of being ungrounded as well. Her worries about how treatment would progress and if the cancer would be beaten were high on her priorities. We decided to make a long-term objective for treatment, building hope for her future. Once the short-term and long-term objectives were created, we were able to determine which art therapy directives were the most appropriate to accomplish her goals.

Sessions

During our first art therapy session, I presented the directive of working with small cubes of polymer clay and a small glass bottle. The pharmacy collects small water-soluble medication bottles to be used for this project. Art therapy staff then cleans these bottles and removes the labels. This way the bottle can metaphorically represent the medications the patients are receiving in the clinic and, therefore, the illness itself. We encourage the patients to use the colorful polymer clay to transform the bottle representing illness into something that is hopeful and positive. Working with the clay is also a physical process of squishing, squeezing, blending, smoothing, and shaping that can help bring the focus down into the hands and off of the cycling thoughts that revolve around worry and anxiety. Tamyra was first presented with a variety of small glass bottles. She then had to choose between tall or short, wide or narrow, and clear or translucent brown. Tamyra was then offered a rainbow of colors as well as neutral colors and asked to pick those that she felt were calling to her. She chose dark purple, magenta, magenta with sparkles, and hot pink. I gave her a short lesson on how to manipulate the clay pieces and then instructed her to create something with the clay that transformed the bottle into something that helped her feel hopeful.

Tamyra created a rose extending out of the uncovered bottle (Figure 4.14). She began with the dark purple and wrapped three pieces of the different magentas around the dark purple. Tamyra added an extra petal of dark purple outside of the magenta. She then added a layer of hot pink petals all around the outside of the rose. At this point Tamyra asked for some green to add leaves to her flower, she was presented with two options and chose the lighter green. She created three leaves out of the green clay and placed all three around the flower and then decided she wanted to move one of them down to the bottom of the rose as if it was more of a stem. Tamyra then placed her rose in the bottle as if it was a flower in a vase. I asked her to tell me about her creation to encourage making meaning. She began to tell me about what the different colors of the flower meant to her. The dark purple she called the anxiety and pain, deep at the heart of everything. The magenta shades represented her support system wrapping around her anxiety as a way to try and help her overcome her stress. She mentioned that a little of the dark purple was outside of the magenta, saying that some stress is even beyond the support. Tamyra then turned to the hot pink; she said this color represented the joy and love in her life. The joy and love wrap around it all to relieve the anxiety and pain, as joy can often help her forget about her stress completely and she finds her love in her family. She did not discuss the leaves; it is possible that they were added simply because of the rose shape. Tamyra did talk about the rose's placement in the bottle, she said it was meant to show growing from the treatment and coming out stronger on the other side.

The second time I worked with Tamyra, we decided to focus more on that hope by creating a small hope stone. Through this process, patients are presented with clear glass stones that range from sizes of two and a half to four centimeters. Patients are then given magazines from which to choose a word or short phrase that makes them feel hopeful as well as a picture for the background. This process is meant to allow their subconscious to speak to them; by allowing them to flip through any magazine while focusing on a theme, the mind can gravitate towards words or images that jump out and represent that theme to them. This way the subconscious can point out themes of hope to the conscious mind. Tamyra liked the circular stones the best and chose to look through a magazine that was geared towards pop culture first.

While flipping through this magazine, Tamyra was drawn to a picture of a singer holding their hands above their head, forming a heart shape. She stared at the picture and then determined to use the picture for her stone. She continued to flip through the magazine to find some kind of word or phrase to go with the image. Eventually, she found a page with

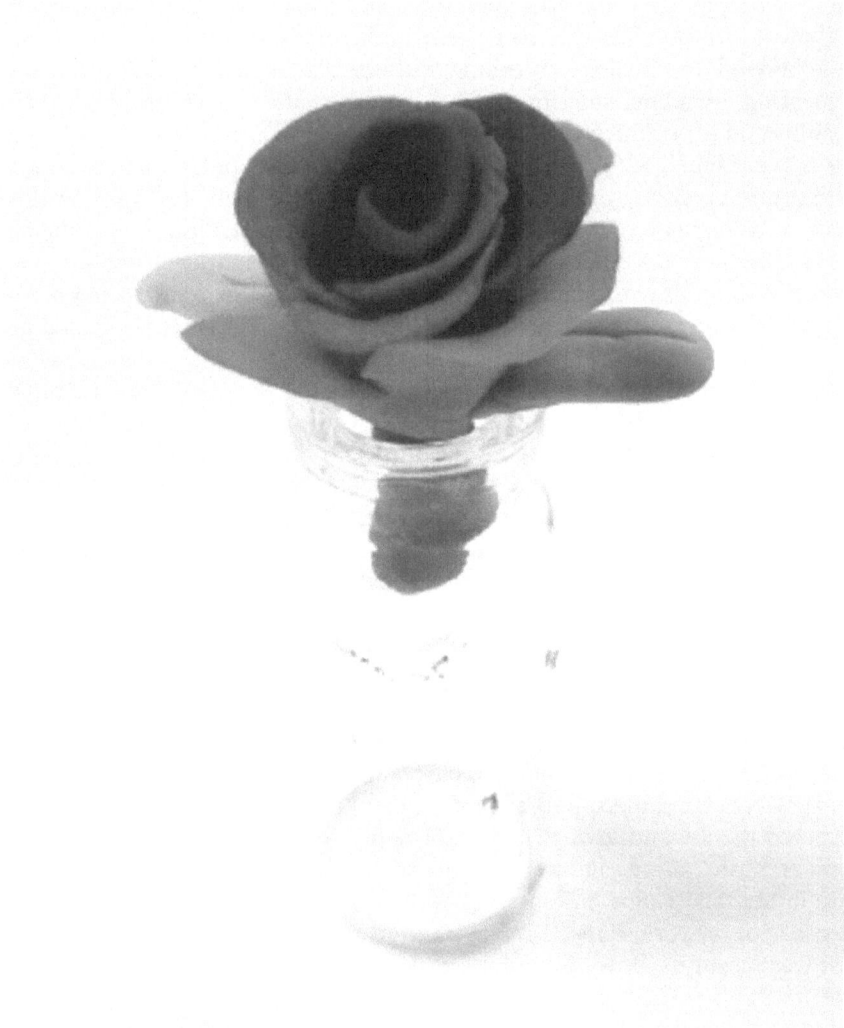

Figure 4.14 Untitled

an elaborate book review and an interview with an actor on the opposite page. The review and the interview were not what caught her attention, instead the words that were located in the title of the book and on a line that was emphasized in the interview. She found the words "Faith" and "Hallelujah". Tamyra was excited about finding these words and immediately cut them out. While trimming the words and deciding where to place them, she began telling me about how faith has played a part in her life, specifically in raising her children. While we glued all the pieces together, she got deeper into the discussion by talking about how much reading the Bible has helped her through all the hard times in her life. She stated it was always a source of comfort. When she completed her stone she smiled and showed me the final product (Figure 4.15). She liked how it turned out and how she was

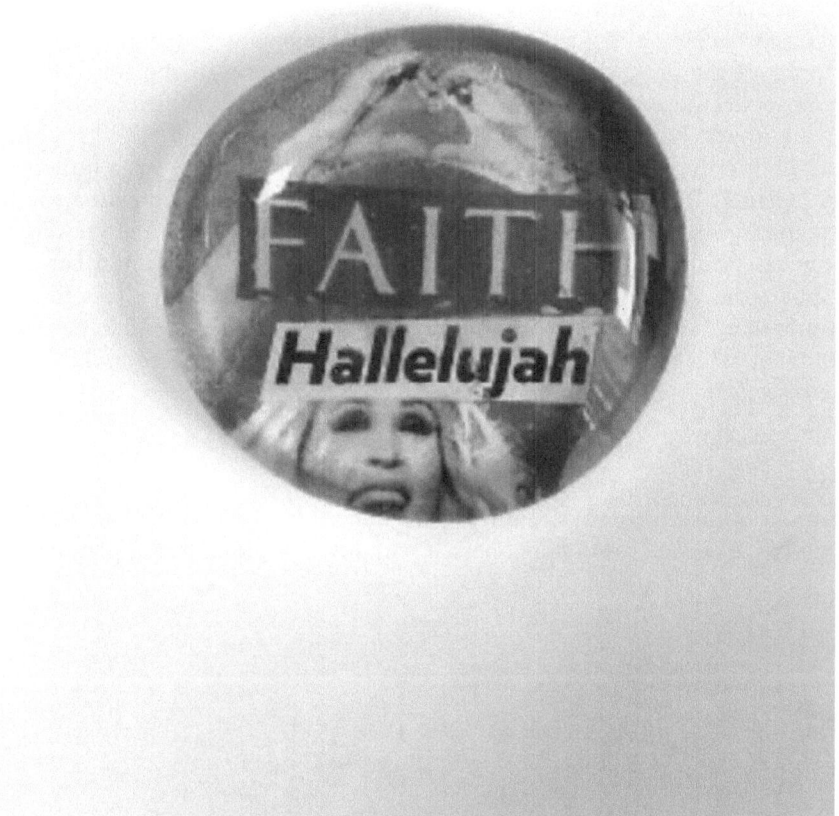

Figure 4.15 Hope Stone

planning to keep it with her as a way to always remember to rely on her faith and on God to help lift her up through the struggle of treatments.

On one of the last times I worked with Tamyra, she came in with a plan. She wanted to create something for her high school age granddaughter as a memento of her grandmother. She mentioned that her granddaughter loved butterflies. We determined the best way to do this was by creating a shrink film keychain that her granddaughter could hang her keys on or display on her backpack. Tamyra showed me a picture of a monarch butterfly on her phone, saying she would like it to look like this but with different colors. She was hesitant to draw this butterfly herself. We decided that the easiest way for her to accomplish her goal would be to print off a black and white version of the image, using the clinic computers so that she could trace the image onto the shrink film. I felt it was important to follow Tamyra's lead on this project as it seemed she had done a lot of thinking outside of our sessions about her goal and how to accomplish it.

We taped the shrink film over the image that I had printed out. I showed her two examples of completed shrink film art, one used permanent markers for color and the other used colored pencils. Tamyra liked the bright colors of the pencils instead of the slightly translucent version with the permanent markers. As she traced and colored in the butterfly, Tamyra talked to me about helping to raise her granddaughter and how proud she was of her. Prom was approaching and Tamyra had just been dress shopping with her granddaughter. She spoke of the granddaughter's intelligence and how well she was doing in school. As Tamyra spoke, there was a big smile on her face and her eyes shined brightly. She chose to make the butterfly blue as it was her favorite color, that way it merged her granddaughter's favorite butterfly with her own favorite color, blue. The result was a little piece of both of them together. When she finished creating the butterfly, I baked it in a toaster oven to complete the shrinking process. I handed the final product back to Tamyra (Figure 4.16), and she smiled. She got quiet for a moment as small tears showed up in her eyes. When Tamyra spoke, she said, "No matter how this turns out, she'll always have this". It was then that I saw that Tamyra was creating legacy work just in case she didn't make it through her treatment. This was a little piece of her that her granddaughter could always have with her to remember her grandmother.

Outcomes

Through the creation of these artworks, Tamyra was able to decode that in order to work through her anxiety, she needed to surround herself with love, joy, and her support system.

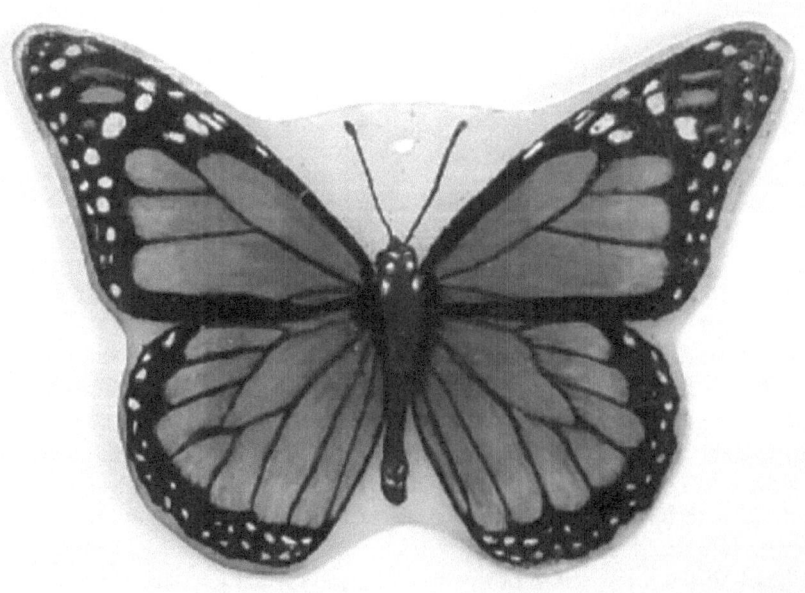

Figure 4.16 Butterfly for Granddaughter

She was reminded that she could always find spiritual connection and hope in her Bible and those in her spiritual community. Tamyra also found a way to always be with those in her family she was most worried about, even if she can't physically be there for them. Through the person-centered approach, she was able to take charge of her therapy sessions and know where she needed them to go in order to achieve the goals that she helped set for herself. She was also able to find these answers on her own, becoming the authority over her own healing journey.

Tamyra did occasionally struggle with this approach. The person-centered approach is meant to encourage the patient to make the decisions about how things will progress and find the answers in their own work. There were times when Tamyra felt unsure of where to start with materials or didn't always know what to say when I asked her to tell me about her creation that day. Sometimes all it took was starting to play with the materials or start to describe the art for the ideas and meanings to start flowing from her. One of the side effects of chemotherapy medications can often be neuropathy, which means that a patient may have nerve damage in their fingers and toes which causes them to not be able to feel or grip things very well. Tamyra did deal with this on a mild level, which caused her a few issues with some of the media tools but she was able to power through it and ask for assistance when needed. There were also days when Tamyra was unable to participate in art therapy at all. Some of the chemotherapy medications or even pre-medications would leave her feeling sick or exhausted and falling asleep. When those days came, Tamyra would often look up at me and say, "I'm so sorry, but I just can't today". To which I would always reply, "No need to be sorry", and that she knows best what her body needs right now.

I have learned in this field to treat each session as though it may be our last for numerous reasons outside of my control. This means that at the end of each session I would talk to Tamyra about what she gained from that session and remind her to always think back on those insights when things got hard. I would then thank her for participating in art-making that day. Tamyra would often end with thanking me, not only for bringing the art to her, but also for listening to her so compassionately. She mentioned that it often seemed hard to find people who would truly listen and let her talk about the things going on in her life. This comment by her really shows the importance and impact behind coming into these sessions with a person-centered approach. Giving her that open and compassionate sounding board to talk and work things through helped her feel as though she was truly appreciated as a person and given the space to work through her anxiety and fears.

After these sessions took place, I stopped seeing Tamyra in the infusion clinic. I asked the nursing staff about her absence. They let me know that on one of the days I was not scheduled to be in the clinic, Tamyra finished her chemotherapy sessions and was declared in full remission. It was reported to me that the nursing staff gave her a referral to a cancer support group for other survivors that she was excited about joining. The nurses also reported that Tamyra had mentioned on her last day that she had talked with them about being grateful for the opportunity to participate in art therapy during her sessions at the hospital.

Concluding Statements

Tamyra was able to leave the infusion clinic cancer-free and ready for the joy in her life to get her back to living it fully. Art therapy helped Tamyra connect to her artwork deeper and encouraged her to find her own path towards her goals, which can be seen in how she came in with a plan of her own for our shrink film session. Creating art acted as a reprieve from her treatments. It allowed Tamyra to take time for her own self-care and gave her time to play again. I have faith that Tamyra took those insights to heart and will continue moving forward with those in mind in order to make the most out of her life.

References

Aburizik, A., Brindle, M., Johnson, E., Provencio, A., Kivlighan, M., & LeBeau, B. (2023). Black women's distress matters: Examining gendered racial disparities in psycho-oncology referral rates. *Psycho-oncology, 32*(6), 933–941.

Barresi, M., & Gilbert, S. (2023). *Developmental biology* (13th ed.). Oxford University Press.

Berg, J. M., Wrzesniewski, A., & Dutton, J. E. (2010). Perceiving and responding to challenges in job crafting at different ranks: When proactivity requires adaptivity. *Journal of Organizational Behavior, 31*(2–3), 158–186.

Biro-Hannah, E. (2021). Community adult mental health: Mitigating the impact of Covid-19 through online art therapy. *International Journal of Art Therapy, 26*(3), 96–103.

Buck, J. N. (1948), The H-T-P test. *Journal of Clinical Psychology, 4*, 151–159.

Cohen, G. D. (2006). *The creative age: Awakening human potential in the second half of life.* Random House.

Csikszentmihalyi, M. (1997). *Finding flow: The psychological engagement with everyday life.* Basic Books.

Curtis-Boles, H. (2017). Clinical strategies for working with clients of African descent. *Best Practices in Mental Health, 13*(2), 61–72.

Dollinger, S., Kzmeierczak, E., & Storkerson, P. (2011). Creativity and self-exploration in projective drawings of abused women: Evaluating the inside me-outside me workshop. *Journal of Creativity in Mental Health, 6*(3), 202–219.

Erikson, E. H. (1950). *Childhood and society.* New York, NY: Norton.

Erikson, E. (1967). *Identity and the life cycle.* W.W. Norton & Company.

Galler, H. (2014). *Heather Galler landscapes modern folk art* [Video]. https://youtu.be/STCVwbquP-s

Gergen K. J. (2015). *An invitation to social contraction* (3rd ed.). SAGE Publications.

Glinzak, L. (2016). Effects of art therapy on distress levels of adults with cancer: A proxy pretest study. *Art Therapy: Journal of the American Art Therapy Association, 33*(1), 27–34.

Good, D. A. (2016) Adult art therapy: Four decades ages 20–60 years. In D. Gussak & M. Rosal (Eds). *The Wiley handbook of art therapy* (pp. 262–271). John Wiley & Sons.

Hammer, E. F. (1958). *The clinical application of projective drawings.* Charles Thomas.

Hass-Cohen, N., Bokoch, R., & Fowler, G. (2022) The compassionate arts psychotherapy program: Benefits of a compassionate arts media continuum. *Art Therapy: Journal of the American Art Therapy Association, 40*(1), 5–14.

Hinz, L. D. (2015). Expressive therapies continuum: Use and value demonstrated with case study. *Canadian Art Therapy Association Journal, 28*(1–2), 43–50.

Hinz, L. D. (2019). *Expressive therapies continuum: A framework for using art in therapy* (2nd ed.). Routledge.

Jenkins, R., Bhugra, D., Bebbington, P., Brugha, T., Farrell, M., Coid, J., ... & Meltzer, H. (2008). Debt, income, and mental disorder in the general population. *Psychological Medicine, 38*(10), 1485–1493.

Kagin, S. L., & Lusebrink, V. B. (1978). The expressive therapies continuum. *Art Psychotherapy, 5*(4), 171–180.

Keselman, M., & Awais, Y. J. (2018). Exploration of cultural humility in medical art therapy. *Art Therapy: Journal of the American Art Therapy Association, 35*(2), 77–87.

King, J. L. (Ed.). (2016). *Art therapy, trauma, and neuroscience: Theoretical and practical perspectives.* Routledge.

Kohlberg, L. (1969). Stage and sequence: The cognitive-developmental approach to socialization. In D. A. Goslin (Ed.). *Handbook of socialization* (pp. 347–480). Ran McNally.

Lachman, M. E. (2004). Development in midlife. *Annual Review of Psychology, 55*, 305–331.

Luzzatto, P., & Gabriel, B. (2000). The creative journey: A model for short-term group art therapy with post treatment cancer patients. *Art Therapy: Journal of the American Art Therapy Association, 17*, 265–269.

Maslow, A. H. (1943). A theory of human motivation. *Psychological Review, 50*(4), 370–396.

Maslow, A. H. (1970). *Motivation and personality.* Harper & Row.

McGoldrick, M., Gerson, R., & Petry, S. (2008). *Genograms: Assessments and interventions.* W.W. Norton & Company.

McNutt, J. V. (2018). Visual narratives as an art therapy treatment in cancer care. In D. Elkis-Abuhoff & M. Gaydos (Eds). *Art and expressive therapies within a medical model: Clinical applications.* Routledge.

Moon, B. L. (2016). *Art-based group therapy theory and practice.* Charles C. Thomas Publisher, Ltd.

Nainis, N., Paice, J. A., Ratner, J., Wirth, J. H., Lai, J., & Shott, S. (2006). Relieving symptoms in cancer: Innovative use of art therapy. *Journal of Pain and Symptom Management, 31*(2), 162–169.

Piaget, J., & Inhelder, B. (1969). *The psychology of a child.* Routledge.

Rogers, C. R. (1979). The foundations of the person-centered approach. *Education, 100*(2), 98–107.

Rogers, N. (2001). Person-centered expressive arts therapy: A path to wholeness. In J. A. Rubin (Ed.). *Approaches to art therapy: Theory & technique* (2nd ed., pp. 163–177). Brunner-Routledge.

Rura, N. (2020). *Following healthy lifestyle habits at middle age may increase years lived free of chronic diseases.* Harvard T.H. Chan: School of Public Health.

Schmanke, L. (2018, November 4). *Use of fairy tale and archetype in art therapy with substance abuse* [Half-day advanced practice workshop]. The 49th annual conference of the American Art Therapy Association, Miami, FL, November 4, 2018.

Schwartz, R. C. (1995). *Internal family systems therapy.* Guildford Press.

Stirnemann, M.V. (1997). *Artist trading cards* [Collaborative Cultural Performance]. INK.art&text, Zurich, Switzerland.

Swan-Foster, N. (2018). *Jungian art therapy: Images, dreams, and analytical psychology.* Routledge.

Thyme, K. E., Sundin, E. C., Wiberg, B., Oster, I., Astrom, S., & Lindh, J. (2009). Individual brief art therapy can be helpful for women with breast cancer: A randomized controlled clinical study. *Palliative Support Care, 7*(1), 87–95.

Toseland, R. W., & Rivas, R. F. (2017). *An introduction to group work practice,* (8th ed.). Pearson Education.

Tripp, T. (2016) A body based bilateral protocol for reprocessing trauma. In J. L. King (Ed.). *Art therapy, trauma, and neuroscience: Theoretical and practical perspectives* (pp. 173–194). Routledge.

Umberson, D., Williams, K., Thomas, P. A., Liu, H., & Thomeer, M. B. (2014). Race, gender and chains of disadvantage: Childhood adversity, social relationships, and health. *Journal of Health and Social Behavior, 55*(1), 20–38.

van der Kolk, B. (2014). *The body keeps the score: Brain, mind, and body in the healing of trauma.* Penguin Books.

Wallas, G. (1926). *The art of thought.* Solis Press.

Wauters, A. (1997). *Chakras and their archetypes.* The Crossing Press.

Weil, A. (1999). *Breathing: The master key to self-healing* (CD). (Audio produced by Sounds True).

Willis, L. R., Joy, S. P., & Kaiser, D. H. (2010). Draw-a-person-in-the-rain as an assessment of stress and coping resources. *The Arts in Psychotherapy, 37*(3), 233–239.

Wolfe, F., Clauw, D. J., Fitzcharles, M. A., Goldenberg, D. L., Katz, R. S., Mease, P., ... & Yunus, M. B. (2010). The American College of Rheumatology preliminary diagnostic criteria for fibromyalgia and measurement of symptom severity. *Arthritis Care & Research, 62*(5), 600–610.

Yalom, I, (1980). *Existential psychotherapy.* Basic Books/Hachette Book Group.

Yalom, I. D. & Leszcz, M. (2020). *The theory and practice of group psychotherapy* (6th ed.). Basic Books.

Chapter 5

Late Adulthood and End-of-Life

Psychosocial development focuses on generativity, passing on knowledge, and contributions to future generations.

Introduction

Developmental Markers

Between the age of 60 and beyond, individuals continue developing and shaping their lives, relationships, and perspectives. Physical changes continue, including age-related declines in sensory abilities, muscle mass, and bone density (Barresi & Gilbert, 2023). Sometimes referred to as seniors, these individuals have increased vulnerability to chronic health conditions and diseases, necessitating greater emphasis on healthcare and lifestyle adjustments.

Psychosocial development focuses on generativity, passing on knowledge and contributions to future generations (Erikson, 1967). Cohen (2006) refers to adults aged 65 to 80 years as summing up. Summing up includes life review, reflecting on accomplishments, and integrating one's life story to find meaning in past experiences. Cohen refers to adults over 80 as being in a stage of encore marking a continued pursuit of new challenges and creativity. Changes in social structures include potential losses of friends and family, and adaptation to changing social roles. Adults in this age range are often undergoing economic changes, adjustment to new routines through retirement, and have time to explore leisure activities and hobbies (Drazic et al., 2023). Storytelling and handing down cultural heritage and traditions often involve community engagement (Levy, 2009).

Neuroplasticity persists during these ages allowing for continued learning and adaptations even in older ages (Hertzog et al., 2008). Older adults may be seen as carriers of wisdom and problem solvers (Baltes & Smith, 2008). Creative outlets serve as a means of coping with life changes and expression of emotions as older adults engage in creative pursuits for personal fulfillment and legacy building (Cohen, 2006). Adults in this age group experience enhanced emotional regulation, increased resilience, and greater emotional well-being derived from life experiences (Hertzog et al., 2008). Reflections on life's legacy and a sense of transition support a deepening of spiritual beliefs, existential reflections, and the search for meaning and purpose (Fowler, 1995).

DOI: 10.4324/9781003324805-6

Setbacks

Between the ages of 60 and beyond, individuals may encounter various setbacks that can impede their developmental progress. Common challenges during this life stage include health issues and physical decline, as well as changes in senses including vision, hearing, taste, and smell (Barresi & Gilbert, 2023). There are increases in susceptibility to chronic illness, mobility issues, and age-related health conditions, including the potential onset of neurodegenerative diseases, such as Alzheimer's or Parkinson's. Neurodegenerative diseases can impact functional abilities and independence (Barresi & Gilbert, 2023).

Coping with unresolved issues, regrets, or unmet aspirations can lead to emotional distress (Levy, 2009). Adjusting to retirement, loss of work-related identity, and finding purpose in the absence of a career can be challenging (Drazic et al., 2023). Financial instability, inadequate savings, or unexpected expenses can cause financial stress and impact overall well-being. Due to both internal and external changing circumstances, older adults have an increased risk of mental health concerns such as depression, anxiety, or existential angst. Older adults are also at risk of experiencing ageism, stereotypes, or discrimination based on age, impacting self-esteem and societal perceptions (Levy, 2009). These challenges can significantly impact individuals' well-being, necessitating supportive interventions, community resources, and coping strategies to navigate effectively through this stage of life.

Case Studies

The settings in this chapter included the clients' homes and complex care centers. The sessions were individually-based, including those given in the open studio at one of the care centers. The clients' ages ranged from 53 to 99 years of age and the length of art therapy services were scheduled from three weeks to four years. Three of the clients were in hospice care, while four of the remaining clients died shortly after their participation in art therapy. A life review (Zieger, 1976) through artmaking was conducted with all the clients whether it was a review including a lifetime of events or in one case a memory of one special family vacation. Art Therapy, Relationship Therapy (Gerlitz et al., 2020), and Narrative Therapy (Dunne, 2016) with a strength-based approach (Blood & Guthrie, 2018) were used with this population.

The loss of verbal communication, identity, and physical abilities, along with social isolation were among the major issues art therapy addressed with these clients. The use of art became a way for clients to express their thoughts and feelings when words began to fail them. Like Matisse, whose artwork changed when he got older, from portrait paintings to cut paper collage (Sooke, 2014), one client, who was once a portrait painter, retained his identity as an artist as he embraced abstract art during his art therapy sessions. His new art style, not hindered by his failing physical abilities, actually improved his ability to hold a paintbrush again. Other clients seen in their homes worked with memories and legacy. In other case studies, art therapy was conducted in an open-studio group setting, included art shows of clients' artwork, and reported client artwork being shared with family members. These are examples of how clients were engaged with others as they let their artwork speak and allowed them to feel less isolated during this stage in their lives.

In some cases, art therapists worked to make the materials accessible to all clients by modifying paint brushes, pencils, and other drawing tools to give clients easier handling. In other cases, they limited the number of materials offered to their clients in order to avoid overstimulation. Many of these clients were able to create artwork independently or as a co-artist with the therapist. When the client was too ill or their energy was too low, their art therapist drew for them. Taking directions from the client, the art therapist used the materials and color palette as well as what the suggested subject matter should be for the artwork. In one instance, the art therapist intuitively drew an image for her client that turned out to have a significant connection to a cherished memory for the client and his family members and kept the client engaged. Art therapy was a major component that helps all these clients to continue to reminisce, communicate, and actively engage with others through their art.

FINDING VOICE IN ART: THE EFFECTIVENESS OF ART THERAPY WITH OLDER ADULTS IN A CARE CENTER

JINNIE JEON

The purpose of the case studies of Vivian, John, and Patricia was to explore the effectiveness of art therapy interventions with older adults in a complex care center during open studio group art therapy sessions. The case studies were in an effort to examine how the creative artmaking process offered an opportunity for older adults to explore their range of play in a nonjudgmental, welcoming, and safe social context. The older adults who participated in these open studios had varying artistic backgrounds, and needs within the group.

Research indicates that active arts engagement can enhance older adults' health and experienced well-being (Groot et al., 2021). By engaging in creative processes and participating in art therapy, older adults can improve motor skills and coordination, stimulate sensory reception, build cognitive function, enhance mood and mental health, and enjoy opportunities for social connection (Banasiak, 2019). Artmaking has also been described as a vehicle for non-verbal communication that gives people with dementia a means to be understood and have their emotions validated by others (Banasiak, 2019; Camartin, 2012).

Allowing older adults to express their feelings by engaging in creative processes offers them distinctive ways to remain active and live fully in the present by expressing their creativity (Bagan, 2009). At the same time, in fostering a creative environment, art therapists must remember to approach older adults as the experts, the leaders, and those in charge of the art therapy session. Older adults determine the course of action and must be supported in their decisions. Whenever possible, they are encouraged to share skills with each other, serving as mentors and support for their peers. They are welcomed into the space to create or observe (Partridge, 2019).

Improving the mental state of older adults will enrich their relationships with the people around them, including staff, family members, friends, and visitors. These enhanced relationships will increase the fulfillment of daily life. The improvement of older adults' mental outlook through the use of art therapy has the potential to improve physical health subsequently.

Through various research studies, professionals working with senior populations have recognized that art therapy effectively enhances older adults' quality of life (Banasiak, 2019; Choi et al., 2013; Li & Li, 2017; Masika et al., 2020; Windle et al., 2018). This is achieved through balancing their physical, cognitive, emotional, and spiritual needs and abilities. In these case studies, as an art therapist, I demonstrated that older adults at a complex care center had the ability to fully engage, find enjoyment, feel accomplished and empowered, and grow within the community of a group art therapy program. Four years of experience in this setting allowed me to work with older adults with various mental and physical limitations.

The following case studies illustrate the need for art therapy in residential facilities for older adults and follow a format guided by these questions:

1. What are the observed expressions, creative arts environments, and relationships within the shared space of group art therapy sessions with older adults and a wide range of physical and emotional levels in the residential care center environment?
2. What are the general diagnoses of older adults at this particular complex care center?
3. What is the overall appearance of the older adults in the group?
4. What is the relationship between the therapist and the older adult in group art therapy sessions?
5. What is the relationship between the older adults in the group?
6. What is the general approach of the older adult in the group?
7. What relationship did the older adults have with the art materials and images?
8. What appeared aesthetically in the older adult's' artworks for themselves and the art therapist?

Clients

All older adult participants were residents of a complex care center on the West Coast of Canada. Older adults decided whether they wished to participate in the open studio art therapy sessions. The time spent in the studio varied based on their daily conditions and schedules. There were two three-hour group art therapy sessions offered on Tuesday and Thursday mornings each week. Most participants were Caucasian and Asian females or males, and there was one First Nations female. All experienced various physical and cognitive challenges, including arthritis, hypertension, hemiparesis, aphasia, dementia, strokes, Parkinson's disease, depression, anxiety, insomnia, and fatigue. Many also suffered from age-related illnesses such as weakened eyesight, decreased ability to speak, loss of hearing, osteoarthritis, osteoporosis, Alzheimer's disease, cardiovascular disease, and diabetes.

Before attending the open studio groups, I obtained appropriate health information from the residential care center records. I selected these clients for the case studies because they were regular attendees who had experienced positive therapeutic changes through engaging in artmaking. Vivian, John, and Patricia diligently and regularly participated in the open studio program for three to four years. They joined the program at different times.

Setting

Because of holidays, special events, illnesses, and other factors, there was some flexibility with sessions. Family members and the care management team encouraged the three older adults to participate in the open studio. However, it was the older adults who made the final decision whether or not to attend. Each older adult who took part in these case studies reflected on their approaches to art materials, the creative process, subject matter, and communication with me. The weekly open studio sessions were conducted in the studio room on the main floor of the residential care center.

Studio participants had access to various materials for different projects. Vivian, John, and Patricia mainly engaged in painting and drawing processes. They used watercolor, acrylic, tempera paints, paintbrushes, canvas, watercolor paper, mixed media paper, and palettes for the painting. For the drawings, they were provided markers, oil pastels, soft pastels, colored crayons, colored pencils, drawing pencils, and colored construction, drawing, and writing paper.

The process was mostly non-directive within the therapeutic framework, and the materials were developmentally appropriate. The program faced some limitations due to varying session times, staff entering the studio during sessions, and the small studio space for five to ten participants who used wheelchairs. Participants were allowed to choose materials and initiate spontaneous artmaking. As the facilitator, I used empathy, warmth, and active listening to build trusting relationships. I was fully engaged, attentive, and aware, both non-verbally and verbally, while participants were engaged in the creative process. I recorded observations and data after each session. I recalled as many details as possible, including the session and participants' processes. I also reflected on the images created.

Vivian

Vivian is a 53-year-old First Nations female born in one of the cities surrounded by the mountains in Western Canada and has lived in this city all her life. Vivian was diagnosed with unspecified hemiplegia, aphasia, an unspecified neck and femur fracture, and unspecified depressive episodes.

Due to her depressive symptoms, Vivian displayed feelings of sadness, tearfulness, emptiness, and hopelessness. She often expressed angry outbursts, irritability, or frustration, even over small matters. Loss of interest or pleasure in most or all normal activities was observed in Vivian's wandering in the building, wheeling her wheelchair, and not being interested in being involved in any activities. From time to time, Vivian seemed to have trouble thinking, concentrating, and remembering things. Vivian also expressed physical pains and headaches related to her diagnoses.

Vivian completed an 11th-grade education and worked as a librarian in the city where she lived. She volunteered to help children with their homework and reading skills. Her family included two daughters and one son. When Vivian first came to art therapy and joined the open studio session, she appeared friendly. She had a nice smile on her face most of the time. She responded to simple questions by nodding because she had lost her ability to speak. According to Vivian's summary report, her favorite pastime activities used to be shopping, needlepoint, and playing bingo.

Intake Sessions

Vivian was referred to the art therapy group by the pastoral counselor at the center who believed that Vivian would benefit from getting support for her depressed feelings and boredom. Even though Vivian was in her 50s, her symptoms brought about issues that often come with advancing years. These challenges were noticed and the people close to her were concerned. Some of her issues included: difficulty accepting life in a care center; feelings of sadness, anger, loneliness, and abandonment; mental states of boredom, hopelessness, anxiety, confusion, and depression; declining self-esteem; and the need for attention. Physically, she had: aches and pains, difficulty seeing or hearing, illness, difficulty speaking, poor memory, and negative physical transformations. Other concerns included loss and death of loved ones and friends, and finances. With encouragement, Vivian was introduced to the art therapy group, where she worked toward meeting some of her needs and enhancing the quality of her life in general.

Vivian was allowed to express and share her inner experiences visually. Through this process her stress was reduced, and she left the studio with smiles, showing gratitude to both the group and me. Vivian focused on her artmaking tasks to experience being fully present in the moment while practicing not worrying about little things during the artmaking process. She experimented and learned new skills in how to use a variety of art materials.

Early Sessions

The Overall Appearance of Vivian

When the pastoral counselor guided Vivian to meet with me, I encouraged her to try painting in the open studio. Surprisingly, she was willing to accept the invitation. She was one of the youngest women residents. According to her records, she became non-verbal due to an accident before being admitted to the center. As sessions passed, I observed powerlessness and sorrowful expressions on Vivian's face. Her sadness often led to tears streaming down her cheeks. Her tears reflected a longing reaction as she recalled memories of her family, especially her husband and daughter.

Relationship with Art Therapist

Since Vivian and I met, she would diligently initiate coming into the studio independently. She was always the first person to enter the studio in the morning, gave me a bright smile, found her favorite space to locate her wheelchair and started painting. Because Vivian had a physical limitation on the right side of her body due to her unspecified hemiplegia, she could only paint with her left hand. Vivian would communicate with me by nodding or shaking her head in response to the questions. Her nodding often returned with a vocal sound. For the most part, Vivian's openness to our relationship depended on her continuous, committed participation in the studio and my acknowledgment of her artwork.

Relationship with Other Participants

Looking out from inside the studio during the art therapy session, Vivian was often observant of people walking around the building. She often looked out the door and would gaze toward the front desk, where many staff and visitors gathered. As sessions progressed, Vivian related more to other participants by expressing her surprise and appreciation by making an expressive vocal sound and through her warm smiles. She showed curiosity to find the artist who created the image. When I pointed out who the artist was, Vivian would make her unique and loud vocal sound toward that participant, expressing her astonishment. From time to time, Vivian would stop painting and look at the person sitting next to her working on their drawing or painting. Again, she smiled to show her reaction toward another person's artwork. This kind of participation demonstrated Vivian's improved engagement and openness within the group. Further, her interest in others' artworks around her showed a positive development in Vivian's interpersonal communication.

Vivian's General Approach

Vivian had no prior art therapy experience. She attended art therapy sessions consistently for four years. During seasonal holidays, art therapy sessions were irregular, and residents would spend time participating in outings and other care center events. I explored providing both directed and non-directed sessions. Vivian responded better to the non-directed approach to art therapy. Her involvement in the art therapy program allowed Vivian to reclaim her freedom as an outlet to express her changing mood every day. While participating in the group, Vivian was provided with opportunities to communicate non-verbally. Every morning, after engaging in the painting process, Vivian left the studio with a contented and fulfilled smile to start her day.

Relationship with Art Materials and Images

Upon arrival in the studio, Vivian often reached for the paint bottles and paint brushes if they were available on the table when she wheeled into the studio and settled in her space. Usually, I would say the name of the color that Vivian selected, and she would attempt to repeat the word after me to practice speaking. Vivian then picked up a paintbrush, got her choice of paint color on her brush, and started painting shapes on the canvas. She often meditatively repeated the same shapes from the top left corner to the bottom right corner of her canvas. She actively used art to express her movements that were fully present. Vivian seemed immersed in her art but was also very interested in her finished products and the images created. When Vivian felt she was done for the day, she would make vocal sounds or stare at me and make eye contact to let me know she was finished. At the end of the painting process, Vivian would have a chance to look at the painting with me and appreciate her artwork.

Later Sessions

Themes Seen in the Art

Various symbols have appeared in Vivian's art, including circle shapes, diamond shapes, letters, and numbers. To explore these symbols emotionally, I verbalized different emotions for Vivian, and she would nod her head and use facial expressions to indicate her feelings. Common feelings reported included sadness, happiness, tiredness, and depressed feelings. Circle shapes were prominent in her artwork, and often symbolized sadness, loneliness, the loss or death of friends, and depression.

By painting various shapes, letters, or numbers, Vivian used her creative expression to communicate with the outside world. Vivian often enjoyed writing a code of numbers and letters on the canvas. Because she lost her ability to speak, she would make sounds that were similar to the words. Art became a powerful way for her to release her inner feelings while stimulating her physical and cognitive functioning. Painting became an active, non-verbal communication that bridged her inner world with the outside world.

Aesthetics of Vivian's Artwork

For Vivian, most art therapy sessions were spent creating spontaneous artworks and patterns of various shapes and colors. Usually, Vivian's attention span engaged in the creative process lasted 15 to 20 minutes. On some days, she would create more than one image, but generally, she completed one picture and left the studio. Most of the time, Vivian created repetitive, circular-shaped images. Her circular shapes were painted in a mixture of thick and thin lines. There were subtle color tones in most shapes except the green circles, which had the most dramatic tonal quality. Vivian used various colors such as sky blue, ultramarine, pink, green, lavender, purple, pinkish red, white, gray, black, brown, and yellow to capture the overall impression of vibrancy.

The overall texture of the forms was rough, and the figures themselves were organically arranged. Forms were asymmetrically placed, yet balance was created by vertically and horizontally placed rows of patterns in these paintings. From time to time, Vivian also added patterns of diamond shapes. Vivian's images carefully and slowly depicted flowing movements. Her paintings were 11 × 17 inches in size and gave subtle, overall impressionistic visions. A sense of unity was achieved through the repetition of randomly chained circular shapes. However, in some of her images, Vivian had aimlessly floating circle shapes that did not touch each other.

There were implied movements depicted between the mildly distorted circles. However, Vivian's soft and vibrant colors and circular shapes were the dominant elements in one particular painting. In this painting, the paints were organically applied. The result was rich, and displayed movement and energy. The use of bright colors and the roundness of the shapes allowed a peaceful mood in Vivian's paintings. Her organically shaped circles created relaxation without searching for perfectionism. Vivian's various ways of depicting shapes developed as the sessions progressed.

John

John, a 74-year-old Korean Canadian male, was born in Seoul, South Korea. He has lived in Western Columbia for 20 years. During his life in Korea, John had a university education and worked in the manufacturing field in a leadership position his whole life. He was married, and his wife was still alive. He also had four daughters, and two of them had children. He was diagnosed with a cerebrovascular accident. He had hypertension, depression, unspecified diabetes mellitus, benign prostatic hypertrophy, and hemiplegia/hemiparesis.

John appeared to be expressionless when he first came to art therapy. His mouth would point downward, drooping with his blank face, and he made no eye contact. His neck appeared stiff, and John would simply respond to a greeting with a rapid and slight voice tone, never turning his head toward the person speaking. However, he actively participated in the painting process and created various images to express his emotions. According to his records, his previous leisure activities included watching baseball, golf, and skating. He had traveled to Europe and the United States.

Intake Sessions

His missionary friend and family referred John to the art therapy group. John faced various challenges that often come with aging, along with his current emotional instability and diagnoses. These challenges were noticed and concerned the family and friends close to John because his anger and frustration seemed to accelerate his symptoms. With strong encouragement from his missionary friend, John was introduced to the art therapy group and explored his major concerns around feelings of anger, hopelessness, and abandonment. The ultimate goal of his artmaking was to support him in finding peace of mind and further enhancing the quality of his life in the care center community.

Early Sessions

The Overall Appearance of John

John has participated in art therapy sessions for over three years. He was struggling with feelings of abandonment when he started participating. He was angry with his family for assigning him to the care center after his major surgery without asking him for his thoughts about coming to the place. He was easily upset and frustrated about living in the care center. He could not accept his situation. The reality was excruciating for John because he could not fully process his thoughts and was unwilling to accept his changes.

Relationship with Art Therapist

As he spent more time in the art studio, he began to express the struggles in his mind through art and began to share his stories verbally. He slowly started to build a sense of belonging within his surroundings. The fact that John and I spoke the same mother tongue, Korean, caused him to remain active in art therapy. It helped him interact openly and helped our relationship-building process. He mentioned that coming to the studio was the only hope left for him, and it was the one activity he looked forward to adding to his reason for living.

Relationship with Other Participants

John rarely initiated greetings in the group. However, he would occasionally acknowledge the person seated next to him by responding to that person's greeting. As sessions progressed, he would sometimes make comments and positive remarks about the works of other studio participants. These acknowledgments were often difficult because of John's physical impediments. He could not quickly turn from side to side to give attention to others.

John's General Approach

John had no prior art therapy experience. His attendance was consistent except during the holiday seasons when he attended special events or when I was away. Although he responded well to both a directed and a non-directed approach to art therapy, John spent most of the sessions creating non-directed, spontaneous artwork. From the beginning, John was able to grasp the concept of art therapy and the purpose of creating art in our safe space after a brief introduction.

Even though it was challenging for John to let go of his tendency to critique and focus on the art process rather than the finished products, he seemed to accept the value of the therapeutic experience in the artmaking process. When John was engaged in painting, he was not afraid to experiment and depict various images and forms. Sometimes, his pictures were realistic. Other times, John's pictures were expressive, which showed abstract forms, and he was confident enough to describe his artwork and share the process. Even though he had physical limitations due to hemiplegia and hemiparesis, John still had normal cognitive functioning and could reflect on his artwork in meaningful ways.

More and more, John began to understand what was expected and helpful to him during this time, even though he struggled some days. Throughout three years of participation in the art therapy group, John became less isolated and more connected to the community and the environment in the care facility. He gradually became involved in other programs despite his challenging ups and downs. For example, he would often enjoy coming down to the art studio to look at his paintings even when there were no sessions.

Relationship with the Art Materials and Images

Initially, John was very cautious about handling various art materials and what to do with them. However, as time passed, he could freely play with multiple types of brushes and colors to convey whatever images, forms, patterns, or symbols he wanted to express. John often began the session by choosing five to eight fine brushes. Then, he would put a wide variety of colors on his palette. John usually engaged in the art process and clearly knew what he wanted to create and what he was expected to do during the session. The way he handled the media was with focus and sensitivity. John often positively described how the art process felt and talked about what it was like to make art.

Later Sessions

Themes Seen in the Art

Many themes appeared in John's art, including flowers, mountains, trees, sky, water, seasons, snow, volcano, clouds, geometric shapes, and patterns. By exploring these themes, John seemed to be able to express his inner feelings, which included anger, loneliness, death, pain, and hope. Many of his artworks were reminiscent as he titled them and told stories about his past. He enjoyed talking about the stories and meaning of his images. Elements in his paintings included depictions of his hometown with little houses and streets, trees, and mountains. He also created many sceneries of nature, blue skies with clouds, mountains, and trees that depicted mountains where he used to enjoy hiking.

Aesthetics of John's Artwork

John's painting process was confident and active. He would start every group art therapy session by making clear choices about the materials he wanted. After John chose his paints and brushes, he would create a warm-up painting. He would then move on to a big piece of paper or canvas, depending on his mood each day. He would complete two to three paintings every session. When he finished an art piece, John would come up with a title for it. Those words were poetic, and they became a part of his artwork. Much of the time, those words completed his painting. John used various colors in his paintings, such as red, blue, yellow, green, brown, orange, black, purple, and white.

His paintings also captured his memories, thoughts, and emotions in an aesthetic sense. One day, he painted his own body image to express the changes that he felt. He shared that every cell inside his body felt as if it was actively moving to recover from his illness. John displayed symmetrical, balanced body forms to show what he felt physically inside. The metaphoric depiction of his hope continued to show in his artwork. Other times he would express things for which he longed. In another image, John attempted to depict a perspective of the countryside road becoming narrower and fading as it extends far into the distance.

John frequently depicted forms with fine and delicate lines. Most of his pictures had medium-to-dark color tones, resulting in somewhat dramatic images. His images had various organic, geometric, angular, and curved shapes. The paintings were created on small (8 × 10 inch) and medium-sized (11 × 17 inch) paper or canvas. A sense of variety was achieved through the types of paintings John created. He explored abstraction as well as realism. John used a variety of images to express personal memories and emotions. The result was a combination of symmetrical, detailed, planned, candid, and spontaneous pictures. The names he gave to each painting demonstrated John's thoughtful reflections on his painting process.

Patricia

Patricia, a 99-year-old Filipino Canadian female, was born and raised in the Philippines. She moved to Canada and has lived there since 1979. Patricia was a homemaker with daughters, grandsons, and a granddaughter, who all lived nearby. Her loving family cared for Patricia by regularly visiting and spending time with her at the care center. Once introduced to art therapy, Patricia actively participated in painting activities and enjoyed creating a nature scene that included an ocean. Her grandson, whenever he visited, would often accompany Patricia to the studio. By engaging in the painting process, Patricia recalled her home country and shared many stories about her hometown and life back then. According to her report, Patricia has traveled to the Philippines and California.

Intake Sessions

Patricia was diagnosed with a transient ischemic attack (TIA), osteoarthritis, type 2 diabetes mellitus, chronic obstructive pulmonary disease (COPD), and diverticulitis. She had an elementary education and had health challenges due to her complex illnesses. When the art therapy studio program officially became available, the care staff referred Patricia as the most potential candidate for the program. Patricia was aging, and what she needed in her life at that point was to be involved in daily activities, to avoid boredom, to be active, and find quality in her everyday life.

Early Sessions

The Overall Appearance of Patricia

Patricia had certain routines that she followed before every art therapy session. In the morning, every Tuesday and Thursday, Patricia would wait for me in the neighboring lounge area next to the single armchair, where she was able to see people walking down the hallway. I would ask Patricia if she wanted to come and spend time making art together, and she would say yes. Often, when I asked her how she was doing, Patricia would, with her loud voice, say, "I cannot see well". Despite her response, she always pleasantly accompanied me to the studio with excitement and anticipation.

Relationship with Art Therapist

Patricia and I did art therapy together in a group setting for three years at the complex care center. When I first met Patricia, she communicated verbally. Patricia's words were direct. She understood and responded to concrete questions. However, it took much work for Patricia to understand abstract questions. Through diligent repetition, Patricia became familiar with the art space and the people.

During the art therapy sessions, she met some expectations by being part of the community, despite her failing eyesight and diminished hearing abilities. Patricia appreciated the fact that I remembered her and helped her join the art therapy sessions every time the studio was in progress. Early in the sessions, I would check in with Patricia by observing her appearance and, at the same time, asking her how she was doing that day.

When I returned after being away for a week, Patricia always asked, "Where did you go?" Then, when I took her back to her place after the sessions, she would ask, "When are you coming back?" Her questioning helped relieve her anxiety. Holding up the number of fingers representing days until the next open studio made Patricia feel assured, knowing when I would return to greet her and invite her to the studio. This was something that she would look forward to as we built a trusting relationship.

Relationship with Other Participants

Patricia was a friendly, welcoming member of the group. As soon as she entered the studio, she would loudly say, "Good morning", to all the participating artists who were already in the studio. During the creative process, she primarily focused on her own painting, rarely noticing other people around her or observing what they were making.

Patricia's General Approach

Patricia had no prior art therapy experience. However, she has attended art therapy sessions consistently. Patricia's time spent in the art therapy sessions remained irregular to some extent. When working in the studio, Patricia preferred to take a spot where her back faced the window in the space. It was because the sun was too bright on her eyes. In the early stages of her participation, Patricia had difficulty determining which paint colors, paintbrushes, and paper size to choose. However, as sessions went by, she got better at expressing her needs, and she was able to make clear choices about art materials.

Patricia became confident enough to engage in painting and showed a focus on her creativity when all the supplies were set up for her. In the beginning, she was unsure about what to paint. She often criticized her work, saying, "It is not good". Her painting process was fast and she completed more than one piece in each session. Because of Patricia's physical limitations and diminutive size, she struggled to reach the art supplies on the table. I helped her by bringing the paint bottles close to her face so she could see them. At the same time, I would speak loudly, giving Patricia the opportunity to make choices for herself. Once she selected the color, I would open the cap, set up the palette, mix colors as needed, load the brush, and hand the brush to Patricia. Then I gently directed her to the canvas where she could start making marks to create her images. She required a little more assistance some days. Patricia painted every brushstroke herself once she received a little initial help.

Relationship with Art Materials and Images

Within the safety of the art therapy studio, Patricia painted rough, vibrant, exotic, earthy, energetic acrylic paintings of landscapes, seascapes, and more. Most images showed traditional paint colors: sky blue for the sky, green for grass and trees, brown for ground or mountains, and rich blues for oceans. Patricia used mostly flowing, bold, and thick lines for her images. The overall tonal quality of her paintings was somewhat dramatic. Her painting surface had rough and uneven textural brushstrokes that resulted in organically created pictures. Some unity was achieved by including the dominant elements of sky blue and ultramarine in every artwork representing the sky and ocean in her paintings.

Patricia created a sense of balance in one of her images by painting two houses on a hill, placing one to the left and the other to the right. There was implied movement in the curved lines of the sky and the two houses' rooftops. This painting also included the dominant elements of sky blue and ultramarine. Patricia's attention span and focus on engaging in the painting process increased as the sessions went by. She was able to stay active for 30 to 40 minutes without interruption. Patricia would call when she needed more colors, and when she completed a piece, she would loudly say, "finished". I often encouraged her to share anything she would like to say about her painting or the process. Patricia would then say, "I do not know". I helped her share by creating simple questions that allowed Patricia to describe what images she had in her picture. She would name most of the images in her artwork one by one. Most of the time, Patricia shared an airplane flying and a car driving to the town where she used to live. When Patricia had an image of a house, she talked about the place in which she used to live. Her most recent paintings included oceans, sailboats, a swimmer, fish, flowers, and trees. The place was called "Baguio" in the Philippines. It clearly shows that she had a yearning for her hometown yet was able to reminisce her stories in a beautiful narrative.

Later Sessions

Themes Seen in the Art

Patricia expressed a combination of receptive and expressive responses about the images she depicted in her artwork. Many themes appeared in Patricia's art: sky, mountains, ocean, earth, flowers, boats, fish, swimmers, airplanes, suns, and houses. Through these prominent images, Patricia was able to recall, describe, and share how her hometown looked and what she used to see and do. Her routine involved painting blue skies at the top of her canvas. She would then add a mountain, ocean, trees, flowers, soil, fish, boats, swimmers, and more.

Hospitalization

After three years of being part of the art therapy group, Patricia had to be hospitalized for a few days. Once she returned to the care center, she could not return to the group immediately. Then Patricia had to go back to the hospital again. After the second trip to the hospital, she looked much better and came to the studio. Patricia, as usual, spent the time creating paintings. Although she looked to have recovered well, she could not get up the following week. I stopped by her room to see how she was doing. The next day at the facility, I revisited Patricia and brought a picture she had painted earlier. It was a single boat with a red flag that was sailing in the deep ocean. I told Patricia that it was a present for her. I placed her painting in a beautiful wooden frame. Patricia promised that she would get well and come back to the studio. Sadly, she never was able to paint again. Shortly after my visit, Patricia passed away. Throughout the last stage of her life, she received caring support from her family. Her grandson was always by her side. Patricia was one of the older adults who confirmed and demonstrated to other staff members and me how art and the creative process contribute to the quality of life in aging adults.

Outcomes and Conclusions

After working approximately four years in group art therapy through the open studio setting with older adults at the complex care center, I witnessed that the art therapy program contributed to an overall improvement in the quality of life of the residents. The art therapy program allowed participants the opportunity to express and share inner and outer experiences visually. Through this process, older adults could revisit their values and find meaning and purpose in their lives. They experienced peace and joy in the moments through the creative process they were engaged in using the art materials as therapeutic tools. Most of the time, participants were able to reduce stress and leave the studio, displaying smiles and showing gratitude to both the group and me.

Despite the challenges faced during artmaking, whether due to physical, emotional, or mental conditions, each participant became deeply involved in the painting and drawing process. Artmaking became both a calming and stimulating activity. As a result, participants focused on their artmaking tasks to experience being fully present in the moment.

The art process and experiences allowed them an opportunity for creative self-expression and personal growth. Participants experimented and learned new skills in how to use a variety of art materials. They had a chance to explore their range of play by exploring artmaking in a nonjudgmental, welcoming, and accepting safe space. Through artmaking, they had a chance to come into contact with past memories, their imaginations, and develop individualized expressive language.

Being with others, participants developed relationships and created a sense of belonging to a community and culture. They identified areas of concern, developed talents, and acknowledged their strengths through the gentle and sensitive support I provided. They valued each other as part of the community by sharing art materials and space, kindly greeting one another, generously taking turns with the art materials, and giving positive attention to each others' artworks. They learned not to criticize but to accept their own and each others' expressions. I often demonstrated this action by describing each individual's unique art process, engaging in an aesthetic analysis, and letting them understand how all their artworks are different and original.

The participants were cooperative and excited about their artwork being exhibited and displayed throughout the care center. They enjoyed sharing their artwork with family, friends, staff, and visitors. Through this experience, they raised their self-esteem by successfully completing their painting projects and witnessing their own artistic accomplishments. Participants also had an opportunity to be selected as the artist-of-the-month to showcase their work at the care center. They were also included in a monthly news article and artist-of-the-month mini-gallery. The participants were acknowledged, empowered, heard, and respected through these events.

The artmaking process was positive, encouraging, and stimulating for all participants, including Vivian, John, and Patricia. The open studio demonstrated that creating art is an empowering tool to enhance the quality of life and particularly helpful for those with physical, cognitive, and emotional challenges. I realized the potential for learning and growing in later stages of life is vast. The benefits of the arts for all those living and working within a continuing care community are far-reaching. I hope more residential communities incorporate art therapy programs at their facilities.

One of the main goals of the open studio project was to help the older adult participants to understand and experience a purpose and reason to strive, learn, and continue to grow through the art-making process. Each noted participant appeared to have an enhanced quality of life and experienced playfulness in a creative atmosphere.

THE USE OF THIRD-HAND ART THERAPY FOR TRANSPERSONAL: KNOWING IN THE LAST DAYS OF LIFE WITH TWO MEN IN HOSPICE CARE

MIA DE BÉTHUNE

Setting

The two men described in this chapter were seen in their homes through the hospice and palliative care program of a suburban hospital near a major metropolitan area in the Northeastern United States. Art therapy was a grant-funded complementary care service along with reflexology, massage, and Reiki to support wellness and comfort during the last months and weeks of a person's life. Hospice services almost always involve a terminal diagnosis of less than six months to live with which the client must come to terms. Complementary care services were coordinated within a network of doctors, nurses, social workers, and bereavement and pastoral care counselors. Art therapy, in particular, was also a support for family members, children, parents, and siblings of the person who was dying before and after their death.

The first man, Ari, was seen in his bedroom in a spacious suburban home surrounded by trees and a pond. It was otherwise empty, except for a young couple that rented his basement apartment along with their two large dogs. The second man, Charlie, was seen in the living room of his modest suburban home on a cul-de-sac where he lived with his wife. His two adult children lived nearby.

My services were often requested by clients themselves at the start of hospice care or would be recommended by a member of the team, usually the care nurse, because the client had an interest in art or they felt it might be an emotional support for processing grief. Sometimes a family member would relay that the client had been an artist and hoped that art therapy would provide some relief. Very often, I was commissioned with supporting children or siblings of the person who was dying or had already died. Because of the nonverbal expression available with art, it can be particularly useful for processing grief. I sometimes worked with family members for as long as six months after the hospice client had died. With these two cases, however, the relationships were a matter of weeks with Ari and only a few days with Charlie. For these men, a brief relationship with me, as an art therapist, seemed to provide a crucial support and connection as they contemplated their last days of life and wished to express their hopes and fears while time seemed to evaporate for them.

Approaches

Resonance and Attunement in a Relational Approach

As an art therapist working in hospice and palliative care, I came to expect the unexpected or to be comfortable with the unknown and the liminal space between life and death. Prior to becoming an art therapist, I was a Reiki practitioner. Reiki is an indigenous Japanese form of energy healing as well as a spiritual practice. It often involves sensing into another person's body to intuit stress, pain, or illness in a form of non-verbal knowing and communication (Stein, 2021). Another modality I use is Somatic Experiencing (Levine, 2010) using a core method to both observe and query an individual about their somatic sensations and to *resonate or attune to their physical, emotional, and energetic state* (Somatic Experiencing International, 2022). Attuning is defined when "two or more persons share an inner-emotional state when interacting" (Krøier et al., 2022, p. 33). Attunement is increasingly being recognized as an essential competency for health and psychological providers (Dall'Alba, 2023). It is also a key component of relational therapy which supports a dialectic between client and therapist in which they both contribute to an "interactive process of continuing dialogue" (Gerlitz et al., 2020, p. 1). Relational dialogue with art therapy addresses "inner and outer realities [and] generates aesthetic knowledge" (Gerber, 2016, p. 1) that can lead to change through mutual negotiation (Gerlitz et al., 2020).

Relational Approach and Transpersonal Knowing at the End of Life

With the elderly and those who have chronic or life-threatening illness, a relational and attuned approach is crucial. Loss of ability for communication due to a disease or the aging process at the end of life can lead to social isolation and more rapid decline. Interpersonal communication can be conceptualized as "being in communication (rather than 'doing' communication)" (Krøier et al., 2022, p. 33). It has been described as how caregivers attuned "to patients' feelings and took on their perspective" (Alsawy et al., 2017, p. 1793). Non-verbal communication such as "gestures, facial expressions, tone of voice, eye gaze and sound", (Krøier et al., 2022, p. 33) done in a turn taking-style, become essential when normal function declines with illness and aging.

There may also be a need for an expanded consciousness with clients as they near the end of life. A transpersonal therapeutic approach allows for an understanding of "intuitive, spiritual, and transcendent states of consciousness" (Boorstein, 2000, p. 409). The word *transpersonal* can be defined as sensing outside our physical selves into the environment and into another person's thoughts and sensations. Reiki is a transpersonal system based on access to a "universal life energy" that is shared by all (Fabbo, 2020, p. 185). Reiki is often used in hospitals and hospice as a form of alternative or integrative medicine (Fabbo, 2020). *Nonlocality* is another transpersonal concept that refers to consciousness outside of the body, such as out-of-body experiences or the use of prayer to heal others (Berger, 2010). People who are very ill and near death often report such out-of-body or nonlocality experiences.

The Use of Active Art Therapy and the Third-Hand Support

For clients whose physical and mental capacities have become diminished, a more active relational role as art therapist may be required (Gerlitz et al., 2020). This can involve co-creating or outright creation of art for clients who can no longer use their hands or even tell us what they would like. This way of working fits with Kramer's concept of *third-hand support* (Consoli, 1992, p. 48), but also moves beyond it. Franklin (2016) outlines a transpersonal form of art therapy which involves "context, content, and process" (p. 103) and requires a mindful presence of the art therapist who is aware of their own inner process as they work with the inner process of their client. Franklin further articulates a silent holding that "the client is a divine being" (p. 103) beyond their diagnosis or illness. Transpersonal art therapy also considers engagement with images and artmaking to be work of the soul and to be particularly appropriate for end of life (Franklin, 2016). The individual is seen as in a transition between life and death (Berger, 2010) and a process of allowing images to emerge from the unconscious or the collective unconscious is valued (Franklin, 2016). Art therapy can meet the existential need to tell the story of those with a life-threatening illness (Roikjaer et al., 2019). This storytelling or life review is a narrative technique that is often used by people at the end of life for resolving unaddressed conflicts and easing their conscience as they approach death (Keisari & Palgi, 2017).

Case Studies

Ari: Longing for Homeland

Ari was a physically large man, who still had a full head of dark hair despite his 70 plus years. He had been a contractor who built luxury homes for people over the course of his career. At the time we worked together, he lived alone in a cavernous, suburban home surrounded by trees and a pond with a fountain. He and his wife were amicably divorced and had grown children. The dogs from the young couple who lived in his accessory apartment often came to visit Ari in his room. He was otherwise alone, except for a care nurse who attended to him 24/7. His ex-wife was often there helping out, and I was told that his children visited, but I never met them. Ari was no longer able to walk except to a nearby bathroom with the use of a walker. He spent most of his time in a hospital bed with long legs propped up due to swelling in his calves and ankles. He had late-stage brain cancer and could not see well or use his hands much. His wife had requested art therapy because Ari had been a hobby painter and she felt painting would boost his mood and give him something to do other than watch television.

Intake and Assessment

In my initial meeting with Ari, he lay in his bed in a front room of the house with the television on. His wife was there and had brought lots of paint and canvases so that my supplies were not needed. His legs were propped up and his attention was on the news. He was polite but showed little interest in artmaking until his wife coaxed him to turn the news off. He looked warily at the paper, paints, and colored pencils I had placed on a tray before him, but agreed to try. Though he chose colored pencils to use, his hands were stiff and he seemed uncomfortable. I demonstrated what the pencils could do by sketching a few lines of color and he said, "You do a drawing Mia". I agreed and began sketching the landscape outside his window, which was a vista of birch trees, ferns, and maples beyond a stone wall. As I sketched, I asked him to select the colors and where I should make the marks. He commented on my process and seemed to relax. As he watched, he seemed to reminisce about scenes from childhood and described the beautiful waters around a coastal village where he was born in a country on the Adriatic Sea.

Sessions

Over the course of six weeks, Ari continued to work with me in a similar manner. He graduated to pastel and then acrylic paint and I would spend a good deal of time mixing a palette of colors at his direction. It seemed important to him to feel the brushes and choose exactly the right one, then he would make a few tentative marks with the brush before getting tired. I then engaged him in directing me where to put the paint and what color to use. The image was usually the same landscape out his window. I also brought in photographs of the Adriatic Sea as he had described it. These prompted memories of his grandparents and parents all buried a half a world away, as well as his brother. He pointed out pictures and other artifacts around his room that recalled his early life in a poor village far from his suburban enclave. He also spoke, with great sadness, of a son who had died. There were pictures of grandchildren and though he spoke with pride of his daughter, who was a professional, I never saw her. Only his wife came occasionally as he became weak and less able to sit up in bed, and the dogs who seemed to bring him great comfort. I reflected on how hard it must have been to lose his son and he reached for my hand to hold it. After this, he told his nurse that "she is a good one".

Outcomes

One of Ari's wishes had been to go sit out in his beautiful yard by the pond when we did our art work. We talked about this during most sessions, but it never came to pass. The nurse would shake her head and say, "I'm afraid not today. It's a little chilly and he's just too weak". Toward the end, Ari just liked to watch me as I drew or painted his landscape continually filling in a replica of the vista out his window of sunlight and leafy trees, or he would ask to hold my hand and tell me again the stories of his parents, his dead son, and the country he left behind. From one week to the next Ari declined rapidly. The last time I visited he was resting with an oxygen tank and not aware of my presence. I stayed for a few minutes to hold his hand one more time and say goodbye.

Charlie: Parting Messages

Charlie had been a fireman his entire life as well as an inveterate smoker. He was near death from emphysema and lung cancer when we met. He lived in a modest house on a cul-de-sac with his wife of 50 years. His two grown children lived nearby. Both were very present on the days that I came. The 40-year-old son took after Charlie and was tall and lanky with the buzz cut typical of firemen. His son was the only one tall and strong enough to lift Charlie off of the couch and back into his hospital bed. His daughter was in her 30s and hovered nearby in case her father or I needed anything. Her six-month-old baby was always on her hip. Charlie's wife seemed quiet and sad and kept a low profile. I had little interaction with her.

Intake and Assessment

When I first arrived on a hot Thursday morning in July, the entire family including the infant and the hospice social worker were jammed in the small entryway to the door of their ranch style home. They waved me away and said, "You know it's bad timing. He's not in a good mood and it's probably best to try another day". Something told me that there might not be another day and so I persisted and just asked if it was okay to try and introduce myself. The social worker looked doubtful, and said, "He's pretty angry right now, mostly at me, but why not?" The two kids and their mother stepped aside to let me in. His daughter pointed out where Charlie was and then left us alone for privacy.

He was a tall, thin, gray looking man with drawn features. He had an oxygen tube attached to his nose and the green tank was on a stand by his leg where he sat on a long white couch that took up most of the living room. A hospital bed was across the room near the kitchen table and a leather recliner was at the far end of the room on the edge of what looked like a dark formal dining room. Charlie was hunched over on himself and looked exhausted. He occasionally coughed or gasped for air. I approached slowly and stood by him but didn't say a word. Without looking at me he said, "I'm so damn angry. I know I'm dying! I don't need somebody to tell me that. Who does she think she is?" This took a lot out of him and he began to cough.

I crouched near and asked if I could just sit next to him and hold his hand. He nodded and I slipped my hand into his and explained, "I'm the art therapist from hospice and you don't have to say anything to me. I can see how upset you are. If it's okay, I'll just sit with you for now". At this Charlie began to weep quietly. I asked if I could place a hand on his shoulder as well and he nodded. After a while, I could feel that his breathing had slowed and he'd relaxed a little. "There are just so many things I want to tell my two kids before I die", he said and sobbed.

I told Charlie that if he wanted, I could help him write some of those things down and be his scribe, but we both agreed that he was much too tired after his meeting with the social worker and that I would come back the next day. On the way out, I talked briefly with his daughter about this plan. She appeared tearful and expressed thanks for my agreeing to help her father. I observed his son lift him off of the couch and place him back in the hospital bed as his wife followed with the oxygen tank.

Session

Schedules and Charlie's doctor visits conspired to keep me from returning until Sunday. By this time, he was on pain medication and less physically available. I found him lying on his recliner near the darkened dining room and he greeted me warmly. He was calmer, but had no strength to relay stories or messages for his kids as we had planned. I had packed paper, colored pencils, and pastels and offered to make a drawing with him. Charlie could not use his hands so I asked what he'd like me to draw, but he just nodded his head "no" as if half asleep. Using intuition, I began a pastel rendering of a highway somewhere in the mountains. I showed him, as I worked, what I was doing. I placed a car on the road surrounded by towering pine trees. Suddenly he seemed more awake and said, "Hey that's the road to...". He tried to remember someplace in Vermont where he and his family had gone for vacations. He called for his daughter to come over, still with the little girl on her hip.

"What is it, pops?" she asked and he said, "What's that place in the mountains we used to go? Doesn't it look like that?" She nodded in agreement and named the place as she looked at the picture. They smiled at each other and she squeezed his hand and said, "Yeah it does. Remember when we'd go there?"

I then suggested another drawing of a tree and conferred with Charlie, who was now more alert. He helped me choose the colors and the shape of the tree, a towering oak with large roots, but with red and orange leaves falling as if in autumn. We worked together for about 40 minutes until he became tired. Then he thanked me and I said goodbye.

Outcomes

I did not need to be told that this would be the last time I saw him. He died the following day. Before I left, I stood with his two children in the hallway by the door. His wife had gone over to sit with him. I told them how angry he had been and sad about stories he had wanted to share with them; about how he was really too tired to be able to tell those stories. I gave them the two pictures I had made with Charlie: the one of a memory in Vermont and the other of an oak tree in autumn. They were both in tears and thanked me. I encouraged them to sit with him and talk to him as much as they could in what time was remaining.

Discussion

With both Ari and Charlie, I took a very active relational approach to art therapy out of necessity (Gerlitz et al., 2020). Neither man had the energy or physical agility to manipulate art materials, yet they had plenty of memories to spare. With Ari, there had been more of an opportunity to develop a relationship and attune to his needs over the course of several weeks (Dall'Alba, 2023; Krøier et al., 2022). My training in both Reiki (Stein, 2021) and Somatic Experiencing (Levine, 2010) made attuning a natural way for me to assess hospice clients in addition to engaging with them verbally. Ari still has some manual dexterity and the visual and tactile elements of art-making (e.g., gazing at his view, and testing his brushes and paint colors) seemed to engage him in an aesthetic knowing and dialogue (Gerber, 2016). This dialogue was negotiated between us through the use of the third-hand support (Consoli, 1992, p. 48) as I continued to consult with Ari about color and line choices in my active doing for him. The act of looking and making seemed to ease his ability to talk about painful memories and emotions that he seemed to be tackling internally as he faced his terminal diagnosis (Keisari & Palgi, 2017). This work seemed to follow the "context, content, and process" of transpersonal art therapy (Franklin, 2016, p. 103). It also seemed important for me to listen to his stories as a life review (Keisari & Palgi, 2017) which helped to provide meaning (Roikjaer et al., 2019) for this stage of his life and to ease his passing. His longing to go outside each week seemed to mirror a longing for home, his family, and the beautiful waters of the Adriatic Sea which he would never see again, perhaps representing a form of nonlocality (Berger, 2010).

With Charlie there was no opportunity to develop a relationship over time. I needed to act quickly and my intuitive or transpersonal knowing kicked in even before I walked into the house and met him (Berger, 2010; Boorstein, 2000). Reiki's "universal life energy" is said to have its own intelligence and know where it is needed for healing (Fabbo, 2020, p. 185). A part of me must have intuited that pushing to meet him despite his anger and the doubts of the family was the right thing for that moment. My training as a somatic therapist has taught me ways in which simple touch and attention to the body can help the nervous system settle after an upset (Levine, 2010). My somatic therapy training also taught me to approach Charlie in the wake of the deeply disturbing, but necessary news that his diagnosis was terminal.

Yet it was the images that emerged spontaneously through our visual dialogue in what Franklin (2016) would call transpersonal art therapy that allowed for both communication and transformation to occur. Our dialogue about drawing was relational and mutual (Gerlitz et al., 2020) in spite of the need for me to be Charlie's third hand (Consoli, 1992). There was the outer reality of Charlie being too tired, medicated, and weak to draw or even recall an image he wanted me to draw, but there was also the inner reality of his unconscious thoughts (Gerber, 2016). In this transition between life and death, images seemed to emerge from the collective unconscious (Berger, 2010) to be interpreted by me as an expression of Charlie's soul (Franklin, 2016). The images that emerged allowed for aesthetic knowing (Gerber, 2016) through shape, color, and story that facilitated a form of life review and emotional exchange with his daughter that might not have otherwise occurred in his deteriorating state. The choice of a tree seemed more conscious for me, but also a collective choice reflecting an organic sense of self, wholeness, and strength in the face of the natural process of mortality. Another form of nonlocality (Berger, 2010) if you will. The choice of the tree also indicates the holding of Charlie as a "divine being" (Franklin, 2016, p. 103) beyond his deadly cancer and emphysema. I sensed that art therapy provided both Charlie and his family a small measure of peace. Even though messages he had hoped to tell them were lost to time, the image of the oak spoke of his towering importance and impact on their lives.

Conclusion

This work with clients at the point of leaving life has given me enormous respect for aspects of knowing that we can't control as well as for intuition, transpersonal knowing, and the images and energies that emerge between client and therapist in session. I believe this is always true, and as an energy and body-focused art therapist, I am always oriented to be noticing in an attuned, subtle bodily way. It is with these clients at the end of life where the need for subtle awareness and knowing become more urgent and apparent because time is literally measured in minutes and seconds.

ART THERAPY, ARTIST IDENTITY, AND PARKINSON'S DISEASE

EMILY SHARP

Art therapy can be a helpful intervention for people struggling with Parkinson's Disease (PD); it helps clients address physical, mental, and emotional symptoms (Cucca et al., 2021). As I worked with Eddie, a formerly self-identified artist diagnosed with PD, I noted how such a complex disease also deeply affected his identity. Creating an art therapy intervention for my client using a strengths-based approach allowed him to re-engage in a consistent art practice. Together we focused on celebrating his strengths, rather than focusing on deficits. This allowed for a shift in his mentality around what type of art he created. In our work together, Eddie worked through physical and mental limitations to re-engage with a consistent practice of art-making and shift his identity from a traditional portrait painter toward an abstract artist.

Setting

Eddie had always identified as an artist. He spent years attending classes in schools and community programs throughout New York City, developing his skills for realistic portraiture using oil on canvas. The living room in his apartment began to resemble a small gallery. Beautiful, carefully executed portraits lining the walls, reflecting a different time and a different artistic ability. When I first met Eddie, he would use a walker to move around, but soon after he became confined to his wheelchair. As the years went on, Eddie's bedroom became his new studio. Eddie's bedroom was stacked with books about art marked with notes and his own drawings. He liked to study these still paintings and create images in his mind, even though he had taken a break from physically painting before we met. In contrast to the rest of his home, his bedroom walls were bare. Slowly over our years of working together, we created a gallery wall celebrating his new artwork and his shift into identifying as an abstract artist.

The art materials that Eddie was drawn to in the past were oil paints and canvas. Since we had the art therapy sessions in his bedroom, the use of oil paint containing toxic fumes was not advised. In order to keep the integrity of his desires to create paintings, we added a large set of acrylic paint, canvas, and other sketching materials to his supplies. Because Eddie was initially hesitant about making art, we eased into the process by using a photo transfer technique to create a self-portrait outline on wood canvas. We also experimented with chalk pastels, pencil, oil pastels, watercolor, and acrylic paint.

As Eddie's Parkinson's progressed, he found himself frustrated by stiff, unsteady hands that would not do what his mind and his eye were telling him to do. There were years when he put his art to the side, and his artist identity lay dormant. During this time, his interest in art remained. When his case manager reached out for an art therapist to begin working individually with Eddie for home visits, it was to reconnect Eddie with his passion for art-making and his identity as an artist.

Early Sessions

Parkinson's Disease impacts a patient's physical, mental, and emotional well-being. People diagnosed with PD may experience a broad array of motor symptoms as part of their condition including slowness, stiffness, tremors, postural abnormalities, poor balance, and walking impairment. This progressive and incurable neurodegenerative disease can manifest itself with several non-motor features, including cognitive and behavioral changes (Bloem et al., 2021). While available medications can address some of the most common motor problems, at least for the first years of the disease, many non-motor symptoms are, unfortunately, devoid of effective treatments. People with PD may frequently experience difficulties in concentration, attention, and multi-tasking. Occasionally, memory impairment, especially short-term recall, can occur. From a behavioral viewpoint, people living with this condition can experience apathy, anxiety, mental fatigue, and mood changes. These problems, coupled with progressive physical disability, persistent negative feelings, and stigma, may conspire to reduce patients' functional independence, thus favoring a progressive physical and psychological withdrawal which in turn may further accelerate the disease progression (Bloem et al., 2021).

Research shows evidence that art therapy can be an effective psychosocial treatment for patients facing such a complex disease. Art therapy has been seen to reduce depression and anxiety. Continuing research results also demonstrate increases in brain connectivity and reduction in symptomatology of PD (Cucca et al., 2021). In a study done in 2021 exploring the potential rehabilitative effects of art therapy with patients diagnosed with PD, researchers found that following art therapy practice, certain areas of clients' brains underwent a rewiring process boosting their perception and some of their cognitive skills (Cucca et al., 2021).

At first, Eddie refused to begin making art. He simply explained to me that his hands did not work as they did before he was diagnosed. Eddie used to be an artist, but that was some time ago, and since his hands could not keep up with what he envisioned, he decided to stop making art. During my initial, informal assessment, I used the time to learn more about Eddie's interests. It is important using a strengths-based approach to take the time to really listen to what the client is saying without imposing desires or outcomes (McGovern, 2015). Using this approach with Eddie focused on abilities, rather than disabilities.

Eddie expressed a great deal of self-doubt when we began working together, so it was my job to assess any physical or mental limitations or beliefs that we could work through slowly together. This process helped to develop trust. During our weekly one-hour sessions of creating art together, our first short-term treatment goal was to build the therapeutic relationship. Our long-term treatment goals addressed improving self-esteem and reclaiming an artist identity. Additional goals looked to increase mood, physical activity, and social interaction.

We spent our first few sessions talking about art, looking at books, and listening to music, in order to build rapport. Before PD interrupted his abilities, Eddie was a traditional portrait painter. Introducing him to abstract art helped to loosen the bounds of perfectionism and encouraged strengths in expressing ideas. He was very opinionated about what he liked and what he did not, and he would easily critique the work he did not like. I continued to encourage strength-based and supportive opinions. After looking through art books, old sketches, and paintings, I began to understand his style. I slowly began to introduce both old and new materials to Eddie. I suggested testing out some of the materials, even if it did not turn into a finished piece. Eddie slowly started to experiment, but his resistance and uncertainty were still apparent. An art intervention to help this transition from a detailed portrait artist was necessary.

About a month after we began, I wanted to help Eddie create a version of a self-portrait that felt accessible but authentic to his past style. I created an acetone photocopy print on a wooden canvas. It was a recent photo that I took of Eddie, reflecting his current state and appearance. In my experience, the power of utilizing a wide variety of art materials in sessions can allow for trial and error to see where clients are drawn. It is important for art therapists to remain flexible, meet the client where they are, and maintain awareness of personal biases in material and process choices.

The photo transfer resembled a detailed coloring page, like a black and white image with the contrast turned up. The defined structure of a coloring page was elevated using the artistic style of a wooden canvas applied directly with an acetone transfer. I applied the acetone transfer at another site and brought it to Eddie to prevent potentially harmful fumes. Eddie was then able to use the elevated art materials of a wooden canvas, watercolors, and professional brushes to make art within the structure he needed to build confidence. If I would have simply handed this to Eddie to color in, he might have been offended; he was an artist with years of history and experience. In addition to the use of elevated materials, adaptive tools were necessary to help support physical challenges from the PD. To help with holding the paintbrush, Eddie and I created an adaptive device using a tennis ball with a hole through it to act as a grip. I gave him a tray of watercolors to add layers on top of the image,

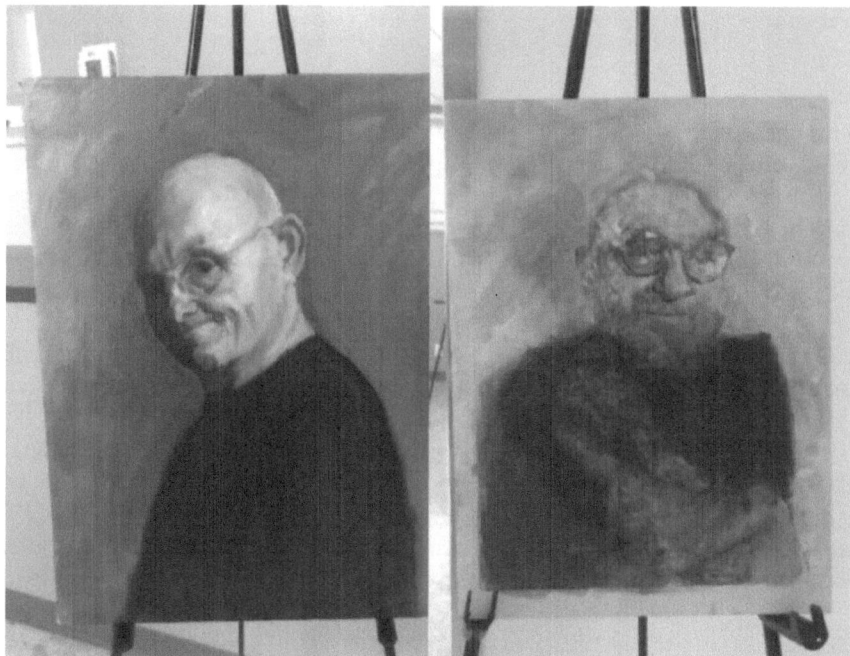

Figure 5.1 Eddie's Self Portraits: Then and Now

and just like that, Eddie was creating again. This technique was the first shifting point toward resurrecting Eddie's artist identity. We worked on this portrait for several weeks to come, and he was really pleased with the results (Figure 5.1).

Later Sessions

Art prompts were used to provide Eddie freedom to follow the directions he wanted to take. This semi-structured approach allowed Eddie to feel in control of our sessions and create an element of me being there as his assistant. There were times he would refer to me as his teacher, and I think this was his way of referencing art classes and experiences from the past.

An important part of helping Eddie reawaken his artist identity was to make art more accessible, attractive, and satisfying. The re-establishment of Eddie's artist identity began with our work together to create habits around re-engaging with the process of art-making. Once consistent, predictable habits and small changes were in place, Eddie had proof, through action, that he was someone who makes art.

> Every action you take is a vote for the type of person you wish to become. No single instance will transform your beliefs, but as the votes build up, so does the evidence of your new identity. This is one reason why meaningful change does not require radical change. Small habits can make a meaningful difference by providing evidence of a new

identity. And if a change is meaningful, it is actually big. That's the paradox of making small improvements.

(Clear, 2018, p. 38)

During Eddie's art therapy sessions, comfort was a priority. The time of day, medication routine, sleepiness, and light, were all considerations. I also wanted to be conscious of some cognitive memory decline that was taking place. Daily fluctuations in alertness, attention, and interactivity are common in people suffering from PD (Blood & Guthrie, 2018). Cognitive performance may sometimes worsen towards the last part of the day or when medications wear off. The possibility for motor worsening and fatigue may limit the client's capability to undergo mental and motor tasks at certain times of the day. Therefore, I made sure we met in the morning. Eddie preferred sitting in a chair with good support and a cushion. For smaller projects he would work on a small rolling table that could be locked in place. For larger painting projects, a large easel was brought into the room.

As an identifying artist, Eddie had many paint brushes, boxes of charcoal, pencils, and sketchbooks that were familiar to him. To build excitement about his new work, I introduced many new art supplies, all good quality to match his previous expertise and tastes. I would carefully arrange the art supplies so that they appeared attractive and intriguing to Eddie, and he was always surprised, thankful, and willing to give them a try, once we developed rapport.

To help make Eddie's art experiences increasingly satisfying, I took the time to learn his style and preferences as they evolved. I did my best to listen and understand what Eddie preferred, rather than trying to tell him what to do or control the speed at which he produced. This is a key element to providing person-centered, strengths-based art therapy for clients, as based on strengths-based social work models (Blood and Guthrie, 2018). Giving options to older adults in stages of decline provides some degree of autonomy. The art projects suggested were based on Eddie's interest and stories. They were intended to make the process as satisfying as possible so that he would not get lost in frustration.

Months went by, and artmaking became the process he asked for and wanted to continue. Sessions were increased to twice a week at the request of his case manager. Sketchbooks, charcoal, and pencils were left with Eddie to practice sketching for homework. Home health attendants reported that art-making helped to engage him between appointments. The availability of artmaking between sessions reduced Eddie's anger and frustration. Artmaking became a regulating and soothing practice for him.

Even though we were experimenting with mediums and subjects in our work together, Eddie would always come back to painting portraits. He would ask to set up a mirror to draw or paint self-portraits, and sometimes painted portraits of me. Despite his cognitive decline and worsening symptoms of PD, working with his hands improved mobility and reduced the need for adaptive devices. Over the course of art therapy, his dexterity improved and he was able to hold brushes, pencils, or charcoal.

Eddie's experience with art in his last years of life was a mix of remembering what was familiar and learning what felt new. Eddie certainly experienced the loss of being able to paint with photographic realism. While that ability faded, Eddie began re-engaging with artmaking and the idea of continuing to see himself as an artist. He began to see new abilities coming forward like using mixed media (Figure 5.2).

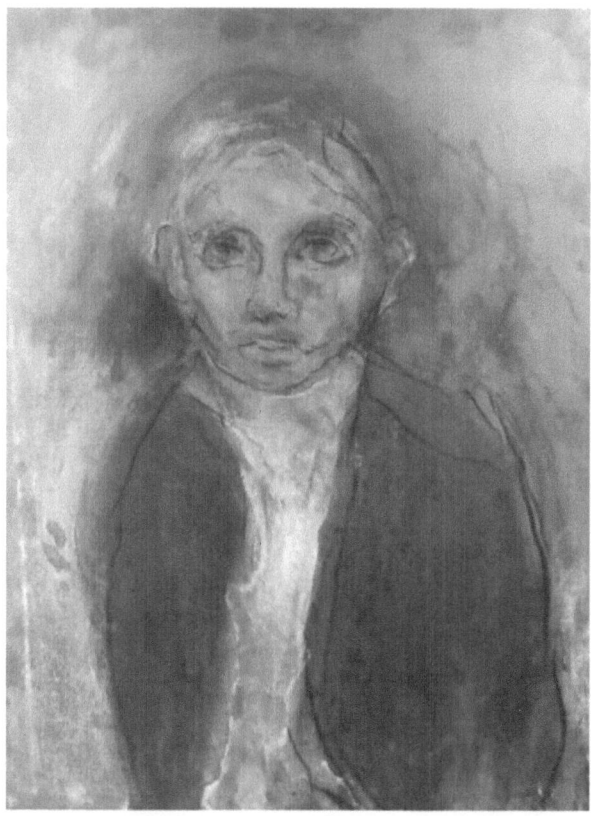

Figure 5.2 Mixed Media Self-Portrait

Outcomes

It was through life-long portrait painting that Eddie claimed his artist identity. First in his younger years, as a traditional portrait artist. After facing physical and mental limitations, Eddie took a break from making any art at all. Later in life, through art therapy, he explored new styles and a revised artist identity. In sessions, he worked on reframing the changes with dexterity and photo-realism in portrait painting. He studied abstract portrait painting and spoke often about artist identity and how styles can change over time. Unlike the health decline of PD, art was an added aspect of quality to the end of life. Reframing his deficiency into a strength helped Eddie to build confidence and re-engage with artmaking, which had physical, mental, and emotional benefits.

When a person with PD goes to the doctor, they are faced with assessments and tools to measure how much they have lost, as compared to the last visit. Medications can help preserve a patient's quality of life and slow the progression of the disease, which is essential for treatment. Including non-medical treatments like art therapy into a protocol for patients living with PD can help them experience a new sense of confidence. Patients with PD who have participated in art therapy develop a sense of voice and a creative identity. There are no medications able to provide this result (Cucca et al., 2021).

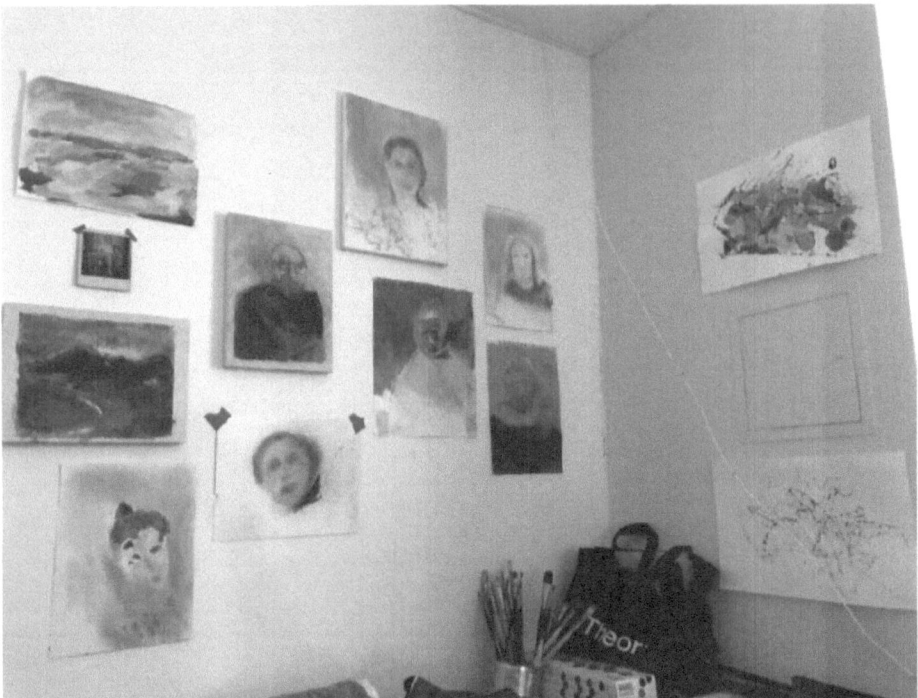

Figure 5.3 Eddie's Gallery Wall of Recent Art

Conclusion

In the final stages of working with Eddie, his family began planning an art show. The timing was prescient, as it was right before New York City shut down due to the pandemic in the spring of 2020. This was also Eddie's last art show, as he passed away that same spring. This was an incredible opportunity for him to celebrate art across his lifespan. His family created a beautiful exhibit and reception in the community space of the building he lived in for years. The artwork that lined the walls of his apartment (Figure 5.3) had a chance to be seen by visitors.

I remember how proud Eddie seemed that day. Though he always began with humility, he expressed amazement to see his paintings exhibited in such a professional way and took joy in getting to share this moment with his community. This was the final shift in his new artist identity, an art exhibit that celebrated both old and new styles, and his previous and current artist identity.

SPONTANEOUS LIFE REVIEW

PEG DUNN-SNOW

Setting

The therapy setting was a small nursing and rehabilitation center located in a small rural town near a state capital city in the Northeast region of the United States. At the time I was an art therapy student and saw many of the elderly residents at the center. One resident stood out among the others and my experience with this man, who I will refer to as Abe, convinced me I was correct in following my new career path of becoming an art therapist. This experience took place during the first year of my graduate studies, after having a long teaching career with special needs students of all ages. Like Abe, most of the residents at the center were elderly with presenting problems, including physical limitations that did not allow them to live at home independently. I was not the first art therapy student to work at this facility and the designated area to do my work was either bedside or in the hair salon at the facility. When working in the salon, the art therapy area was set up behind a screen during the time residents were not scheduled for hair appointments. The facility also provided the art materials that were limited to paper, markers, graphite and colored pencils, erasers, oil pastels, a watercolor palette, and brushes.

Approaches

Being a student in my first experience working as an art therapist, my approach with Abe was to follow my professor's advice, "Trust the art-making process and follow the lead of your client". After my work with Abe was completed, I later realized Abe had conducted his own life review during our art therapy sessions together (Ravid-Horesh, 2004; Zieger, 1976). Abe's life review included all aspects of his life from childhood memories to his residency at the center. It was not apparent at first that a life review was taking place because Abe did not appear to present the events in his life in any sequential order. Although looking back at his timeline, it was sequential in reverse, from present to past rather than past to present.

With no accessibility, considerations focused on the fact that Abe was wheelchair-bound and he exhibited slight tremors in both his hands. There was a table where his wheelchair could fit under, and drawing pencils and brushes were altered with rubber grips or wrapped in masking tape for easier handling.

Intake Session

During our first session, Abe wheeled himself into the hair salon and introduced himself. Although physically challenged, his mind was sharp. He said very little about himself during this first session, but instead, asked me many questions about myself. When asked if he was interested in drawing, he said yes. He then proceeded to quickly draw and label a detailed map of the center (Figure 5.4). He said he was drawing it for me to help me find my way around, since this was the first time I had been to the center. He continued to select the art tasks he created during his art therapy sessions. He came each week with a clear idea of what he wanted to draw or paint, followed by a discussion that Abe led. He also directed the sessions when he only wanted to talk. When I asked him how he spent his time at the center, he said, "I write letters to my congressman", indicating that he had a great interest in state politics.

Early Sessions

During our next session, Abe rolled into the hair salon and greeted me with a smile. He talked about other residents he thought I should be working with during the summer. He

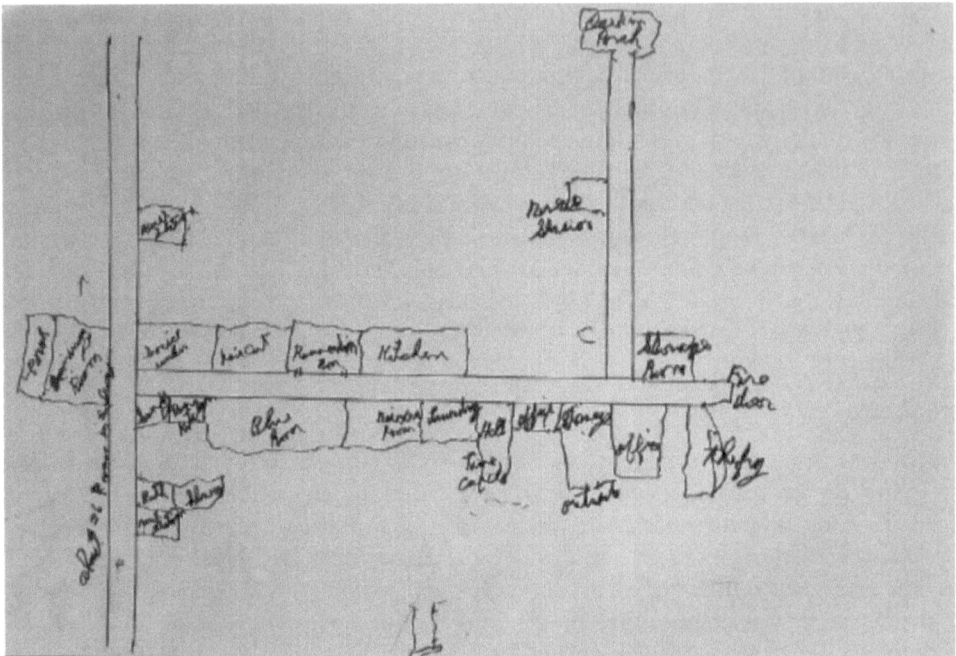

Figure 5.4 Map of the Center

then got busy drawing another map for me, listing the names of all my potential patients on this map and where their rooms were located in the building. Abe explained this was to help me navigate the corridors of the facility. For the next few sessions, Abe began to tell me more about his own life. In one session, he drew his log cabin home that he built himself and on the back of the drawing he wrote detailed steps on how to build his cabin, including a list of the tools he had used. In another session, he drew a wonderful Jersey cow. Abe was once a dairy farmer and had a herd of cows. He explained how each cow was cataloged on the farm with a number and a name. He named the cow in his drawing Peggy Jane (Figure 5.5). During my supervision session that week, my supervisor speculated there might already be some positive transference happening between Abe and myself. The very next session I had with Abe, he brought in a plaque he received in 1987, winning the Green Pasture Award in the state. In a later session, Abe did a drawing of his plaque and colored it in with watercolor paints.

Later Sessions

In many of the later art therapy sessions, Abe just wanted to talk. I learned about his wife who had recently died and his children who lived out-of-state. He told me he only left his home state a few times in his life, including a visit to one of his children in upstate New York. He also told me about other jobs he had held, including the position of county clerk in his small rural town.

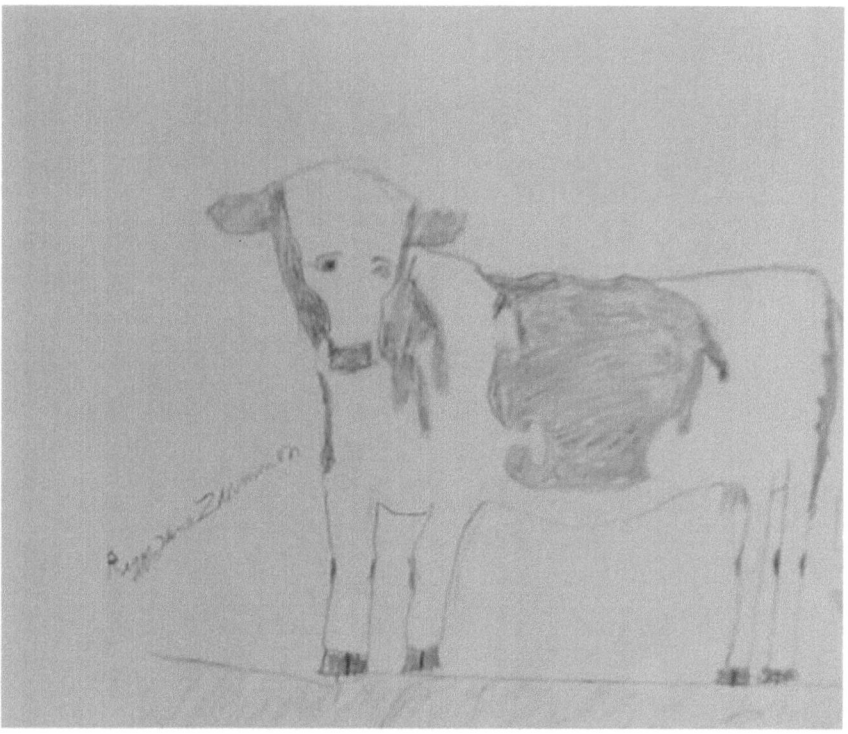

Figure 5.5 Peggy Jane the Jersey Cow

In one of our last sessions, Abe came into the session holding a page from a recent newspaper that showed a vintage, black and white photo of a snowplow in winter. But unlike the snowplows of today, this one was made of wood and pulled by a team of horses. Abe called it a "snow roller". He told me this was how he remembered the snow being plowed as a small child when he and his friends would run behind it on the newly plowed roads. Abe then decided to make a drawing of the photograph (Figure 5.6).

Outcomes

Abe was a kind and articulate man, whose behavior illustrated he was concerned for others as well as himself. With gentleness and humility, he took pride in telling me about his experiences, skills, and accomplishments during his lifetime. In addition to the last session, a goodbye party was given for me at the center and all the residents I worked with were invited. Abe came to the party and seemed to enjoy the cake and conversation.

Conclusion

Abe's ability to tell his story through words and images was evidenced through his conversations and the several drawings he completed during art therapy sessions. His physical

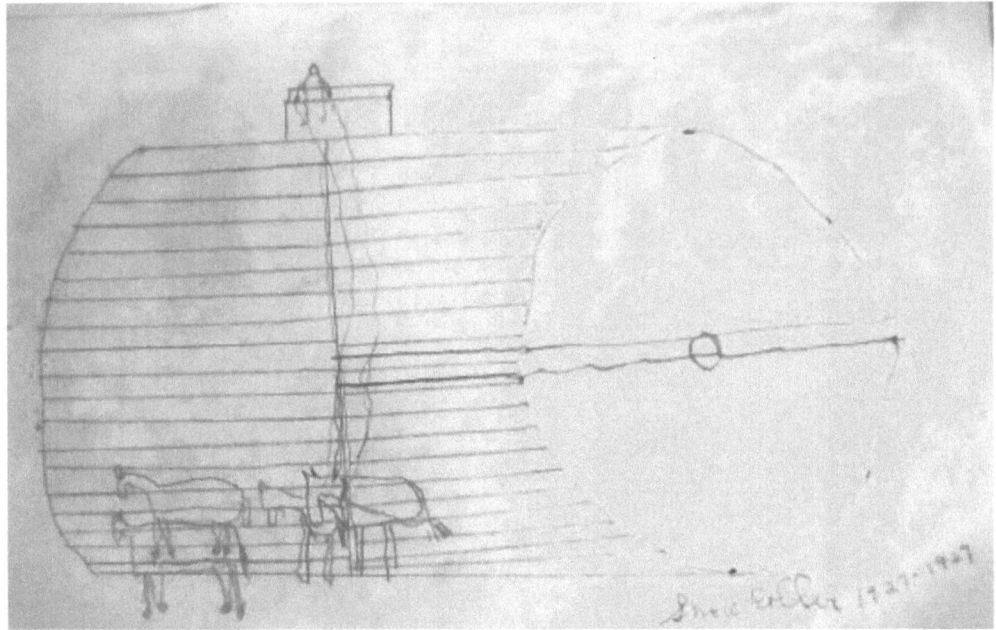

Figure 5.6 The Wooden Snow Roller

limitations did not stop him from participating in the activities at the center and engaging in his continued interest in the news, especially local and state government affairs. He read the daily newspaper and frequently wrote to his state senators and representatives. Abe taught me more than I taught him about living a full and productive life as well as about the value of art therapy.

LIVING AT THE END OF LIFE: CO-CREATION OF NARRATIVE COLLAGE IN HOSPICE CARE

MIA DE BÉTHUNE

Setting

The setting for this case study was the home of a client. It was part of a Complimentary Care Program of a hospice and palliative care center in the suburbs of a major North American city. As the sole art therapist, my mandate was to provide bereavement support and palliative care activities for children and older clients in hospice as well as their families. I went to the home of this client once a week from February until November of the year that she died. All materials were brought into the site in addition to photos and magazines from the family to support resonance with her memories.

Approaches

This case used collage-making exclusively in a narrative and relational approach to support the process of end-of-life review for a woman with terminal cancer. Co-creation of collages helped to enhance her experience and investment in living, at a time when her body and mind were in rapid decline. Collage allows for experimenting with pictures that can lead clients to more flexible images of themselves (Landgarten, 1993; Riley, 1999). In my work with elder clients, facing mortality due to life-threatening diseases and disabilities, I have found collaging can provide new vitality, an embodied sense of self (Chilton & Scotti, 2014), and the telling of stories at a time when life review is an important task (Safrai, 2013; Stallings, 2010).

Client

Irma was 99 years old when she was diagnosed with terminal stomach cancer and her doctors determined she had two months to live. She was a tall, thin, elegant woman with wispy white-blonde hair and bright curious eyes. She was from an upper-middle-class family and had been a leading child therapist in her day. I met her two months after her diagnosis when she had beaten the doctor's predictions and was still quite vigorous. The hospice nurse suggested art therapy as something she might enjoy and that could occupy her time. She was still intellectually curious, although somewhat disorganized in her thinking, and yet did little more than watch TV from the confinement of her wheelchair. Other team members were a personal aide, a social worker, and a reflexologist. Her adult daughter and grandchildren tried to be present and doting but led busy professional lives. We all did our part to increase the functioning of this vital individual who might have otherwise sunk into isolation. Art therapy, in particular, seemed to help communicate Irma's thoughts, wishes, and concerns at the end of her life as she gradually lost language.

Intake Session and Assessment

Irma was polite but reserved when I first went to her home. She sat by her bed with the television on while I explained what I did. I described the materials I could bring: paint, pastels, and possibly fiber crafts, like weaving. Irma nodded at this and said she very much enjoyed working with yarns and fabrics. She spoke haltingly, often searching for words, but seemed able to communicate her ideas. I agreed to return the following week with just such items. When I returned, she looked at me with disdain as I presented yarns and a loom. She asked, "Why am I doing these crafty projects?" As a former therapist, she seemed dismayed to find herself on the other end of a therapeutic directive.

Fortunately, I had also brought colored pencils and paper and Irma drew a small, but delicate flower garden that day. She even wrote out a poem in a scratchy hand, yet these efforts seemed taxing and the words were barely legible. The following week, I brought coloring pages of flower designs and some markers. Irma had trouble distinguishing between the different spaces on the coloring page. Even choosing which colors went where seemed like an effort as did pushing markers across the page to fill in color. I needed to prompt her to try a new color and hand her the marker. She often seemed to look up as if surprised to still find me there and perhaps hoping that I would disappear. She did not seem able to tell me she did not want to do this activity and instead quizzed me about how I worked with children as if to test out my knowledge. Eventually, she asked her aide to take her to the bathroom. It was a tactic I would learn that she used when she wished to avoid activity and couldn't say "No". Before I left, her aide advised me that Irma loved to cut up paper if given a pair of scissors. I also assessed that she was easily overstimulated and needed limited materials as well as those that interested her but did not infantilize her.

Early Sessions

The following week I brought images from a book about early twentieth-century life, from about the time Irma was born. I hoped these might capture her imagination and prompt memory. She seemed captivated by women in bustles and men with handlebar mustaches and top hats riding big-wheeled bicycles. I offered her scissors to cut out her own images while I cut more and placed them on her table tray. The transformation in demeanor was almost immediate. Rather than seeming irritable and exhausted, she had a gleam in her eye as she worked slowly, but carefully with the scissors. When we looked at the images together, Irma began to recall that her father had worn a mustache and hat like the ones she saw. She began speaking about her mother and a flood of childhood memories followed. Her whole face appeared to soften and to become young as if once again inhabiting the child's body in her mind.

Collaging as a Team

Over those early weeks, I continued to bring collage material as well as construction paper as a base. I began to offer Irma two or three options and invite her to choose a background color for each collage. This broader type of decision-making seemed to empower and be less taxing than choosing markers for pre-made coloring pages. Irma chose quickly and seemed to drink in the bright color onto which I laid out her cut images. I learned not to overload her visual field with too much on her table tray lest she become confused. If I offered two or three choices, she would generally love one or two and then reject another.

As we continued to look at the images on her tray, I would move them into various configurations and check in with Irma about how the changes felt. Her hands were shaky and she could not manipulate the edges of small pieces to pick them up, but she was able to approve a layout or she would ask me to move them again. Often she seemed to frame her design decisions based on emotional relationships between the images (e.g. "She needs to do as she is told", or "Her mother might not approve of that"). Irma's childhood family dynamics appeared to unfold through the collage, and seemed a way of working through relational issues with her parents as well as giving meaning to her current state entirely at the mercy of her caregivers and family for when and what she ate, what was on the TV, and even getting into and out of the bathroom. Though she lived in the home of her daughter and had helped raise her grandchildren, she was now often isolated. She was confined to her wheelchair and losing her ability for language. In our interactions, she struggled to articulate words. I came to understand certain silences, gestures, or expressions (e.g., furrowed or raised brows) to indicate fatigue, disapproval, or just contemplation.

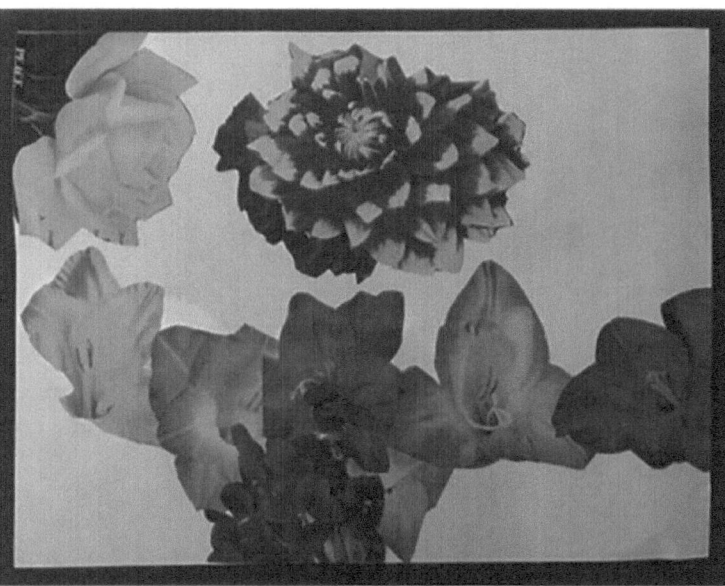

Figure 5.7 Dahlias

Later Sessions

In an effort to maintain the connection with Irma, I continued to search for vintage magazines that might stimulate memories. I was offered a cache of magazines from the 1940s by
the family. One was a seed catalog featuring bright images of flowers and vegetables. Irma
was elated and clapped her hands when she saw them. She had begun to look forward to
my visits and even started to thank me. She eagerly agreed to cut out the picture of a large
pink dahlia while I worked on a yellow one. As we arranged the flowers against a bright
pink background, she appeared animated (Figure 5.7). Perhaps it was their brightness, but
Irma was quite vocal about where the flowers should be on the page. Once we settled on the
design, I pasted the images with a glue stick and Irma pressed them down. I took the dahlia
collage and stood back to create distance for her. Irma clapped again and said, "I love it".
She insisted it should be placed on her bookshelf so that she could look at it all the time.

We continued with this method of working together for the next six months and created
over 15 collages. We looked at *Good Housekeeping* issues from the 1940s which she pored
over reliving old times. Animal pictures from *National Geographic* elicited strong physical
and emotional responses. Irma would identify with the physicality of a seal underwater or
the trepidation of a baby otter waiting for its mother to rescue him, and the regal elegance
of a camel resting from a long journey. One image of a man standing in the waves of the
ocean led her to imagine the feel of salt water up her nose (Figure 5.8). Irma would continue
to stare at her collages and speak to herself about them even as I left. When I arrived each
week, she was always eager and happy to begin "our" work. Photos of a woman and a man
with a horse evoked an entire love story worthy of a Hollywood script. Each collage seemed
to have a story related to her past relationships and I wrote these down along the margins
of the picture.

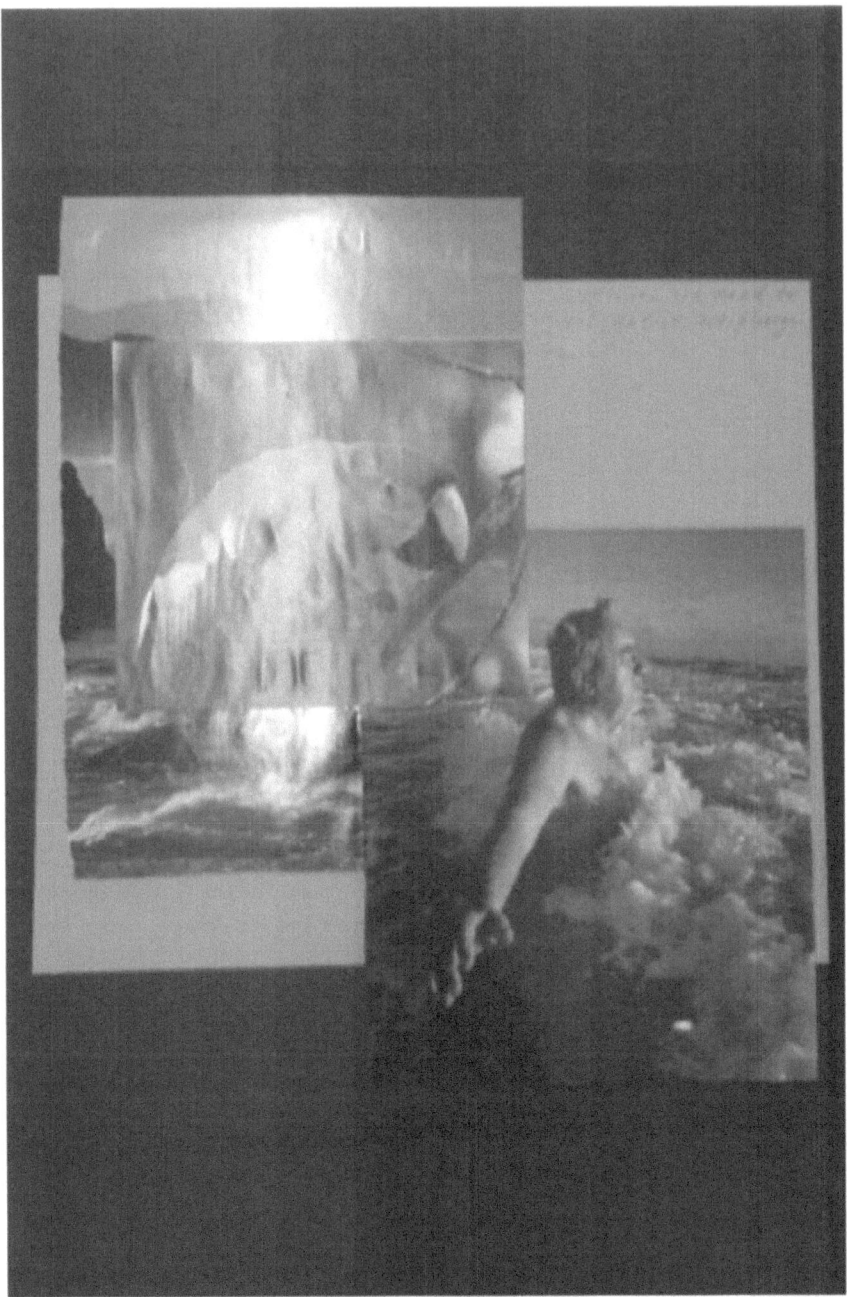

Figure 5.8 Man in the Waves

Creating Connections with Family

At the end of each session, I placed the current collage on Irma's table so she could continue to look at it after I left. She showed these collages to other hospice staff, her aide, and her family, and I would often find them on her bookshelf where she could see them. Her daughter and grandchildren began to comment on her connection to the images and how alive they seemed. Her family seemed surprised at what we produced during our sessions together and also were impressed with her abilities. Even if visiting from the city, the grandchildren made sure not to interfere with our sessions because they regarded them as an important part of her week. Eventually, I compiled all of her collages into one album and we began to review them each session before making a new one. During the summer Irma turned 100, her family held a party to which I was invited along with my colleagues from the hospice team. The album of collages was featured prominently on the table of photos.

Outcomes

Near the end of our time working together, Irma was quite weak and confined to her bed. She was less able to cut images or even talk, so looking through the album became an important activity. She continued to create a few more collages that were all cut out and arranged by me. Her second to last collage was of a garden walkway framed by a wooden gate around which I arranged, with her guidance, small cut-out flowers to create a bower (Figure 5.9). I had heard from the nursing aide that she was in decline and chose the gateway image instinctively. Sure enough, Irma described this gate as a passage to another place as if preparing herself for her own passing from life. Her final collage was of flowers created from jewels cut out of a luxury catalog. Irma struggled with words, but she was able to indicate where she felt each piece should go by pointing and nodding, and I was able to decipher that she said, "The jewels are filled with light". When I repeated this statement, she nodded. I had the palpable sense that she felt transported somewhere else as she reached out to touch the finished collage. She held her hand there for a long while as if trying to reach into the light of the image. The following week she was unable to open her eyes to work and five days later she died – a full nine months after her cancer diagnosis. The hospice team was invited to her service and the collage album was once again prominently displayed as a testament to her vigor up until the end. The family attributed Irma's extraordinary vitality in the final year to the care and support of the hospice team including me as the art therapist.

Conclusions

My role as an art therapist appeared as a conduit for Irma's life story to continue rather than be stifled as she waited for death. With voice and the ability to relate experience comes vitality and a will to live. As communication breaks down, humans can become cognitively stagnant (Coors, 2013) and creating alternative communication channels becomes crucial. Rather than ask Irma what she might like to work with, I took an intersubjective stance (Schwarz et al., 2018) and imagined what would stimulate her. Images from the Victorian era seemed to capture her imagination and prompt memory (Loizeau et al., 2015). Providing the cutting activity, brightly colored background papers, and discussion about the images seemed to constitute an "enriched environment" that fostered "neurogenesis" and supported language use even at a time of decline (Pike, 2013, p. 159).

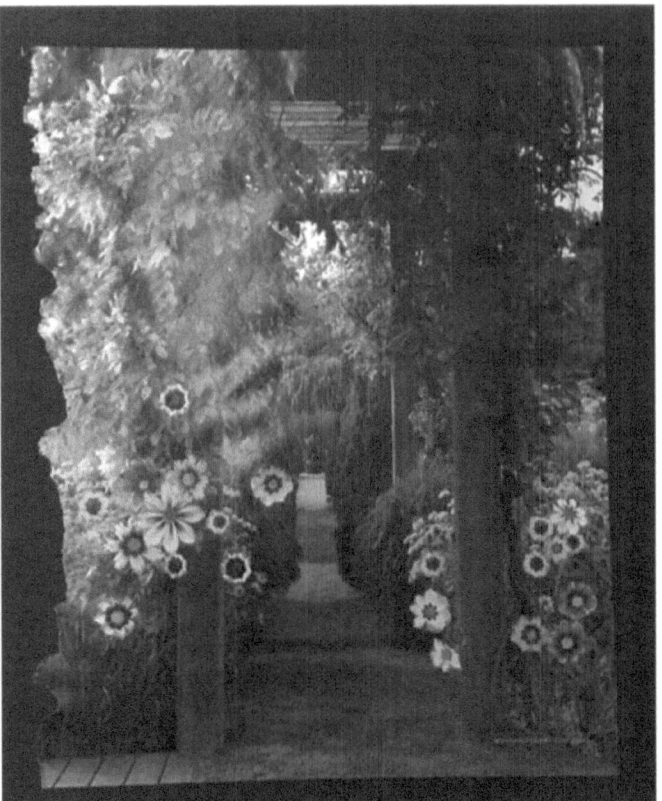

Figure 5.9 The Garden Gate

Additionally, images of animals and eventually other people, especially a man standing in ocean waves (Figure 5.8) appeared to allow Irma an embodied experience of physicality despite her restricted movement. This embodiment related to the sensory experiences depicted (Chilton & Scotti, 2014) and seemed to increase her vitality. It's likely that parallel treatment in reflexology enhanced bodily feeling and allowed fuller access to her imaginal experience. Prompting the stories seemed to give her an opportunity to explore her emotional connections (Chilton & Scotti, 2014) and access a part of herself that remembered physical love, sexual attraction, and the sensation of pleasure in her body (Loizeau et al., 2015).

As Irma's health and strength declined, looking over her work in the album enabled her to move out of a diminishing body into a space of her own reckoning (Merleau-Ponty, 1964). My role as co-creator became more important (Schwarz et al., 2018) as the inter-relational work continued. My instinct to provide the image of a garden gate (Figure 5.9) seemed intuitive of her progression toward a liminal state (Sibbett, 2005). Irma appeared to confirm this with her verbalization of it as a passage to another place as if preparing emotionally for her own passing from life.

The notion of retained skillfulness (Chilton & Scotti, 2014), a sense of wholeness (O'Callaghan et al., 2018), and joyfulness (Harrison & Grasdal, 2003) seemed facilitated through the process of co-created collaging and added to her family's ability to continue to see Irma as a remarkable, capable being, despite her decline and impending death (Loizeau et al., 2015; O'Callaghan et al., 2018).

References

Alsawy, S., Mansell, W., McEvoy, P., & Tai, S. (2017). What is good communication for people living with dementia? A mixed-methods systematic review. *Internationa Psychogeriatrics*, *29*(11), 1785–1800.

Bagan, M. (2009). *Expressive arts: Aging, Alzheimer's, and Parkinson's A manual for artists, art educators, health professionals, and others who work with older adults*. Charles C. Thomas Publisher.

Baltes, P. B., & Smith, J. (2008). The fascination of wisdom: Its nature, ontogeny, and function. *Perspectives on Psychological Science*, *3*(1), 56–64.

Banasiak, J. (2019). Art therapy for older adults: A systematic review. *Journal of Gerontological Social Work*, *62*(1), 1–18.

Barresi, M., & Gilbert, S. (2023). *Developmental biology* (13th ed.). Oxford University Press.

Berger, A. S. (2010). Practicing death: Alternative views. *The Journal of Transpersonal Psychology*, *42*(1), 48–60.

Bloem, B. R., Okun, M. S., & Klein, C. (2021). Parkinson's disease. *The Lancet*, *397*(10291), 2284–2303.

Blood, I., & Guthrie, L. (2018). *Supporting older people using attachment-informed and strengths-based approaches*. Jessica Kingsley Publishers.

Boorstein, S. (2000). Transpersonal psychotherapy. *American Journal of Psychotherapy*, *54*(3), 408–423.

Camartin, K. (2012). The use of art therapy with persons with dementia. *Canadian Art Therapy Association Journal*, *25*(2), 7–15.

Chilton, G., & Scotti, V. (2014). Snipping, gluing, writing: The properties of collage as an arts-based research practice in art therapy. *Art Therapy*, *31*(4), 163–171.

Choi, H. J., Lee, Y. H., & Seo, Y. J. (2013). The effects of group art therapy on depression, anxiety, and quality of life in psychiatric patients: A meta-analysis. *Korean Journal of Adult Nursing*, *25*(6), 637–646.

Clear, J. (2018). *Atomic habits: Tiny changes, remarkable results: an easy & proven way to build good habits & break bad ones*. Avery.

Cohen, G. D. (2006). *The creative age: Awakening human potential in the second half oflife*.Random House.

Consoli, J. J. (1992). The art therapist's third hand – reflections on art, art therapy and society. *Art Therapy*, *9*(1), 48–49.

Coors, M. (2013). A dementalized body? Reconsidering the human condition in the light of dementia. *Geriatric Mental Health Care*, *1*(2), 34–38. https://dx.doi.org//10.1016/j.gmhc.2013.04.004

Cucca, A., Di Rocco, A., Acosta, I., Beheshti, M., Berberian, M., Bertisch, H. C., Droby, A., Ettinger, T., Hudson, T. E., Inglese, M., Jung, Y. J., Mania, D. F., Quartarone, A., Rizzo, J. R., Sharma, K., Feigin, A., Biagioni, M. C., & Ghilardi, M. F. (2021). Art therapy for Parkinson's disease. *Parkinsonism & Related Disorders*, *84*, 148–154.

Dall'Alba, G. (2023). Toward responsive attunement as health professionals. *Studies in Continuing Education*.

Drazic, I., Schermuly, C. C., & Busch, V. (2023). Empowered to stay active: Psychological empowerment, retirement timing, and later life work. *Journal of AdultDevelopment*, 1–18.

Dunne, P. (2016). *The narrative therapist and the arts* (2nd ed.). Possibilities Press.

Erikson, E. (1967). *Identity and the life cycle*. W.W. Norton & Company.

Fabbo, L. (2020). The shared spiritual experience of reiki and early psychoanalytic practice. In M. Jaffe, W. Nicola, J. Floersch, & J. Longhofer. (Eds.). *Spirituality in mental health practice : A narrative casebook* (pp. 182–197). Taylor & Francis Group.

Fowler, J. W. (1995). *Stages of faith: The psychology of human development and the quest for meaning.* HarperSanFrancisco.

Franklin, M. A. (2016). Essence, art, and therapy: A transpersonal view. In D. E. Gussak & M. L. Rosal (Eds). *The Wiley handbook of art therapy* (pp. 99–111). John Wiley & Sons.

Gerber, N. (2016). Art therapy education: A creative dialectic intersubjective approach. In D. E. Gussak & M. L. Rosal (Eds). *The Wiley handbook of art therapy* (pp. 794–801). John Wiley & Sons.

Gerlitz, Y., Regev, D., & Snir, S. (2020). A relational approach to art therapy. *The Arts in Psychotherapy, 68,* e-Article 101644.

Groot, L. J., Schers, H. J., Burgers, J. S., Schellevis, F. G., Smalbrugge, M., Uigen, A. A., van de Ven, P. M., van der Horst, H. E., & Maarsingh, O. R. (2021). Optimising personal continuity for older patients in general practice: A study protocol for a cluster randomised stepped wedge pragmatic trial. *BCM Family Practice, 22,* 207.

Hertzog, C., Kramer, A. F., Wilson, R. S., & Lindenberger, U. (2008). Enrichment effects on adult cognitive development: Can the functional capacity of older adults be preserved and enhanced? *Psychological Science in the Public Interest, 9*(1), 1–65.

Keisari, S. & Palgi, Y. (2017). Life crossroads onstage: Integrating life review and drama therapy for older adults. *Aging & Mental Health, 21*(10), 1079–1089.

Krøier, J. K., McDermott, O., & Ridder, H. M. (2022). Conceptualizing attunement in dementia care: A meta-ethnographic view. *Arts & Health, 14*(1), 32–48.

Harrison, H., & Grasdal, P. (2003). *Collage for the soul: Expressing hopes and dreams through art.* Rockport.

Landgarten, H. (1993). *Magazine photo collage: A multicultural assessment and treatment technique.* Routledge.

Levine, P. (2010). *In an unspoken voice.* North Atlantic Press.

Levy, B. (2009). Stereotype embodiment: A psychosocial approach to aging. *Current Directions in Psychological Science, 18*(6), 332–336.

Li, W. C., & Li, C. H. (2017). Effects of art therapy on patients with dementia: A systematic review and meta-analysis. *Journal of the American Medical Directors Association, 18*(7), 604–613.

Loizeau, A., Kündig, Y., & Oppikofer, S. (2015). "Awakened art stories" – Rediscovering pictures by persons living with dementia utilizing TimeSlips: A pilot study. *Geriatric Mental Health Care, 3*(2), 13–20.

Masika, R., Reid, D., Gao, W., & Kyle, R. G. (2020). The impact of creative arts on symptoms of anxiety and depression in adults with mental health disorders: A systematic review and meta-analysis. *BMC Psychiatry, 20,* 534.

McGovern, J. (2015). Living better with dementia: Strengths-based social work practice and dementia care. *Social Work in Health Care, 54*(5), 408–421.

Merleau-Ponty, M. (1964). *The primacy of perception.* Northwestern University Press.

O'Callaghan, C., Byrne, L., Cokalis, E., Glenister, D., Santilli, M,, Clark, R, McCarthy, T., & Michael, N. (2018) "Life within the person comes to fore": Pastoral workers' practice wisdom on the use of arts in palliative care. *American Journal of Hospice & Palliative Medicine, 35*(7), 1000–1008.

Partridge, E. (2019). Art therapy with older adults. Jessica Kingsley.

Pike, A. A. (2013) The effect of art therapy on cognitive performance among ethnically diverse older adults. *Art Therapy: Journal of the American Art Therapy Association, 30*(4), 159–168.

Ravid-Horesh, R. H. (2004). "A temporary guest": The use of art therapy in life review with an elderly woman. *The Arts in Psychotherapy, 31*(5), 303–319.

Riley, S. (1999). *Contemporary art therapy with adolescents.* Jessica Kingsley.

Roikjaer, S. G., Missel, M., Bergenholtz, H. M., Schønhau, M. N., & Timm, H. (2019). The use of personal narratives in hospital based palliative care interventions – an integrative literature review. *Palliative Medicine, 33*(10), 1255–1271.

Safrai, M. B. (2013). Art therapy in hospice care: A catalyst for insight and healing. *Art Therapy, 30*(3), 122–129.

Schwarz, N., Snir, S., & Regev, D. (2018). The therapeutic presence of the art therapist. *Art Therapy: Journal of the American Art Therapy Association, 35*(1), 11–18.

Sibbett, C. (2005). "Betwixt and between": Crossing thresholds. In D. Waller & C. Sibbett (Eds). *Art therapy and cancer care* (pp. 12–37). Open University Press.

Somatic Experiencing International (2022). *Somatic Experiencing Beginning Year Module 1 Manual.*

Sooke, A. (2014). *Matisse: A second life.* Penguin Books.

Stallings, J. W. (2010). Collage as a therapeutic modality for reminiscence in patients with dementia. *Art Therapy, 27*(3), 136–140.

Stein, J. B. (2021). Energy healing: Reiki, therapeutic touch and healing touch in the United States and beyond. In D. Lüddeckens, P. Hetmanczyk, P. E. Klassen, & J. B. Stein (Eds). *The Routledge handbook of religion, medicine, and health* (pp. 229–243). Taylor & Francis Group.

Windle, G., Gregory, S., Newman, A., Goulding, A., O'Brien, D., Parkinson, C., & Tischler, V. (2018). Understanding the impact of visual arts interventions for people living with dementia: A realist review protocol. *Systematic Reviews, 7*(1), 1–10.

Zieger, B. L. (1976). Life review in art therapy with the aged. *American Journal of Art Therapy, 15*(2), 47–50.

Final Thoughts

While writing and editing this book and after reading each of these case studies several times, it was clear to us, as the editors, that our guest authors of the case studies clearly illustrated the length and breadth of how the profession of art therapy has developed itself over the last 70 years. Collectively, these authentic case studies provide a window into the work achieved by exemplary art therapists who showcased the efficacy and effectiveness of why art therapy is a valued therapeutic service in the helping professions.

It was not so long ago that when art therapy was mentioned in a sentence the most familiar response was, "What is that?" Today, it is clearly a respected profession and therapeutic approach for healing and rehabilitation. Art therapy can and is used with everyone throughout the lifespan. Art therapy services are found in a variety of settings too. Patients and clients in these case studies received art therapy services in: hospitals, medical clinics, schools, correctional facilities, through virtual means, as part of home-health care programs, and in private practice.

Art therapy is also a profession that collaborates well with other health care providers including but, not limited to, medical doctors, psychiatrists, psychologists, mental health counselors, family therapists, social workers, school psychologists, guidance counselors, teachers, spiritual care providers, law enforcement, correctional personnel, and others. Again, we thank the case study authors who contributed to this collection, and the students who motivated us to develop this book. We look forward to creating the website that will expand the material in this text.

Glossary

The following glossary terms include developmental and learning theories, creativity and artistic theories, other therapeutic approaches complimentary to art therapy, along with art therapy formats and settings illustrated in the case studies featured in this book.

Acceptance and Commitment Therapy (ACT)   a form of mindfulness-based therapy that helps clients to stay in the present and encourages them to simply accept their thoughts and feelings rather than ignoring them.

Adverse Childhood Experiences (ACEs)   looks at the impact of various physical, emotional, and familial negative traumas and the impact those experiences have on lifelong health and well-being.

Artistic Development (2-D)   Lowenfeld and Brittain (1986), the oldest and widely referenced theory of artistic development in drawings. Includes five stages: Scribble Stage (ages 18 months to 4 years); Preschematic Stage (ages 4–7 years); Schematic Stage (ages 7–9 years); Gang Age: The Dawning Realism Stage (ages 9–12 years); Adolescent Art: The Period of Decision Stage (ages 14–17 years).

Attachment Theory   is about relationships. Both Winnicott and Bowlby write about attachments. Bowlby emphasized and wrote about external environment attachments and advocated that each young child must have one primary caregiver in order to feel safe and experience normal social and emotional development. Winnicott emphasized and wrote about internal attachments within oneself and what the person believed about himself through his relationship with others.

Cognitive Development Theory   Piaget developed this comprehensive theory. His ideas cover the nature of knowledge and how we learn and acquire such information. Piaget's four-stage process of learning includes sensorimotor, preoperational, concrete-operational, and formal-operational.

Cognitive Behavioral Therapy (CBT)   rooted in the work of Aaron Beck, CBT challenges a client's negative self-concept to change unhealthy behaviors that can help treat mood disorders such as depression. Its premise is thoughts precede feelings followed by actions.

Critical Theory,   largely developed by Max Horkhiemer in the 1930s, is orientated in human emancipation and power. Its focus is to prevent the loss of truth, past knowledge and history. It believes science should make society better and current values and beliefs should be challenged together with examining current social issues that influence the behaviors and beliefs held by the dominant culture of the day.

Diagnostic Drawing Series (DDS), developed by art therapist Barry Cohen in 1982, the three-drawing art therapy assessment (free drawing, tree drawing, and feeling drawing) is given to clients to assess their cognitive, symbolic and affective abilities. The assessment is designed to identify clients' defenses and strengths to help in the planning of treatment.

Ecological Systems Theory developed by Urie Bronfenbrenner, focused on the quality and conditions of children's environments. When the child's environment becomes more elaborate the complexity helps promote the child's physical and cognitive growth. As a scientific approach to studying lifespan development it emphasizes the interrelationship between cognitive, social, and biological growth in which children are active participants in their own development.

Existential Theory beliefs include personal freedom and therefore the responsibility to determine their own meaning, existence, and purpose in life. Therapy approaches compatible with existential theory include humanistic, experiential, depth, and relational psychotherapy.

Expressive Therapies Continuum (ETC) developed by art therapists Lusebrink and Kagin, the ETC explains human interaction with creative media through a bipolar, neurological system including levels of Sensory/Kinesthetic, Perceptual/Affective, and Cognitive/Symbolic. Creativity is seen to exist throughout every level.

Eye Movement Desensitization and Reprocessing (EMDR) and Brain Spotting are called power therapies because they produce fast results. The EMDR, developed by Francis Shapiro, uses bilateral eye movements to stimulate the brain, to help access stored, non-verbal information and heal traumatic memories. Brain Spotting, developed by David Grand, stimulates brain functioning by asking the client to hold an eye position connected to a specific conscious memory. Each approach is reported to process and relieve a client's pain from past traumatic experiences.

Flow and Happiness Theory Mihaly Csikszentmihalyi developed a happiness theory based on the belief that people are happiest when they are in flow, which is a type of intrinsic motivation including both challenge and skill. It involves being fully focused on the situation or task in the present.

Gestalt Theory of Development The premise of this theory states that areas of human development happen simultaneously in contrast to other stage developmental theories that focus on different aspects of human growth. Learning is based on viewing and understanding environmental stimuli in concert with one another and not separately. Each aspect of human growth informs the other. The whole is more than the parts is a quote often used to explain this concept.

Hierarchy of Needs developed by Maslow, explains the motive behind human behaviors. This pyramid model includes levels of needs that build upon each other, starting with the need for safety and ending with the need for self-actualization.

Instinctual Trauma Response (ITR) Tinnin and Gantt developed this approach to treating the root causes of trauma while addressing the events that trigger related painful memories. Clients revisit and re-code traumatic events by integrating into consciousness awareness both body and brain memories through drawing, narrative therapy, and parts work, helping clients to place the trauma in the category of past experience.

Internal Family Systems (IFS) developed by Richard Schwartz. This approach to psychotherapy identifies a family of personality parts within everyone, including young, exile parts that hold painful memories, protective parts that try to shield painful experiences, and the healthy core-self parts of each personality. The goal of this approach is successful when all parts work together to allow core-self parts to be in charge of clients' decisions in life with a corrected understanding of their past traumatic experiences.

Kintsugi   is the Japanese art of repairing the cracks in broken pottery with a urushi lacquer, containing powdered gold.

Media Dimension Variables (MDV)   developed in the late 1960s by Sandra Graves, are composed of three continua in which art materials are placed according to the following inherent qualities in a given medium which may be utilized in a therapeutic setting to help clients currently communicate through their art in the best way possible. The three continua included resistant vs fluid, structured vs unstructured, and simple vs complex.

Moral Development   is a process where clients develop their beliefs about what is right and what is wrong. Lawrence Kohlberg's theory focused on the development of moral reasoning and was based on Piaget's general theory of cognition. Kohlberg identified six stages of moral development including: obedience and punishment, self-interest, interpersonal accord and conformity, authority and maintaining social order, social contract, and universal ethical principles. Carol Gilligan later expanded on Kohlberg's work and addresses moral development from a feminist perspective, as Kohlberg's research was only done with boys.

Narrative Therapy   was developed by Michael White and David Epston and based on the Social Construction Learning Theory. The premise is that storytelling helps clients re-story their lives once they understand where they have been and where they are heading. Clients are motivated to reconstruct their lives continuously and consider alternative life experiences for the future.

Open-Studio Approaches   began with the work of artists working in psychiatric hospitals in the 1940s. As the profession of art therapy developed, some art therapists embraced this approach and refined it as an art-centered structure within the therapeutic work in the field. Today, the art therapy open studio is used in a variety of settings with a diverse population of clients.

Personal Construct Theory   is a constructivist approach to therapy, focusing on the belief people construct a personal view of the world and how it works. The environment is consistent but each individual responds differently based on their own ideas formulated by past experiences. George Kelly developed this theory in the 1950s and believed people understand their world by the way they anticipate events rather than by the ways they react to them.

Polyvagal Theory   describes the automatic stages of the nervous system (ventral vagal, sympathetic, and dorsal vagal) in response to traumatic events. Stephen Porges developed this new theory of neurological development that presents two defense systems that respond to danger and safety beyond mobilization i.e. fight or flight.

Psychodynamic Therapy   emphasizes the unconscious mind and how it influences behavior. The goals of this therapy focus on clients understanding how their forgotten past influences their present actions. Sigmund Freud's work from the 1890s through the 1930s developed ideas that informed the premise of the psychodynamic approach to psychology.

Psychosocial Developmental Theory   explains how human personalities develop based on the resolution of existential crises. Erikson identified several developmental crisis stages starting with trust vs. mistrust, followed by autonomy vs. shame and doubt, initiative vs. guilt, industry vs. inferiority, identity vs. role confusion, intimacy vs. isolation, generativity vs. stagnation, ego integrity vs. despair, and support vs. criticism.

Radical Acceptance is defined as rejecting suffering with a willingness to completely accept the reality of one's situation in life, using intellect, physical abilities, and spiritual-emotional understanding.

Racial and Cultural Identity is a developmental theory model originated by Derald Wing Sue and David Sue. They wanted others to understand the struggles minorities experience growing up within a dominant culture that is not their own. The authors write about five stages in this theory and how it can inform the counseling process. The stages include conformity, dissonance, resistance and immersion, introspection, and integrative awareness.

Relational-Cultural Theory (RCT) was developed from the work of Jean Baker Miller in the 1970s and 80s. The roots of the theory included Carl Rogers' person-centered therapy, multiculturalism, feminism, and Freud's psychoanalytic theory. The premise of the theory states that healthy and enjoyable relationships with others are essential for emotional health and stability.

Sanctuary Therapy Model, created by a team led by Sandra Bloom in the 1980s. The model expanded the definition of trauma and noted that all people have adverse traumatic experiences. It includes a roadmap to promote client-facing change in organizations and clinical settings. The model modifies clients' behaviors and symptoms by asking the question "What happened to you?" instead of "What is wrong with you?" This model uses the acronym SELF: safety, emotion management, loss, and future is the framework the model uses to develop treatment plans to help clients heal.

Sandtray Play Therapy (not to be confused with Jungian Sandtray) is a form of play therapy. It is used often with children who have experienced traumatic events. A sandtray scene is believed to be a metaphor that illustrates the current state of a person's emotional reaction to a traumatic event. When the sandtray scene is completed, children can be helped to understand their creation by a therapist reflecting, but not interpreting, the scene. Reflections can include child-selected miniatures, how miniatures were arranged, and what children said about the sandtray scene.

Social/Constructionist Learning Theory developed by Lev Vygotsky, the primary principle of the theory is the belief that learning takes place only when new concepts and ideas can be related and connected to something the learner already knows. Learners are not passive recipients, but instead are active organizers of their understanding. Constructivists also believe new concepts are best introduced through examples that complement a client's learning style.

Sociocultural Theory is both a psychological and sociological theory developed by Lev Vygotsky. It focuses on the influence a person's society and culture has on their development. Vygotsky believed cognitive development is guided by social interactions, that we are born with four mental functions, attention, sensation, perception, and memory, and within our social environment these functions developed into higher mental functions.

Solution Focused Brief Therapy (SFBT) was developed in the late 1970s by Steve de Shazer and Insoo Kim Berg. SFBT focuses on future goals and solutions versus past problems. The therapy incorporates positive psychology principles and practices that encourages clients to examine their experiences and resources to re-construct a viable solution.

The Spiritual Development Model was developed by James Fowler who believed spiritual understanding is developed in concert with other models of human development, including motor skills, cognitive and emotional development, and social actions. Fowler's seven stages of faith complement Maslow's hierarchy of needs and include primal undifferentiated, intuitive-projective, mythic-literal, synthetic-conventional, individuative-reflective, conjunctive, and universalizing or enlightenment.

Strength-Based approach to therapy developed in the 1950s by Donald Clifton is a form of positive psychology that explores clients' internal strengths and resources with the belief they can heal themselves.

Trauma-Based Therapy, sometimes referred to as trauma-informed therapy, is a generic term that refers to any approach to therapy focused on helping clients reframe and recover from a strong emotional reaction caused by a traumatic experience in their lives.

Transference/Countertransference is defined as projecting thoughts and feelings related to a particular person toward another. In a therapeutic relationship between therapist and client, transference refers to a client projecting their feelings about another onto their therapist, and countertransference is when the therapist projects their feelings about another onto the client.

Index